Textbook of Pharmacognosy

(As per Education Regulation 1991)

Textbook of Pharmacognosy

(As per Education Regulation 1991)

GK Singh M Pharm, PhD
Senior Lecturer, LM College of Science and Technology
Jodhpur 342 003 (India)

Anil Bhandari M Pharm, PhD
Senior Lecturer, LM College of Science and Technology
Jodhpur 342 003 (India)

CBS

CBS Publishers & Distributors Pvt Ltd

New Delhi • Bengaluru • Chennai • Kochi • Kolkata • Mumbai
Hyderabad • Jharkhand • Nagpur • Patna • Pune • Uttarakhand

Textbook of Pharmacognosy
(As Per Education Regulation 1991)

ISBN-13: 978-81-239-0692-8
ISBN-10: 81-239-0692-7

First Edition: 2000
Reprint: 2003, 2004, 2005, 2006, 2007, 2008. 2011, 2014, 2016, 2017, 2018, 2019, 2022 **2024**

Published by **Satish Kumar Jain** and produced by **Varun Jain** for

CBS Publishers & Distributors Pvt Ltd
4819/XI Prahlad Street, 24 Ansari Road, Daryaganj, New Delhi 110 002, India.
Ph: 011-23289259, 23266861, 23266867
Fax: 011-23243014
Website: www.cbspd.com
e-mail: delhi@cbspd.com; cbspubs@airtelmail.in.

Corporate Office: 204 FIE, Industrial Area, Patparganj, Delhi 110 092
Ph: 011-4934 4934 Fax: 011-4934 4935
e-mail: publishing@cbspd.com; publicity@cbspd.com

Branches

- **Bengaluru:** Seema House 2975, 17th Cross, K.R. Road, Banasankari 2nd Stage, Bengaluru 560 070, Karnataka, India
  Ph: +91-80-26771678/79 Fax: +91-80-26771680 e-mail: bangalore@cbspd.com
- **Chennai:** 7, Subbaraya Street, Shenoy Nagar, Chennai 600 030, Tamil Nadu, India
  Ph: +91-44-26680620, 26681266 Fax: +91-44-42032115 e-mail: chennai@cbspd.com
- **Kochi:** 42/1325, 1326, Power House Road, Opp KSEB, Ernakulum, Kochi 682 018, Kerala, India
  Ph: +91-484-4059061-65,67 Fax: +91-484-4059065 e-mail: kochi@cbspd.com
- **Kolkata:** 147, Hind Ceramics Compound, 1st Floor, Nilgunj Road, Belghoria, Kolkata-700056, India
  Ph: +91-9096713055/7798394118, 9836841399 e-mail: kolkata@cbspd.com
- **Mumbai:** PWD Shed, Gala no 25/26, Ramchandra Bhatt Marg, Next to JJ Hospital Gate no. 2, Opp. Union Bank of India, Noorbaug Mumbai-400009, Maharashtra, India
  Ph: +91-22-66661880/89 e-mail: mumbai@cbspd.com

Representatives

- Hyderabad 0-9885175004
- Jharkhand 0-9811541605
- Nagpur 0-9421945513
- Patna 0-9334159340
- Pune 0-9623451994
- Uttarakhand 0-9716462459

Printed at Glorious Printers, Jhilmil Industrial Area, Delhi, India

PREFACE

It is our great pleasure in bringing out the first edition of "*Textbook of Pharmacognosy*". This book has been prepared as per the syllabus of Diploma in Pharmacy in Pharmacognosy courses according to Education Regulation 1991 of Pharmacy Council of India. In this book, upto date information is given on all aspects of natural products used as crude drugs based on recent investigations. Another feature of this book is the inclusion of large number of neat and well-labelled diagrams. Due emphasis is given to vernacular name, biological source, geographical distribution, preparation, collection, salient features, chemical constituents, tests for identity and therapeutic uses of each drug. Pharmacognosy is the only one branch of science which provides comprehensive, accurate, scientific information of biological and chemical nature of crude drugs. We hope that this book will be useful to the students of D.Pharm and B.Pharm. We are highly thankful to *Prof. (Mrs.) Brinda Singh* for her valuable suggestions on various aspects such as morphological and anatomical features of plants. We extend our thanks to our teachers, colleagues, students and management of *L.M. College of Science and Technology, Jodhpur,* who have given us encouragement and suggestions for this assignnment. Suggestions, critics and errors from our readers will be appreciated for improvement of the future edition. Finally we are highly thankful to *Sh. Satish Kumar Jain*, CBS Publishers and Distributors for his interest and co-operation in bringing out this book in a short duration.

We have every hope that this edition will be enthusiastically received by our students and teachers.

Dr. G.K. Singh
Dr. Anil Bhandari

SYLLABUS

PHARMACOGNOSY

1. Definition, history and scope of pharmacognosy including indigenous system of medicine.
2. Various systems of classification of drugs of natural origin.
3. Adulteration and drug evaluation; significance of Pharmacopoeial standards.
4. Brief outline of occurrence, distribution, outline of isolation, identification tests, therapeutic effects and pharmaceutical applications of alkaloids, terpenoids, glycosides, volatile oils, tannins and resins.
5. Occurrence, distribution, organoleptic evaluation, chemical constituents including tests wherever applicable and therapeutic efficacy of following categories of drugs
   - (a) Laxatives : Aloes, Rhubarb, Castor oil, Ispaghula, Senna.
   - (b) Cardiotonics : Digitalis, Arjuna.
   - (c) Carminatives and G.I. regulators : Umbelliferous fruits, Coriander, Fennel, Ajowan, Cardamom, Ginger, Black pepper, Asafoetida, Nutmeg, Cinnamon, Clove.
   - (d) Astringents : Catechu.
   - (e) Drugs acting on nervous system : Hyoscyamus, Belladonna, Aconite, Aswagandha, Ephedra, Opium, Cannabis, Nuxvomica.
   - (f) Antihypertensives : Rauwolfia.
   - (g) Antitussives : Vasaka, Tolu balsam, Tulsi.
   - (h) Antirheumatics : Guggul, Colchicum.
   - (i) Antitumour : Vinca.
   - (j) Antileprotics : Chaulmoogra oil.
   - (k) Antidiabetics : Pterocarpus, Gymnema sylvestris.
   - (l) Diuretics : Gokhru, Punarnava.
   - (m) Antidysenterics : Ipecacuanha
   - (n) Antiseptics and disinfectants : Benzoin, Myrrh, Neem, Curcuma.
   - (o) Antimalarials : Cinchona.
   - (p) Oxytocics : Ergot.
   - (q) Vitamins : Shark liver oil, Amla.
   - (r) Enzymes : Papaya, Diastase, Yeast.
   - (s) Perfumes and flavouring agents : Peppermint oil, Lemon oil, Orange oil, Lemon grass oil, Sandal wood.

(t) Pharmaceutical aids : Honey, Arachis oil, Starch, Kaolin, Pectin, Olive oil, Lanolin, Beeswax, Acacia, Tragacanth, Sodium alginate, Agar, Gugar gum, Gelatin.

(u) Miscellaneous : Liquorice, Garlic, Picrorhiza, Dioscorea, Linseed, Shatavari, Shankhpushpi, Pyrethrum, Tobacco.

6. Collection and preparation of crude drugs for the market as exemplified by Ergot, Opium, Rauwolfia, Digitalis, Senna.

7. Study of source, preparation and identification of fibres used in sutures and surgical dressings : Cotton, Silk, Wool and regenerated fibres

8. Gross anatomical studies of : Senna, Datura, Cinnamon, Cinchona, Fennel, Clove, Ginger, Nuxvomica and Ipecacuanha.

CONTENTS

Preface v

Syllabus vii

1. History, Definition and Scope of Pharmacognosy 1-6
History, Definition, Scope of Pharmacognosy, Indigenous system of Medicine, Ayurveda, Homeopathic system of medicine, Unani system of medicine.

2. Classification of Natural Drugs 7-10
Alphabetical classification, Taxonomical classification, Morphological classification, Pharmacological classification, Chemical classification.

3. Plant Morphology and Anatomy 11-25
Leaves, Stomata, Trichomes, Leaf constants, Stem Roots, Wood, Bark, Inflorescence, Flowers, Fruits, Seeds, Organized and unorganized drug.

4. Collection and Preparation of Crude Drugs for the Market 26-29
Collection, Harvesting, Drying, Garbling, Packing, Storage and Preservation of Drugs.

5. Adulteration and Evaluation of Drugs 30-38
Adulteration, Evaluation of Drugs, Organoleptic evaluation, Microscopic evaluation, Physical evaluation, Chemical evaluation, Biological evaluation.

6. Different Chemical Groups of Natural Drugs 39-62
Introduction, Alkaloids, Terpenoids, Glycosides, Volatile oils, Isolation of volatile oils, Resins, Fixed oils, Fats and Waxes, Tannins, Carbohydrates

7. Natural Drugs and their Therapeutic Efficacy 63-197

7-A **Laxative :** Aloes, Rhubarb, Castor oil, Ispaghula, Senna, Senna pod 63-74
7-B **Cardiotonics :** Digitalis, Digitalis Lanata, Arjuna 75-79
7-C **Carminatives and G.I. Regulators :** Umbelliferous fruits, Coriander, Fennel, Ajowan, Caraway, Dill, Cumin, Anise or Aniseed, Cardamom, Ginger, Black pepper, Asafoetida, Nutmeg, Cinnamon, Clove 79-99
7-D **Astringents :** Pale Catechu, Black Catechu 100-102
7-E **Drugs acting on Nervous system :** Hyoscyamus, Belladonna, Datura, Aconite, Ashwagandha, Ephedra, Opium, Cannabis, Nux vomica 103-120
7-F **Anti-hypertensive Drugs :** Rauwolfia 120-122
7-G **Anti-tussives :** Vasaka, Tolu balsam, Tulsi 123-126
7-H **Anti-rheumatics :** Guggul, Colchicum 127-130
7-I **Anti-tumour Drugs :** Vinca 130-132
7-J **Anti-leprotic agent :** Chaulmoogra oil 132-134
7-K **Anti-diabetic Drugs :** Pterocarpus, Gymnema sylvestrie 134-136

7-L	**Diuretics :** Gokhru, Bara Gokhru, Punarnava	136-140
7-M	**Anti-dysenterics :** Ipecacuanha	140-142
7-N	**Antiseptics and Disinfectants :** Benzoin, Myrrh, Neem, Curcuma	143-148
7-O	**Antimalarial :** Cinchona	148-151
7-P	**Oxytocics :** Ergot	151-154
7-Q	**Vitamins :** Shark liver oil, Amla	154-157
7-R	**Enzymes :** Papaya, Diastase, Yeast	156-160
7-S	**Perfumes and Flavours :** Flavouring Agents, Peppermint oil, Lemon oil, Orange oil, Lemon grass oil, Sandal wood oil	161-166
7-T	**Pharmaceutical aids :** Honey or Mel, Arachis oil, Starch, Kaolin, Pectin, Olive oil, Lanolin, Beeswax, Acacia, Tragacanth, Sodium alginate, Agar, Guar gum, Gelatin	166-186
7-U	**Miscellaneous Drugs :** Liquorice or Glycyrrhiza, Garlic, Picrorhiza, Dioscorea, Linseed, Shatavari, Shankhpushpi or Shankhavali, Pyrethrum, Tobacco	187-197

8. Gross Anatomy of Crude Drugs 198-208

Senna leaf, Datura leaf, Cinnamon bark, Cinchona bark, Fennel fruit, Clove bud, Ginger rhizome, Nux-vomica seed, Ipecac root

9. Fibres, Surgical Dressings and Sutures 209-218

Fibres, Absorbent cotton, Jute, Flax, Silk, Wool, Viscose Rayon, Surgical Dressings, Sutures

Glossary

Botanical Terms 219-222

Medical Terms 222-226

Index 227

CHAPTER 1

HISTORY, DEFINITION AND SCOPE OF PHARMACOGNOSY

From the ancient times plants and animals are used as source of food. Later on plants and animals were differentiated according to their use. Initially the plant was differentiated into poisonous and non poisonous plants. Gradually man tried to develop and explore the knowledge of naturally occurring drugs for the treatment of various ailments and diseases. First of all, they transmitted their knowledge of natural drugs orally from one generation to other and later on in written form as papyri parchment and herbal manuscripts.

HISTORY

The history of Indian medicinal plant is very old e.g., before 3500 B.C. The curative value of plants have been mentioned in the **Rigveda** and **Atharvaveda** (3500-1500 B.C.) In the **Ayurveda** a good number of plants and their curative values are described. **Charak Samhita** and **Susruta Samhita** are well treatise of Ayurveda. **Papyrus Ebers** is an old document written in 1500 B.C. in which Egyptians have mentioned about the use of medicinal plants and animal and also about human anatomy. The great Greek Physician **Hippocratus** father of medicine(460-370 B.C) described human anatomy and physiology. **Aristotle**, a renowned Philosopher and a student of **Pluto** (384-322 B.C.) is known for his studies of animal kingdom. **Theophrastus** (370-287 B.C), a student of Aristotle is well known for the study of plant kingdom. A Greek physician **Dioscorides** (78 A. D) described thousands of medicinal plants and their properties in **"De Materia Medica"**. Natural history is compiled by **Plini** (23-70 A.D) in 37 volumes. A great

Greek pharmacist **Galen** (131-200 A. D) described various methods of preparation containing active constituents from plant and animal sources and it is known as glanical pharmacy. Later on all the detailed information's were compiled to form **Materia Medica** that was utilised by the physicians. Naturally occurring drugs may be obtained from plants, animals and minerals.

A German scientist **Seydler** introduced the term pharmacognosy in 1815 in his work entitled **"Analecta pharmacognostica"** The word pharmacognosy is derived from the Greek word **pharmakon**- a drug and **gignosco**- to acquire the knowledge of" Recently pharmacognosy deals with the crude drugs and their natural derivatives. Crude drug means simple drug which exist in natural form.

Table : 1.1 Some important crude drugs and their natural derivatives.

Crude drug	Natural derivatives
Digitalis leaf	Digitoxin
Senna leaf	Sennoside
Glycyrrhiza	Glycyrrhizin
Vinca	Vinblastine, Vincristine
Belladonna leaf	Atropine
Opium latex	Morphine, Codeine

Pharmacognosy is closely related with various branches of science like Botany, Biotechnology, Phytochemistry, Pharmacology, Zoology, Pharmaceutics,, etc.

DEFINITION

In broad sense phamacognosy is defined as the scientific and systematic study of physical, chemical and biological characters of crude drugs including their history, cultivation, collection and preparation for the commerce.

Generally the crude drugs are obtained from plants. But a limited number of drugs are also obtained from animal and mineral origin. The entire plant or part of plant is used as crude drug. Some crude drugs are also obtained by simple physical process e.g.- Catechu, Agar. (extraction with water), Opium, Papain (insions) .There are several other economic substances affecting health of human beings and animals like allergens (Mold, spores, pollen grains), antibiotics (Penicillin, streptomycin, tetracycline), immunizing agent (Antitoxin, sera, vaccines), insecticides (Pyrethrum, tobacco), flavouring agent (fennel, vanilla),spices (asafoetida, clove, coriander),vehicles (Castor oil, Honey, Theobroma oil), etc.

SCOPE OF PHARMACOGNOSY

Pharmacognosy is important not only as an academic exercise. It is the infrastructure on which evolution of novel medicines depends. Several crude drugs are utilised for the preparation of galanicals. Several crude drugs provide essential intermediate for final synthesis of bioactive molecule. Eighty percent of world population depends on crude drug and folklore medicine. All over the world, the demand of herbal drug increased enormously. Pharmacognosy has a wide and broad scope in the field of pharmacy and it's allied branches. Some of them are very important which are described below.

1. **Cultivation and domestication of Medicinal plants :** India imports many drugs such as Benzoin, Storax, Ipomoea, Tolu Balsum, Copaiba,, etc. If the cultivation of these drugs producing plants are carried out and cultivated in India, a lot of foreign exchange can be saved which will be helpful in the development of the country. Cultivation and domestication of some important plant are also essential to fulfill the demand of phytochemical industries e.g. *Mentha piperata* Linn., *Santalum album Plantago ovata, Ocimum sanctum,*, etc.

2. **Analysis of Phytochemicals :** Many bio-active molecule are extracted and isolated from the crude drugs. These are analysed by modern technique such as paper, thin layer, gas and high performance liquid chromatography.

3. **Preparation of General Tonics and Stimulants :** Despite the many advances made in the field of modern medicine there are a number of diseases for which these medicine has no cure. These medicine provide only symptomatic relief to patients. Liver disorders, arthritis, cancer, AIDS are some of them. Some of Ayurvedic formulations based on crude drugs are very effective in liver diseases and disorder e.g. Liv-52, Livomin, Livergen, etc. Ginseng, Tulsi, Ashwagandha, Shatavari, Brahmi, etc. are used as stimulants and adaptogenic drugs.

4. **In steroid industry :** Many pharmaceutical industries are involved in the extraction of diosgenin from Dioscorea species. It is an important precursor for production of steroidal drugs such as sex hormones, contraceptives, corticosteroids.

5. **Herbal preparation :** Recently herbal preparations are popularized due to their high effectiveness, low cost, easy availability and less side effects. *Adhatoda vasica*

(Vasaka) - Bronchodilater, *Boerhaavia diffusa* (punarnava), and *Andrographis paniculata* (Kalmegh), -Antihepatotoxic Anabolic, *Bacopo monnieri* (Brahmi)- Memory,, etc. are used as herbal medicines.

6. **Preparation of antibiotics :** Antibiotics are prepared from natural sources. These are very useful in maintaining the health of people through out the world. A large number of synthetic medicinal compounds are traced back through naturally occurring substances.

7. **Flavouring agents and perfumes** : There are large number of aromatic plants which are extensively used as flavouring agents perfumes spices and medicines. India produces a large number of essential oils. e.g. Ajowain, Citronella, Eucalyptus, Mentha, Palmrosa, Lemon grass, Turpentine, etc. Mentha oil is used in the production of menthol. Lemon grass oil is used in the preparation of vitamin A. Central Institute of Medicinal and Aromatic Plant (CIMAP) Lucknow is doing significant work in this field.

8. **Tissue culture :** This technique is now a days widely applicable for the production of secondary metabolites. People are using this technique to increase the yield of bio-active molecules. Due to a great demand of herbal medicines scope of pharmacognosy is increasing day by day, but there is need of standardization of herbal medicine. Although it is very difficult because various exogenous and endogenous factors are involved in the production of crude drug but standardization is very essential to maintain the quality of herbal medicine.

INDIGENOUS SYSTEMS OF MEDICINE

Various systems of medicine are practiced in India including Ayurveda, Unani Medicine and Homeopathic system.

Ayurveda

Ayurveda is one of the oldest system of medicine originated from India. The word Ayurveda is made up of two parts *Ayu+Veda*. *Ayu* means life and *Veda* means Knowledge. Thus Ayurveda means "science of life". It deals both physical and mental health and also covers art of living. In Ayurveda health is defined as a well-balanced metabolism and a happy state of being. It deals with all aspects of human life which are emanating from body, mind, external factors and natural intrinsic factors. In this system diseases are cured by using drugs, diets, exercise and surgery. Body (sharira), mind

(Manas) and soul (Atma) are the tripod of life in which equal attention should be given for the achievement of sound health.

Ayurveda classifies the body into three basic biological elements which are known as **Vata, Pita and Kapha**. These elements originate from five basic elements' airs (Vayu), energy (Tej), space (Akash), water (Jal) and soil (Dharti). The biochemical combination of space and air forms Vata. Pitta is composed of energy and water and Kapha is derived from the combination of water and soil. These three Doshas are the regulators of cell function in different ways and thus help in maintaining health. Drug therapy is well developed in Ayurveda. The oldest treatises **Charaka Samhita** and **Susruta Samhita** deals about Ayurveda. Basically Ayurveda has developed from **Rigveda** and **Atharaveda**. It deals with both preventive and curative aspects of life. According to Ayurveda all of the universal objects are made up of Panchbhuta. It is based on **Tridosa** (Three dosa - Vat, Pitta and Cough) theory. Ayurveda pharmacopoeia consists more than 8000 recipes. All the recipes contain crude drugs obtained from natural origin i.e. Plant, Mineral, Animal. There are various formulation of drugs ranging from churna (fine powders), Arka (distillate), Vati/ Gutika (Tablets/Pills), Bhasma (Calcined residue), Pisti (very fine powders), Ghrita and tails (Medicated Ghee and oil) are available. One of the important technique of Ayurveda is called **Samskaera** (refinement) is known as shuddhi (purification). Shuddhi is a process in which the toxicity of the harmful substances is eradicated and usefulness of pharmaceutical manipulation are increased.

Homeopathic system of medicine

This system of medicine was discovered by a German chemist, physician and pharmacist **Samuel Hahnemann** (1755-1843). His principle of treatment was reverse of the allopathic system. In this system only its symptoms are responsible for the cure of disease because there is no normal and natural method of diagnosis of the disease. He started the treatment of a disease with a low dose of the drug which is responsible for production of similar symptoms in normal man. According to homeopathic medicinal system a person will not suffer from any disease till the potency or immunity governing the body is powerful and strong. Anger, under and over diet, narcosis, evils, habits of telling lie ,etc. are the symptoms of mental diseases. These can be cured after collecting the information from the person who is suffering from the disease. Hahnemann worked on cinchona for cure of malaria because, its symptoms are similar to malaria in normal human being. Similarly belladonna was used for the treatment of scarlet fever. He prepared a list of drugs and their effects on healthy persons. Thus Gelsemium root (Yellow jasmine) and Nux-vomica became a useful drug for the cure of common cold and influenza respectively. No side effects are observed in homeopathic system of medicine. It is a cheaper system too. The medicines are used in the form of powder, small pills, mother tinctures ,etc.

Unani system of medicine

The Unani system of medicine was introduced in India in 10th century A.D. When Arabs conquered a great part of the ancient civilized world, they extended their knowledge of Unani medicine from Spain to India. The book **Kitab tafsir isma - al - Aqaqir**. is translated by Manaka, a popular Indian physician, from Sanskrit to Arabic that deals with a list of Indian Herb's and drugs. **Ibn-al-Baytar** (Spanish) prepared rose water and also, recommended the use of cotton oil, Nutmeg, colocynth and pyrethrum.
Arabs introduced many drugs of Indian origin such as clove, betel nut, sandal wood, cassia bark, etc. in Egypt. Arabs purchased dyes, drugs, perfumes and spices from Malabar coast of South India and introduced these articles in Egypt, Turkey and other countries. The Unani system of medicine is based on ancient principle. This system comes under the Tibbi discipline. Tibbi discipline is based on the elemental principle. These principles are Al-Nar (Fine), Al-hawa (Air) Al-ma (water) and Al-ardh (Earth). According to Tibb, human body is made of seven natural principles and components such as :

a. Al-arkan (Elements)
b. Al-akhalt (body fluid)
c. Al-a'za (organs)
d. Al arwah (vital spirit)
e. Al- at'al (Function)
f. Al - mizaj (Temperament)
g. Al - quwa (powers)

All of these are known as Al-Umur Al- tabiyah. These are very important for life and loss of any one of them may cause disease. The main aim of Unani medicine is to combat the disease, preservation and promotion of health through preventive, primitive and curative measures. The medicines are obtained from natural sources like plants, animals and minerals.

CHAPTER 2

CLASSIFICATION OF NATURAL DRUGS

Crude drugs are derived from the natural sources e.g. from plants, minerals and animals. These drugs are used in the treatment of various diseases and ailments of human being. For a systematic and scientific study of crude drugs it is very essential to classify all the drugs in proper system crude drugs can be arranged in different classes.

A. ALPHABETICAL CLASSIFICATION

In this classification crude drugs are arranged alphabetically either in Latin name or in English name. This method of classification is adopted by the following books.

1. **British pharmacopoeia [English titles]**
2. **British pharmaceutical codex [English titles]**
3. **British Herbal Pharmacopoeia [English titles]**
4. **Indian pharmacopoeia [English titles]**
5. **European Pharmacopoeia [Latin titles]**
6. **Pharmacopoeia Internationalis [Latin titles]**

Here drugs are easily traceable as they are arranged alphabetically but does not help in distinguishing the source of drugs whether it is from plant, animal or mineral. This classification does not indicate whether drugs are organised or unorganised.

B. TAXONOMICAL CLASSIFICATION

This is a purely botanical classification. It is based on phytogenetic similarities of plants. In this system crude drugs are arranged in a group according to their division, class,

order, family, genus and species. This system gives in detail an idea about the whole plant but it is not significant because in most of the cases only one part of the plant is used as drug. The whole plant is rarely used as drug. For example Cinnamon bark, Cinchona bark, Nux vomica seed,, etc. This system does not give any idea about the chemical constituents and pharmacological activity of crude drugs.

Table : 2.1 Taxonomical classification of crude drugs

Drug	Division	Class	Order	Family	Genus	Species
Senna	Angiosperm	Dicotyledons	Rosales	Leguminasae	*Cassia*	*angustifolia*
Fennel	Angiosperm	Dicotyledons	Umbellflorae	Umbelliferae	*Foeniculum*	*valagre*
Nuxvomica	Angiosperm	Dicotyledons	Gentianales	Loganiaceae	*Strychnos*	*nuxvomica*
Scilla	Angiosperm	Monocotyledons	Liliflorae	Liliaceae	*Urginea*	*maritima*
Vanilla	Angiosperm	Monocotyledons	Microspermae	Orchidaceae	*Vanilla*	*planifolia*
Ephedra	Gymmosperm	-------------------	Genetales	Ephedraceae	*Ephedra*	*equistina*

C. MORPHOLOGICAL CLASSIFICATION

In this type of classification crude drugs are arranged in various groups according to the part of plant (For example leaves, fruits, flowers, bark, etc.) used as drug. When a drug represents a cellular structure of the plant, it is known as organised drug but when a drug does not represents part of plant or any cellular structure of the plant, it is known as an unorganised drug.

Table : 2.2 Classification of organised drugs

Part of plant	Drugs
Barks	Cinnamon, Cinchona, Kurchi
Entire plants	Ephedra, Chirata, Sankhpushphi,
Flowers	Rose, Clove
Fruits	Cardamom, Fennel, Gokhru.
Hairs & Fibres	Silk, Cotton, Hemp
Leaves	Senna, Datura, Eucalyptus.
Roots	Withania, Rauwolfia, Aconite.

Table : 2.3 Classification of unorganised drugs

Category	Drugs
Extracts	Agar, Gelatin
Fixed oil	Castor oil, Arachis oil.
Fat	Lard
Gums	Acacia, Tragacanth
Gum resins	Myrrh, Asafoetida.
Juice	Aloe
Latex	Opium
Resins	Benzoin, Colophony
Waxes	Beeswax, wool fat

This type of classification does not gives any idea about the chemical constituents and therapeutic values of drugs.

D. PHARMACOLOGICAL CLASSIFICATION

In this system of classification, drugs are grouped according to pharmacological action of their most important constituent. Here drugs having similar action are kept together. It may be possible that the same drug having two different types of pharmacological actions can be classified separately in two groups e.g. Cinchona - Antimalarial & Bitter,Nux vomica - Stimulant & Bitter. This system does not give any indication about morphological and chemical nature of drugs. .

Table : 2.4 Pharmacological Classification of crude drugs

Pharmacological action	Drugs
Anti-cancer	Vinca, Podophyllum, Taxus
Antiasthmatic	Ephedra, Lobelia
Antinflammatory	Colchicum seed, Turmeric
Antispasmodics	Datura, Hyoscyamus
Antiamoebic	Kurchi, Ipecacuanha
Anthelmintics	Quassia, Male-fern
Astringent	Myrobalan, Ashoka bark
Purgative	Senna, Aloe, Rhubarb
Carminative	Coriander, Fennel ,Caraway, Cinnamon
Bitters	Quassia, Nux-vomica, Gentian, Cinchona.
Cardiotonic	Strophanthus,Digitalis,Squill.
Analgesic	Poppy
Expectorant	Liquorice, Vasaka, Balsum
Hallucinogens	Cannabis, Cocaine.

E. CHEMICAL CLASSIFICATION

The plants and animals synthesize a large number of chemicals like carbohydrates, proteins, fats, alkaloids, glycosides, volatile oils,, etc. In these system drugs are classified according to their main chemical category. This system is very useful for the study of crude drugs because it gives logical reasoning for the biological activity. Here it is very difficult to place the drug containing two different types of chemicals. e.g.
(a) Cinchona contains both alkaloid and glycoside
(b) Nutmeg contains volatile oil and fixed oil.

Table : 2.5 Chemical classification of crude drugs

Chemical Constituents	Drugs
Alkaloids	
Amine	Colchicum. Ephedra
Tropane	Datura, Belladonna, Coca
Quinoline	Cinchona
Isoquinoline	Ipecac, Opium
Pyridine & Piperidine	Areca, Nicotiana
Indole	Rauwalfia, Vinca, Ergot
Purine	Coffee, Tea.
Carbohydrates	
Gum	Acacia, Guar gum, Tragacanth
Mucilage	Ispaghula
Glycosides	
Anthraquinone	Aloe, Senna, Rhubarb
Saponin	Dioscorea, Liquorice
Isothiocyanate	Mustard
Cyanophore	Wild cherry bark
Lactone	Cantharide insect
Aldehyde	Vanilla
Lipids	
Fixed oil	Castor, Cottonseed, Almond
Fat	Theobroma, Lanolin
Waxe	Beeswax Spermaceti
Proteins	Gelatin
Resin and resin combination	
Resin	Cannabis, Podophylum
Oleo-resin	Capsicum, Ginger
Oleo-gum-resin	Asafoetida, Benzoin, Myrrh.
Steroids	
Cardiac glycosides	Digitalis, Squill.
Volatile oils	Cardamom, Cinnamon, Clove fennel, Mentha, Orange peel.

CHAPTER 3

PLANT MORPHOLOGY AND ANATOMY

Plants range from unicellular form to highly differentiated higher plants form. The higher plant consists of roots, stems, leaves, buds, flowers, fruits and seeds. The plants are mainly divided into two groups gymnosperm and angiosperm. The gymnospermic plants are naked seed plants in which ovules and seeds are not protected inside the ovary. In the angiospermic plant the ovules are enclosed inside a case called ovary. The ovules mature to form the seeds and ovary forms the fruit. Drug containing plants are not only arranged according to family and chemical constituents but also on the basis of morphological characters such as roots, stems, barks, leaves, buds, flowers and seeds. Generally bioactive molecule are present in the specific part of the plant but sometimes whole plant is used as drug such as Brahmi, Kalmegh, Shankhpushpi,, etc.

Morphological and anatomical descriptions about crude drugs are very important because there are some salient terms and structures found in Pharmacopoeias and allied works.

LEAVES

The leaf is a lateral outgrowth of the stem or an appendage developing upon a node and having a bud in its axil. It is flat, thin and the colour is generally green due to chlorophyll. Its main function is to carry on the process of photosynthesis. Leaves are divided into two types, simple leaves and compound leaves. Compound leaves possess many segments which are known as leaflets. These are the morphological characters by which leaves are identified.

Duration : Caducous (leaf shed soon after the bud opens)

Deciduous (leaf lasts for one season)
Persistent (leaf lasts for several seasons)

- **Shape** : Ovate, lanceolate, acicular, elliptical, oval, oblong, etc.
- **Apex** : Acute, acuminate, apiculate, emarginate, recurved, obtuse.
- **Leaf base** : Symmetrical, asymmetrical, cordate, reniform, etc.
- **Margin** : Entire, serrate, dentate, crenate, sinuate, ciliate, etc.
- **Venation** : Parallel, Reticulate palmate, Reticulate pinnate, etc.
- **Surface** : Glabrous (free from hair), pubescent, spiny, hairy, etc.
- **Petiole** : Long, short, grooved.
- **Texture** : Brittle, papery, fleshy, etc.
- **Phyllotaxy**: Alternate, opposite, etc.

ANATOMY OF LEAVES : Leaves are characterised by several microscopic structures. The leaf is made up of a epidermis, a parenchymatous mesophyll and vascular system.

Epidermis : Epidermis of leaf shows different functions and contains stomata, trichomes, water pores, cell inclusions,, etc.

Mesophyll : It can or cannot be differentiated into spongy mesophyll and palisade tissue. The palisade tissues are present in both lower and upper epidermis. Mesophyll cells are rich in chloroplast. Mesophyll contains parenchyma, collenchyma, sclerenchyma, secretion ducts, mucilage cells and hydathodes (water pores). Sometimes crystals of calcium oxalate are also present.

Vascular system : Phloem and xylem are also associated to form a vascular bundle. Arc shaped vascular bundles are found in leaf. Xylem is found towards upper epidermis and a band of phloem are also found. Collenchyma, a band of pericycle, and medullary rays are also found. The structure of the epidermis and stomata are helpful in the identification of leaf. In *Coca* and *Senna* leaves straight walled epidermal cells are present. Wavy walled epidermal cells are present in *stramonium, belladonna,*, etc.

STOMATA

Stomata consists of a pair of identical bean shaped cells known as guard cells. The stomata are the openings through which gaseous exchange takes place between the inner atmosphere of the leaf and the outside atmosphere. The stomata are surrounded by subsidiary cells which are different in shape. The stomata are divided into five different classes according to the numbers, shapes and arrangement of the subsidiary cells.

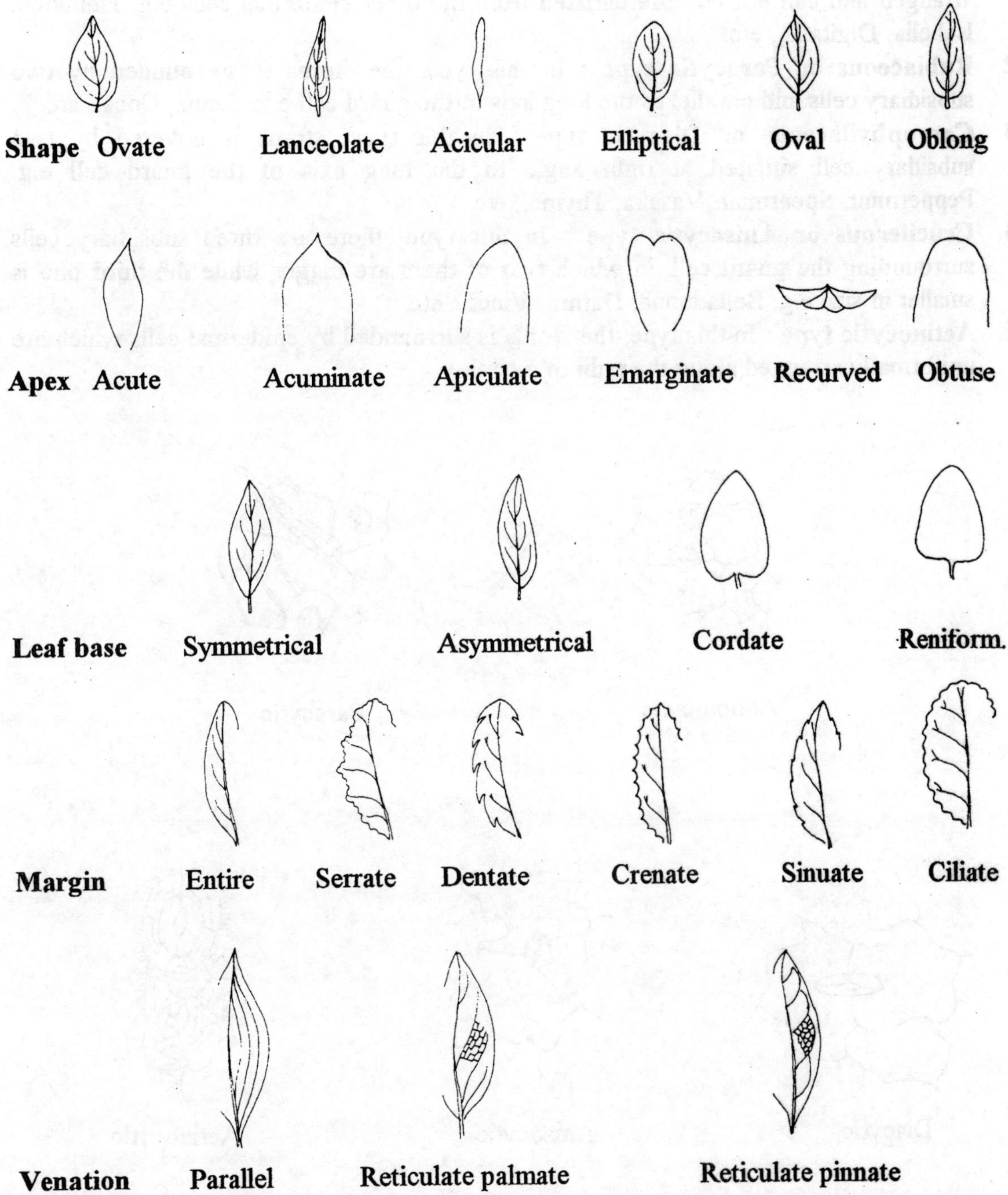

Fig. 3.1 Different types of shape, apex, base, margin and venation of leafy drugs

1. **Ranunculaceous or Anomocytic type** : In this type, the stomal pores are surrounded by unmodified epidermal cells of varying size which are irregularly arranged and can not be differentiated from the other epidermal cells e.g. Hemlock, Lobelia, Digitalis,, etc.
2. **Rubiaceous or Paracytic type** : In this type, the stoma is surrounded by two subsidiary cells and parallel to the long axis of the guard cell e.g. Senna, Coca,, etc.
3. **Caryophyllaceous or Diacytic type** : In this type, stoma is covered by two subsidary cell situated at right angle to the long axis of the guard cell e.g. Peppermint, Spearmint, Vasaka, Thyme,, etc.
4. **Cruciferous or Anisocytic type** : In this type, there are three subsidiary cells surrounding the guard cell, in which two of them are bigger while the third one is smaller in size e.g. Belladonna, Datura, Vinca,, etc.
5. **Actinocytic type** : In this type, the stoma is surrounded by epidermal cells which are uniformally arranged along the radii of a circle.

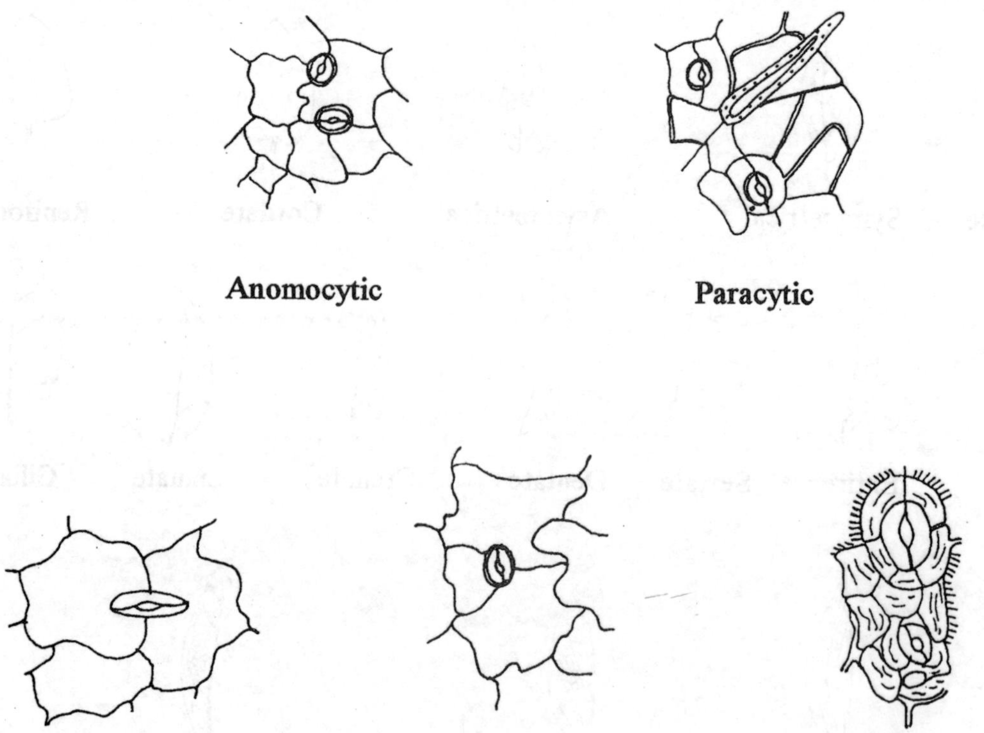

Fig. 3.2 : Different types of stomata

TRICHOMES

Trichomes are outgrowth of epidermal cells. It is also known as plant hairs. It is very important for the identification of the plant. Trichomes also perform secretory functions. It excretes water and sometime volatile oils too. e.g. Peppermint. Trichomes consist of two parts i.e. root and body. Root is found below the epidermis and body outside the epidermis. Trichomes are absent in root and present in most of the aerial parts of the plant, e.g. ,leaves, herbaceous stems, flowers, fruits and seeds. Trichomes are classified into three groups.

(I) **Covering or Non glandular or Clothing Trichomes** : These are simple, non-glandular, covered with cuticle and protective in nature, such as :

(a) **Senna :** It contains short, conical, unicellular, warty trichomes.
(b) **Vinca** : It contains long unicellular warty and bulbous base.
(c) **Nux Vomica seed** : It contains long, thick walled, unicellular, lignified trichomes.
(d) **Datura** : It contains uniseriate, multicellular, conical unbranched trichomes.
(e) **Digitalis** : It contains uniseriate multicellular and warty cuticle.

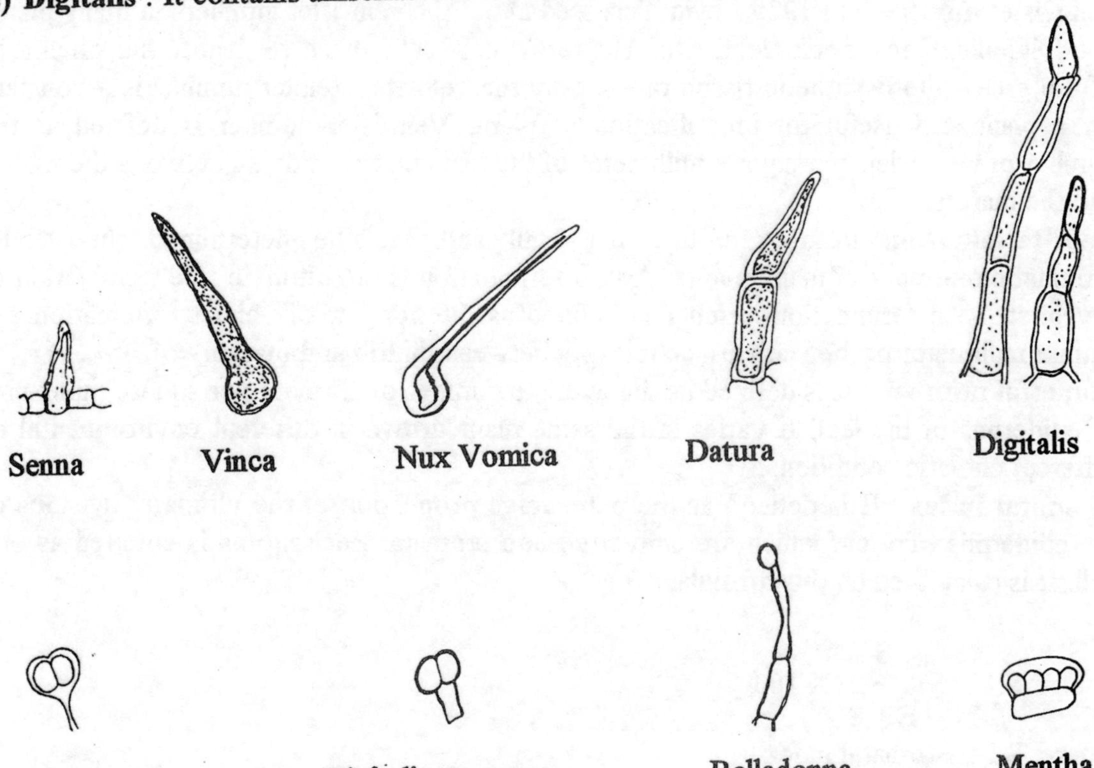

Fig. 3.3 : Different types of Trichomes

(II) Glandular Trichomes or hairs : The presence of glandular cell at the top of the trichomes are the characteristic feature of this type of trichomes. They may be unicellular or multicellular, uniseriate or multiseriate with or without stalk. such as

(a) **Vasaka** : It contains unicellular glandular trichomes in which stalk is absent.
(b) **Digitalis purpurea** : It contains trichomes with unicellular stalk and head.
(c) **Belladonna** : It contains uniseriate multicellular stalk and unicellular head.
(d) **Mentha** : It contains short stalk with multicellular head and unicellular stalk.

(III) Hydathode : It is a special type of trichomes which helps in absorption or secretion of water e.g. *Piper betel.*

WATER PORES : Water pores are modified stomata and are present in the teeth of the margin. e.g. *Digitalis purpurea, Lobelia inflata.*

LEAF CONSTANTS

Vein-islet number : In 1929 Levin discussed about the vein-islet numbers in many plants e.g. Digitalis, Coca, Senna leaf,, etc. The term vein-islet is used to denote the small area of the green photosynthetic tissue out line by the veinlets. Veinlet number is a constant for a plant and useful for identification of plant. Vein-islet number is defined as the number of vein-islets per square millimeter of the leaf surface midway between the midrib and the margin.

Vein-termination number : In 1951 Hall and Melville determined the veinlet termination number of many plants. A vein termination is the ultimate free termination of a veinlet. Vein termination number is defined as the number of veinlet termination per square millimeter of the leaf surface midway between midrib and margin.

Stomatal number : It is defined as the average number of stomata per square millimeter of epidermis of the leaf. It varies in the same plant grown in different environmental or different climatic conditions.

Stomatal Index : It is defined as the percentage proportion of the ultimate divisions of the epidermis of a leaf which are converted into stomata. Each stoma is counted as one cell. It is calculated by this formula.

$$S.I = \frac{S}{E + S} \times 100$$

where, S.I = Stomatal index
S = Number of stomata per unit area.
E = Number of epidermal cell in the same unit area.

Palisade ratio : In 1925 Zoringh and Weiss developed this technique while studied on compositae family. It is defined as the average number of palisade cells beneath each epidermal cell. It is counted for at least four adjacent cells.

STEM

Stem is defined as the aerial portion of the plant which develops from plumule portion of the embryo. It contains nodes, internodes and buds. The stem may be aerial, subaerial and under ground.

Some common technical terms are given below for the description of the stem of a Plant.

Herb : A small, soft textured plant may be annual, biennial or perennial containing little woody tissues. e.g. Fennel, Dill, Brahmi.
Shrub : It is bigger than herb and smaller than woody tree in nature having several main stem but no main trunk e.g. Lemon, Ephedra, Commiphora,, etc.
Tree : Big in size, woody in nature and having main trunk.
Annual : Plant survives for one season.
Biennial : Plant survives for two seasons.
Perennial : Plant survives for more than two seasons.
Creepers or prostate stem : The stem lies flat on the ground without roots are known as creepers. e.g. Mint, grasses,, etc.
Climbers : They are not able to stand alone due to its weakness so they climb on the support with the help of hooks, tendrils, roots or prickles. e.g. *Piper longum*, *Piper betel. Tylophora indica, Asparagus racemosus* ,etc.
Twiners : The stem twine round the support and grow further. They are thin and wiry in nature. e.g. Ipomoea.
Rhizomes : It is underground modification of stem. The stem is prostrate, thick, fleshy and creeps horizontally in side the soil. They posses nodes, internodes, scale leaves, occasional bud in leaf axil, and adventitious roots on the lower surface. e.g. Ginger, Rhubarb, Turmeric,, etc.
Bulb : It is like a biconvex lens with closely set leaves on the other surface and fibrous adventitious roots on the lower surface, e.g. ,Garlic, Squill and Onion.
Corm : It is condensed underground fleshy stem growing in a vertical direction, e.g. Colchicum, Saffron,, etc.
Tuber : It arises in the axil of lower leaf which are positively geotropic in nature. It accumulates reserve food e.g. Potato,, etc.
Stolon : When subaerial branches grow out in all directions and bend upward to become aerial. e.g. Glycyrrhiza,, etc.

Runner : In runners the plant creeps on the ground and roots are found at node. It possesses nodes, leaves and auxiliary buds e.g. Straw berry, Penny wort,, etc.
Offsets : It is a short thick and originated from the axil of the leaf. Rosette type of leaves and cluster of fruit at their bottom are the main characteristic of the plant. e.g. Aloe, Agave, Valerian,, etc.
Sucker : When lateral branches develop from an underground stem and grow obliquely upward to become an aerial stem is known as sucker. e.g. Mentha species, Banana,, etc.

ROOTS

The roots are the downward growth of the plant into the earth. They are positively geotropic and negatively phototropic in nature. They don't show differentiation into nodes and internodes. They do not bear leaves, auxiliary buds and flowers. The primary root develops from the radical of the embryo. The primary root gives secondary lateral branches and after that it is again divided and turns into tertiary lateral branches. All lateral branches arise in a cropetal succession.

WOOD

Many drugs consist of wood so there is need to describe it Wood consists of the secondary tissue produced by the cambium on inner side, secondary xylem and smaller amount of other tissues are present in wood. The cells are highly lignified, the vessels, tracheids, wood fibres and parenchyma are found in wood. In trees, the cells of old wood become coloured due to the presence of tannins and other colouring matters. Mainly two types of **wood** are present **heart wood** or **duramen** and **Sap wood** or **alburnum**. The heart wood consists inner most central region of dicot root or stem. It is dark in colour due to presence of tannin, gums, pigments, resin ,etc. e.g. Sandal wood. Sap wood is the outer region of the wood. It is functional wood which carries food material and water to plant. It is light in colour e.g. Quassia. The transverse section of wood reveals the annual ring which represents season's growth. The wood formed in spring season is called **spring wood** and the wood formed in winter season is known as **autumn wood**. In some plants annual rings are not well marked due to absence of seasonal interruption in growth so they are known as **false annual rings** e.g. Quassia. When spring vessels are arranged more or less in a ring then this type of wood is known as **ring porous wood**. The wood in which spring vessels are arranged uniformly through out spring then the wood is known as diffused porous wood. The nature of wood is also decided by the arrangement of fibres. When the fibres are arranged straight and parallel the wood is described as straight grained wood. But when fibres are arranged at an angle of 30° the wood will not break easily. This results in an irregular and splintery fracture and this type of wood is known as interlocked grain e.g. Guaiacum.

BARK

Commercially bark consists of all secondary external tissues laying outside the cambium in root or stem of dicotyledonous plant. Botanically, the term bark is also known as periderm. Periderm consists of three layer, cork (Phellem);cork cambium (phellogen) and secondary cortex (phelloderm). A young bark is composed of epidermis primary cortex, phloem, pericycle and endodermis. The epidermis is not found in bark due to the excessive growth produced by the cambium thus the external tissue tangentially stretched or torn. Barks are identified through its morphological and histological character. The morphological characters are very essential for the identification of the barks.

Shapes in barks :The shape of the bark depends upon the method of its preparation, type of incision made and the extent of any subsequent shrinkage of the tissues. These are described as follows

a) Flat barks : These are produced from the large trees and dried under pressure. e.g. Arjuna, Quillaia ,etc.
b) Curved barks : These are obtained from small branches. They form concavity on the inner side due to shrinkage of soft tissues. e.g. Cassia, wild cherry, etc.
c) Recurved bark : Concavity is found on the outer side of the bark e.g. Kurchi.
d) Channeled bark : Channel like structure is found due to shrinkage of the tissue e.g. Cassia, Ashoka, *Cinchona ledgeriana.*
e) Quill bark : One edge of the bark covers the other e.g. cinnamon, cascara,, etc.
f) Double quill : Both the edges of the bark roll independently forming quill. e.g. Java, Cinnamon.
g) Compound quill : One quill of the bark put inside other quill e.g. Cinnamon.

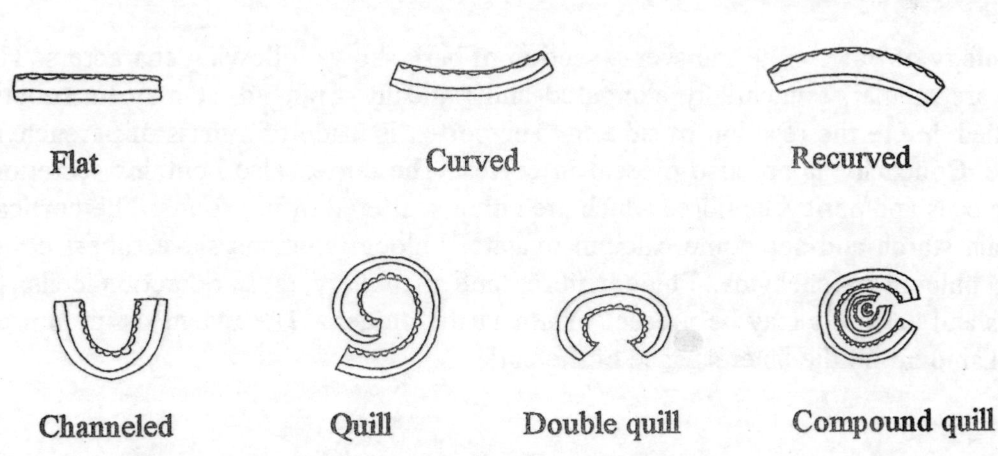

Fig. 3.4 : Different shapes of barks

Fracture : The fracture is the appearance of exposed surface of transversely broken bark. It is also useful in the identification of barks. The descriptions about the fractured barks are given below.

a) Short : Containing smooth fractured surface e.g. Cinnamon, Cassia, Cascara,, etc.
   Granular : It shows small rounded grain like appearance e.g. Wildcherry,, etc.
b) Splintery : The broken surface shows uneven projecting points. e.g. Quillaia.
c) Fibrous : Transversely broken surface shows a number of thread like fibres e.g. Cinchona.
d) Laminated : The exposed surface shows the arrangement of layer one over the other e.g. Quillaia.

Outer surface : These are also important for the identification of barks.

a) Smooth : The outer surface is even e.g. Arjuna bark.
b) Lenticels : The outer surface forms transversely elongated The holes due to lateral pressure e.g. Cascara bark and wild cherry.
c) Wrinkles : It is present on outer surface of bark due to shrinkage of soft tissues e.g. Cascara bark.
d) Cracks and fissures : They are present on the outer surface of bark due to lack of elasticity or increase in diameter e.g. Cinchona bark.
e) Furrows : Troughs are found between wrinkles.
f) Exfoliation : The cork of bark flakes off e.g. wild cherry bark.
g) Corrugations : Inner surface shows transverse wrinkles.
h) Epiphytes : Lichen, moss and liver warts are present on bark. e.g. Cascara bark.

Histology of bark : The transverse section of bark shows following characters. The cork cells are tabular, tangentially elongated and radically arranged. It may be suberised or lignified due to the reaction of suberin. The cortex is made of a mass of parenchymatous tissue. Collenchyma are also present in cortex. The cortex also contains secretion cells, stone cells and pericyclic fibres which are either scattered or in groups. The cortical cell's contain starch and sometime calcium oxalate. Phloem contains sieve tubes, companion cells, phloem parenchyma. Phloem fibres and medullary rays. Secretion cells, phloem fibres and sclereids may be present or not in the phloem. The xylem tissue is present in small amount on the inner surface of the bark.

INFLORESCENCE

It is the arrangement of flowers in various ways. The whole flower or the part of the flower are used medicinally. The inflorescence are classified on the basis of limited or unlimited growth of main axis (Peduncle)length of peduncle, presence or absence of pedicels in the flowers, etc. These are the different types of inflorescence which are used in drug.

(a) Raceme - Mustard, Digitalis.
(b) Panicle - Goldmohar
(c) Cymose - Jasmine
(d) Umbel - Coriander, Carway, Fennel.
(e) Hypanthodium - Fig.
(f) Capitula - Arnica, Sunflower, Pyrethrum.

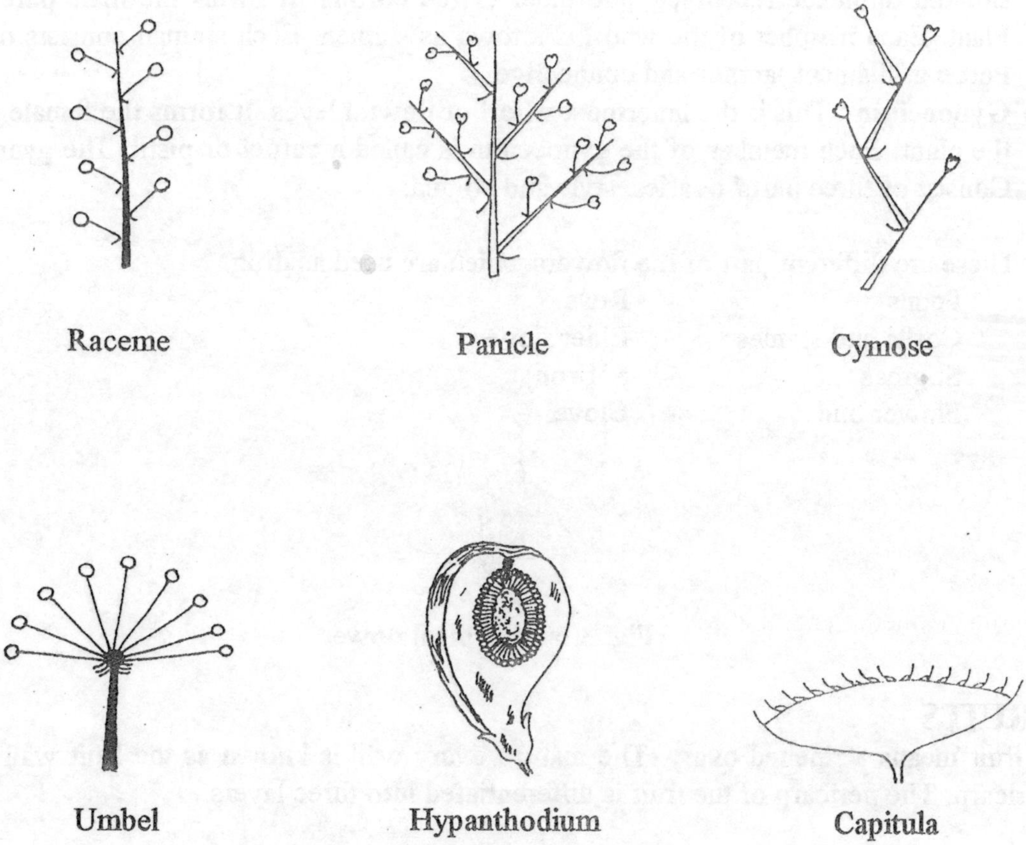

Fig. 3.5 : Types of inflorescence

FLOWERS

Flower is a modified shoot which is concerned with the sexual reproductive process in higher plants. This leads to the formation of fruits and seeds. A typical flower possesses the following parts.

(a) **Pedicel and Thalamus** : The stem of flower is known as pedicel. The swollen tip of the pedicel in which floral leaves are attached, is known as thalamus.
(b) **Calyx** : The outermost whorl of the flower is known as calyx. It is green in colour and flat in structure like ordinary leaves. Each member of the calyx is called sepal.
(c) **Corolla** : The second whorl of floral leaves is known as corolla. It is situated inside to the calyx. It is either white or bright in colour. The individual member of corolla is called petal. It is the most attractive part of the flower.
(d) **Androecium** : The third whorl of flowral leaves is known as androecium . It is situated upon the receptacle and inner to the corolla. It forms the male part of the Plant. Each member of the whorl is known as stamen. Each staman consists of three Part e.g. filament, anther and connective.
(e) **Gynoecium** : This is the innermost whorl of flowral leves. It forms the female part of the plant. Each member of the gynoecium is called a carpel or pistil. The gynoecium Consist of three parts' ovaries, style and stigma.

These are different part of the flowers which are used as drug.

Petals	-	Rose
Corlla and stames	-	Elder flowers
Stigmas	-	Saffron
Flower bud	-	Clove.

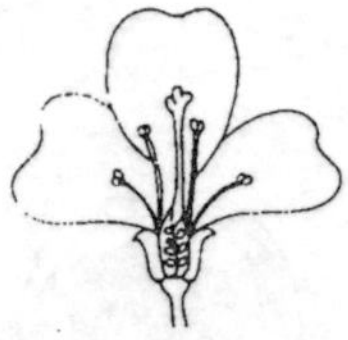

Fig. 3.6 : A typical flower

FRUITS

A fruit means a ripened ovary. The mature ovary wall is known as the fruit wall or the pericarp. The pericarp of the fruit is differentiated into three layers.

(a) **Epicarp** : The outermost covering of the pericarp is known as epicarp. It may be thin, thick or woody in nature.

(b) **Mesocarp** : It is a middle layer present in between epicarp and endocarp. It may be fleshy or consist of spongy parenchymatous tissue.

(c) **Endocarp** : It is the innermost layer of the pericarp it may be thin, thick or woody in nature.

The fruits are classified into three categories which depend upon the number of carpels present in the flowers and other structure.

Simple fruit : It is formed from ovary of a monocarpellary, syncarpous gynoecium with one pistil. Simple fruits may be dehiscent and indehiscent. It may be fleshy or dry fruits.

The classifications of some simple fruits are given below.

(I) Simple dry, Indehiscent fruits.

(a) Achene - Sunflower, Cannabis
(b) Caryopsis - Found in all cereals- (Rice, Wheat, Maize, etc.)
(c) Nut - Cashew nut, Areca nut
(d) Samara - Dioscorea,

(II) Schizocarpic or splitting Fruits : These are dry, multi seeded, bicarpellary fruit which on maturity breaks up into two mericarps. It is classified into two groups.

(a) Lomentum : Acacia, Peanut.
(b) Cremocarp : Dill, Fennel, Caraway, Coriander.

(III) Simple dry, dehiscent fruits : These are dehiscent fruits which develop from monocarpellary or multicarpellary, syncarpous gynoecium. The main types of these fruits which are used as drugs are discussed below.

(a) Legume : Senna, Tamarind
(b) Follicle : Aconite, strophanthus, Rauwolfia, Anise.
(c) Capsule : Poppy, Cardamom, Datura, Cotton.
(d) Siliqua : Mustard, Radish.

(IV) Simple, Fleshy fruits (Succulent fruits) : It contains fleshy fruits and seeds remain embedded in the pulp.

(a) Berry : Capsicum, Colocynth, Bael, Nux-vomica.
(b) Drupe : Mango, Olive, Coconut, Almond.
(c) Pome : Apple, Pear.
(d) Hesperidium : Orange, Lemon.

SEEDS

The fertilized ovule is known as seed. The seed may be developed from orthotropous, campylotropous or anatropous ovules. The seed is surrounded by one, two or three seed coats. The seeds contain seed coats, endosperm and embryo. The endosperm is the nutritive tissue nourishing the embryo. Some seeds don't contain endosperm. The seeds are classified into three types.

Albuminous Seeds or Endospermic : Distinct endosperm is formed during development of the seed e.g. Nux vomica, Isabghula, Linseed, Fenugreek, Castor, etc.

(a) **Exalbuminous seeds or Non endospermic** :The endosperm is fully absorbed by embryo in this. Endosperm is not formed and the embryo become large e.g. Cotton, Soybean, Almond, Peanut, etc.

Perispermic Seeds : The nucleus develops to a greater extent and forms a big storage tissue called perisperm. The seed contains embryo, endosperm, perisperm and seedcoat. e.g. Pepper, Cardamom, Nutmeg,, etc.
The following structures are the main characteristic features by which the seeds are identified.

(a) **Hilum** : A point of attachment of seeds to stalk.
(b) **Chalaza** : Present at the base of nucellus.
(c) **Raphe** : A longitudinal marking which is adherent stalk of anatropous ovule.
(d) **Micropyle** : A small opening in the seed coat through which water is provided for the germination of seeds.
(e) **Aril** : A fleshy growth from hilum covering the entire seed e.g. Nutmeg,
(f) **Arillode** : A covering originating from micropyle e.g. Cardamom.
(g) **Caruncle** : A warty out growth arising from micropyle. e.g. Castor, Croton.
(h) **Wing** : At the base of seed, extension of testa is present e.g. Strophanthus.
(i) **Hairs** : An out growth from apex of seed. e.g. Calotropis, Gossypium.

UNORANISED DRUG : Unorganised drug is obtained from plant or animal but donot contain cell or cellular tissues.

Table · 3.1 : Difference between Organized drug and Unorganized drugs.

Organized drugs	Unorganized drugs
1. These are organs of plants or animals containing cellular structure e.g. Bark, Fruits, Insects, Leaves, etc.	These are obtained from part of plants and animals by physical processes like incision extraction, expression, etc. e.g. Juices, extracts, resins, etc.
2. Microscopically studies are important parameter for identification of organised drugs. e.g. Cinchona, Senna, Fennel ,etc.	Physical standards and chemical tests are important factor for identification of these drugs. e.g. Pepsin, Castor oil, Opium, Aloe, Agar ,etc.
3. These are solid in nature, e.g Cinchona bark, Nux-vomica seed, Ginger, etc.	These are solid, semi solid or liquids in nature e.g. Opium, Oil, Guggul, etc.

CHAPTER 4

COLLECTION AND PREPARATION OF CRUDE DRUGS FOR THE MARKET

The preparation of crude drugs for market depends mainly upon the morphological character, geographical source, method of collection, chemical constituent, drying, garbling, storage, etc. For commercial purpose the drugs are collected from wild and cultivated plants. After collection some important changes are required. In vanilla pod, fermentation of the drug is very essential because the fresh drug is devoid of odour and the aromatic fragrant constituent. In this case vanillin is formed only after fermentation. But such type of changes are undesirable in glycosidal and non-glycoside drugs because it deteriorates the quality of drugs e.g. In case of Digitalis enzymatic hydrolysis takes place, thus drug loses its cardioactive principle. Care should be taken during the treatment of drugs so that its morphological appearance should not be affected.

COLLECTION

The drugs may be collected from wild or cultivated plants and this task is done by casual, unskilled labour or by skilled workers or even by botanists. Drugs are collected when they contain maximum concentration of active chemical constituents. Proper time, suitable season, environmental conditions and age of the plant are also taken into consideration during the collection of the crude drugs for maintaining quality and better morphological appearance. Some examples are given below.

Roots and rhizomes : These are collected in autumn season, when the drug contains optimum bioactive molecules. The roots are sliced either transversely or longitudinally which facilitates better drying. Rhizomes are collected when they store ample reserve food material.

Bulbs : Bulbs are collected in late autumn season, long after flowering of the plant.

Leaves : Leaves are collected just before they reach their flowering stage. During rainy season, leaves should not be collected e.g.. Belladonna, Senna, Digitalis, Vinca, etc.
The Aloe leaves are collected when they become sufficiently fleshy to get optimum constituent. The leaves of solanaceous drugs are collected in morning.

Barks : Barks are usually collected in spring or early summer when the cambium is active as it is easy to separate most readily from the wood. Some times it may be collected in autumn season e.g. wild cherry. Cinnamon is collected during rainy season because it contain maximum active constituent at that time.

Flowers : Flowers are collected just before pollination in dry weather during the mid day e.g. saffron, arnica, etc. The clove flowers are collected in the bud condition.

Fruits : Fruits are collected when they fully grow up and ripened e.g. umbelliferous fruits. Some times unripe fruits are also collected e.g. Black pepper, Cubeb.

Seeds : Seeds are collected when they fully mature but before the indehicsence of the fruits. e.g. Fox glove, Black mustard, Strophanthus, etc.

Resin, gums and lattices : These are collected in dry weather when they ooze out of the plant.

HARVESTING

Harvesting is an important operation in the cultivation of crude drugs. The task of harvesting should be performed by skilled workers or botanist because it reflects the economic aspects of crude drugs. Leaves of Digitalis, Tea, Vinca, Senna and bark of Cinchona are mainly harvested by hand picking method by skilled workers. Roots, rhizomes, tubers, bulbs and other underground drugs are harvested by mechanical devices such as plow, diggers or lifters. The underground drugs are thoroughly washed with water for removal of adhered dirt, soil and other foreign materials. The aerial parts of the plant are harvested by binders. Flowers, small fruits and seeds are harvested by using a special device known as seed strippers. The Coriander and Dill are mowed, dried, thrashed and the fruits are separated by winnowing. Some times reaping machines are also used for their harvesting. Peppermint and spearmint are harvested by mower, partially dried and sent for distillation of the volatile oil. The Cochineal insects are collected from branches of cacti by brushing. Agar-Agar and other sea weeds are harvested by long handled forks.

DRYING

Drying is a process by which sufficient moisture content of the crude drug is removed. It prevents moulding, action of bacteria, enzymatic reactions and chemical or other possible changes. It facilitates pulverizing, grinding and milling of crude drugs. Control of temperature and regulation of air flow are the main principles of drying. Slow drying at a moderate temperature is essential for encouraging enzymatic reactions e.g. Vanilla pods, Cocoa seeds, Orris rhizome, etc. Glycyrrhiza, Calumba, Scilla, etc. are dried after slicing and cutting into smaller pieces. There are two processes of drying (i) Natural or sun drying (ii) Artificial drying.

Natural drying : There are two processes of natural drying.
(a) Direct sun drying
(b) Drying in the shade.

When the contents of drugs are not affected by temperature and sun light, they are dried directly in the sun light e.g. Gum Acacia, Fruits, Seeds, etc. For maintaining natural colour and retaining volatile principle of the drugs, drying in the shade is preferred.

Artificial drying : Trays, stove, oven, hot water pipe, spray and vacuum dryer are the main devices of the artificial drying. Leaves and aerial parts of the plants are dried by tray method at temperature between 40 to 60°C. Barks and roots are dried between temperature 35 to 60°C. e.g. Cinchona bark, Belladonna roots, Tea and Rasp-berry leaves and Gum. In vacuum dryers the sensitive drugs are dried at higher temperature e.g. Digitalis leaves and tannic acids. The drugs which are highly sensitive to temperature and atmospheric conditions are dried by spray drying method e.g. Papaya latex, pectin, milk, tannin, etc. Rapid drying and prevention of enzymatic reactions are the main advantages of artificial drying. Flowers and leaves retain their colour and aromatic drugs retain their aroma by rapid drying.

GARBLING

After drying garbling is the next step for the preparation of crude drugs. In this step dirt, sand, vegetable debris, foreign organic matters and other parts of the plant are removed. These are removed by several ways and means e.g. excess stems are removed from leaves of lobelia and stramonium. In case of clove buds, stalks are removed. Rhizomes are separated from roots and root-lets. The dirt and sand from roots and rhizomes are removed by washing thoroughly in water by passing air current. Magnet the removal of iron dust in case of castor seeds before crushing.

PACKING

Morphological conditions, storage, climatic conditions, chemical nature, transportation and ultimate use of the drug by manufacturer are important factors of packing. The packaging of the drug should be done in such a way that helps in saving space during transportation, storage and provides sufficient protection to the drugs. Leaves or herbs are baled with pressure by power balers into a solid compact mass. Bales vary in weight among 100 to 700 lb.e.g. senna leaves, stramonium, vinca, etc. The drugs that have deteriorated by moisture should be packed in moisture proof containers. Gums, resins and extracts are packed in barrels, boxes or casks while vanilla beans are packed in tin lined boxes. Aloe is packed in goat skin and in a 55 gallon steel drums. Liver oil should be packed in such containers which are not affected by sunlight. Balsam of tolu and colophony are packed in kerosene cans. Roots and seeds are packed in gunny bags, which are internally coated with polythene.

STORAGE AND PRESERVATION OF DRUGS

The storage of the drug should be done in light proof, moisture proof, air tight, closed containers (covered by metal bins), and amber glass containers. Drug should not be stored in wooden boxes or in drawers and never in paper bags because the drug will deteriorate by moisture and also attack by insects, rats and mice. Few drops of chloroform and carbon tetrachloride are very useful for preventing insect attack. It should be added to the container from time to time. Digitalis and ergot need low moisture content so it should be kept with calcium oxide which are nonliquifying, inert and dehydrating substance. The drugs containing volatile oil should be stored in well closed, air tight, dark coloured containers in cool and dark place. Ergot contains alkaloid, chitin and fixed oil which becomes rancid in the presence of moisture, high temperature, light, air and bacteria and liberate ammonia therefore it should be stored in well filled closed container at low temperature in dark and cool place. In some drug's sterilization is important before storage because it prevents microbial contamination and development of other living organisms. The ware-houses should be cool, dark, well ventilated, fire proof, moisture proof, steel or brick constructed ware-house is preferred. All the biological products should be stored at a temperature between 2 to 8°C.

CHAPTER 5

ADULTERATION AND EVALUATION OF DRUGS

ADULTERATION

Adulteration means incorporation of impurities in genuine or standard drugs. Adulteration may be accidental or deliberate. In few cases dealers mixed the substandard and spoiled drugs with genuine drugs due to scarcity and high price of drugs in the market to cheat the customer. Adulteration may occur due to improper collection, drying, preparation and storage of crude drugs. In this way adulterated drugs are inferior in quality, containing less amount of bioactive molecules and more amount of foreign matter. There are various methods used for adulteration of drugs.

1. **Substitution of exhausted drugs** : This type of adulteration normally take place with costly drugs. Many drugs are extracted on large scale to isolate their active constituents or volatile oil. These exhausted materials are used entirely or partly as a substitute for the standard drugs. i.e. Used tea leaves are collected, dried and mixed with genuine drug and send to the market. Volatile oil containing drugs like caraway, fennel, etc. are used to extract volatile oil by steam distillation then exhausted drugs are mixed with standard drugs due to similar appearance.

2. **Adulteration by artificial substitutes** : Artificial substitutes are prepared for some drugs which resemble with genuine drugs in form and appearance e.g. Paraffin wax is yellow in colour and substituted for yellow bees wax, artificial catechu is prepared from clay and tannin and adulterated with genuine catechu, etc.

3. **Adulteration due to common vernacular name** : This type of adulterant is caused by common vernacular name of different plants. In different region of India, same plant is known by different vernacular name. i.e. *Trianthema portulacastrum* and

Boerhaavia diffusa are two different plants but having common vernacular name e.g. "*punarnava*."

The plant *Herpestis monniera* (L.) H, B & K is known as *Brahmi* in plant states of India where as the plant *Hydrocotyl asiatia* L. is known as Brahmi in the other states of India. Both the plants are sold in the market by the name of Brahmi. The plant *Evolvulus alsinoides* Linn, *Convolvulus microphyllus* sibe and *Clitoria ternatea* Ls are Known as " *Shankhpushpi*". Similarly roots and rhizomes of *Acorus calamus*, *Alpinia officinarum Anacyclus pyrethrums* are sold in the market by the name of "*Boch*".

4. **Substitution by different plant material** : In place of standard drugs, some substituted plant materials are sold in the market which resemble in appearance with genuine crude drugs e.g. Ashoka bark is obtained from *Saraca indica* L. but this crude drug is substituted with *Trema orientalis* Blume bark. Similarly kurchi bark is obtained from *Holarrhena antidysenterica* but it is substituted with *Wrightia tinctoria* R. Br. Senna leaves are obtained from *Cassia acutifolia* and *C. angustifolia* Delile but these leaves are replaced with *Cassia auriculata* Linn.

5. **Adulteration with other materials** : In this type of adulteration, standard crude drugs are partially adulterated with other similar plant materials such as Black Catechu with Aloe, black pepper with papaya seed, *Cinnamon cassia* with *C. zeylanicum*, mustards seed with *Argemone mexicana* seed.

6. **Adulteration with faulty collection** : The optimum bioactive molecules are present in a crude drug at a particular season, time and age of the plant. When the drugs are not collected during that specific period, the quality and quantity of the drug may be reduced. When these drugs are mixed with standard drug they cause adulteration. i.e. coriander fruits and linseed should be collected when they are fully grown and ripened. Belladonna roots are collected when the plant is 3-4 years old. Solanaceous drugs are collected during flowering season. Wild cherry bark and male fern are collected in autumn season while colchicum corms are collected in summer season. Sometimes less valuable part of the plants are collected and adulterated with genuine drugs. e.g. Clove buds are collected with stalks whereas buchu leaves and senega roots are collected with stems.

7. **Adulteration due to imperfect storage** : A number of drugs are spoiled due to imperfect storage or some times these are destroyed by the action of enzymes, microorganisms, moisture, light, temperature, etc. Thus the drugs are not useful for human consumption. So this type of drugs is considered as adulterated drug. i.e. when cod liver oil is not protected from light the decomposition of vitamin A takes place. When digitalis, stramonium and belladonna leaves are not stored in moisture

proof container and in a dry place, enzymatic hydrolysis takes place and decomposes the active constituents. If volatile oils are not stored in well closed containers and not protected from light and high temperature, evaporation of volatile constituents take place.

EVALUATION OF DRUGS

Evaluation means determination of identity, quality and purity of drugs.

Identity : It refers to the exact biological source of the drug.

Quality : It refers to the concentration of therapeutically active constituents.

Purity : It refers to the absence of foreign materials, either organic or inorganic.

There are different method for evaluation of crude drugs.

ORGANOLEPTIC EVALUATION

In this type of evaluation, drugs are evaluated with the help of sense organs. It includes gross morphology and sensory characters like colour, odour, taste and texture of crude drugs.

Morphological characters : Morphological features of various part of plants are very useful in the identification of crude drugs. They also give idea about presence of adulterants in crude drugs. Organised drugs are classified on the basis of the part of the plant used as drug.

Barks : Barks are the tissue present in woody roots or stems outside the inner fascicular cambium, e.g. Cinchona, Ashoka, kurchi, Quillaia, etc.

Underground structure : They may be roots, rhizomes, bulbs, corms and tubers.The crude drugs are often swollen due to storage of carbohydrate and other chemicals. e.g. Rauwolfia, Ginger, Turmeric, Dioscorea, Liquirice, Garlic, etc.

Leaves : They are the lateral outgrowth of stem or an appendage developing upon a node and having a bud in its axil. It is usually flattened and green. They are the photosynthetic organs. These drugs are identified on the basis of shapes, margin, base, apex and venation of leaves. E.g. Senna, Digitalis, Tulsi, Vasaka, etc.

Flowers : The flower is the structure that is concerned with the sexual reproductive process in higher plants. It is composed of four basic parts calyx,corolla, androecium and gynoecium. The flowers help in the formation of fruits and seeds i.e. Pyrethrum, Saffron, Banafsha, etc.

Fruits : It is a ripened ovary and contains seed i.e. Cardamom, Fennel, Amla, Harde, Bahera, Almond, etc.

Seeds : Seeds are developed from the ovules in the carpels of the flowers and are characterised by the hilum, the micropyle and some-times by raphe. e.g. Ispaghula, Nux-vomica, Psoralia, etc.

Herbs : Herbs are small soft textured plants. They contain little woody tissues. They may be annual, biennial or perennial. Sometimes the whole aerial part of the plant is used as drug e.g. Brahmi, Kalmegh, Pudina, Chirata, etc.

Sensory characters : Sensory characters like colour, odour, taste and texture are the important factors for the evaluation of crude drugs. If the drugs are dried in shade they contain dark colour than that of sunlight exposed drugs. Drugs stored in well-closed containers retain bright colour otherwise they may fade when exposed for a longer time. Volatile oils containing drug give characteristic odour i.e. Clove, Cinnamon, etc. different species of mentha leaves are also characterised by their smell. Deteriorated ergot and cantherides give undesirable ammoniacal odour due to improper storage. Garlic also gives alliaceous odour. Drugs like glycyrrhiza and honey give sweet taste whereas gentian and chirata produce bitter taste. Capsicum and ginger contain pungent taste whereas ispaghula contains mucilaginous taste. Aconite has a horny-fracture due to gelatinization of starch whereas glycyrrhiza possesses hard and fibrous fracture due to the presence of woody tissue and fibres.

MICROSCOPIC EVALUATION

Microscopically evaluations of drugs are very useful in the identification of different varieties of a drug and its adulterants. The drug is examined under a microscope. This can be performed by powdering, cutting a thin section (LS/TS) or preparing a macerate of the crude drug. After this, different reagents and stains are used to distinguish the arrangement of cellular structures. The microscopic evaluation also includes the study of chemical constituents by application of chemical tests. The arrangement of tissue is clearly visible in transverse section of drug. The basic arrangement of tissues in stems roots, leaves, barks, seeds, etc., is fairly constant. Sometimes considerable variation may exist due to different climatic conditions, extent of lignification, detailed appearance of the cells, etc. Fibers, sclereids, tracheids vessels, etc. are least affected by drying. Starch, calcium oxalate crystals, epidermal trichomes, lignin and fixed oil should be examined carefully in a crude drug. Sometimes the absence of certain cells or cell contents may be useful for the identification of crude drugs. e.g. absence of cork from bark, absence of starch from root and rhizome, absence of stamen in a flower, etc. The characteristic of cell wall, cell content, fiber, trichomes, sclerieds vessels, stomata ,etc. are examined in details e.g. lignified trichomes in nux-vomica.

Microscopically examination is very essential for the identification of powdered crude drugs. In powdered drugs, the fragments either composed of plant cells or group of cells. Cell content either in free state or present within the cells should be observed carefully. During microscopical study, drawings are very essential for the identification of a crude drug. It has significant role in the study of qualitative and quantitative evaluation of crude drugs and adulterated powder drugs. This can be achieved by counting a specific anatomical feature such as stomatal index, stomatal number, vein-islet number, palisade ratio, vein termination number. Calcium oxalate crystals, starch grains, phloem fibres ,etc. are measured with the help of ocular and stage micrometer. Lycopodium spore methods are used for the determination of starch grains in wheat or ginger powder. It is also used for calculating the number of pollen grains in pyrethrum powder.

PHYSICAL EVALUATION

It is very essential for the determination of quality and purity of drugs. In this evaluation, physical constants are determined wherever possible e.g. viscosity for drug containing gums, froth number for saponin containing drugs, swelling factor for mucilage containing drugs. Extractive value and solubility in different solvents, refractive index, optical rotation, density, specific gravity, ash-value, volatile oil content, boiling point, melting point, freezing point, moisture content, spectroscopic analysis, radioimmuno assays, etc. are useful parameters for evaluation of drugs. Some of them are described below.

1. **Moisture content** : The presence of excessive moisture content in a drug will deteriorate its quality due to activation of certain enzymes and growth of micro-organisms. The moisture content can be determined by a standard procedure i.e. Karl Fischer methods. Pharmacopoeias prescribe standard limits for crude drugs are as under :

Drugs	Moisture content (%) w/w should be not more than
Digitalis	5
Tolu Balsam	4
Aloe	10
Starch	15
Acacia	15

2. **Melting point** : It is a useful parameter for determining the purity of crude drugs. Pure phytochemicals and other chemical compound give a very sharp and constant

melting point. It is very helpful for the evaluation of solid fixed oil and waxes.

Drugs	Melting point (°C)
Cocoa butter	30 - 33
Bees wax	62 - 65
Wool fat	34 - 40

3. **Refractive index** : It is a ratio of the velocity of light in vacuum to velocity in the substance. It depends upon wavelength of incident light, temperature and pressure. It is a physical constant and very useful for standardization of volatile and fixed oil. It is measured by means of refractometer.

$$R.I = \frac{\text{Velocity of light in vacuum}}{\text{Velocity of the light in substance}}$$

4. **Optical rotation** : Many substances obtained from biological origin have a capacity to rotate the plane of polarised light. If the rotation of plane of polarised light is towards right it is known as dextrorotatory (+) and if it is towards left, called levorotatory (-). Optical rotation is determined with the help of polarimeter. Most of the volatile oils and fixed oils are optically active, and thus it is a very important parameter for determining their purity.

5. **Rf values** : Thin layer chromatography and paper chromatography are important techniques by which qualitative and quantitative estimations of the drugs are performed. Rf means *Relative flow*. It is a constant which is determined by ratio of distance covered by the solute to the distance covered by solvent.

$$Rf = \frac{\text{Distance covered by the solute}}{\text{Distance covered by solvent}}$$

Rf value for a compound is a constant for particular solvent system. This value is used for the identification of compound and is compared with the reference standard.

6. **Volatile oil content** : Volatile oil content present in the crude drugs like clove, cardamom, rose, cinnamon, etc. is determined. A weighed quantity of drug is boiled with water in a round bottomed flask and fitted with *Clevenger* apparatus. The

content of volatile oil is determined by direct reading because the oil floats on water in a graduated tube. Volatile oil containing crude drugs are evaluated on the basis of their volatile oil content e.g. Clove contains not less than 15% volatile oil whereas cardamom seeds contain not less than 4% volatile oils.

7. **Foreign matter** : It is very difficult to get a crude drug (vegetable origin) in pure condition. Foreign matter like other parts of the plant, animal excreta or any other organic matter are present with crude drugs. The maximum limit for the foreign matter is defined in the monograph of crude drugs. If the crude drug exceeds the limit then it is said to be substandard.

8. **Extractive value** : Crude drug contains a large number of chemical compounds. There is a lot of diversity in the chemical nature and properties of crude drugs. Sometimes extractive value is determined for evaluation of crude drugs. Extract of crude drugs are prepared in different solvents likes water, alcohol, ether, chloroform, etc. by using maceration, percolation or soxhlation method. Water is used as a solvent for glycosides, tannins and sugar containing drugs. Alcohol is an ideal solvent for extraction of various crude drugs and is used as a solvent for the extraction of crude drugs e.g. Rhubarb, Aloe, Asafetida, Benzoin, etc.

   Ether soluble extracts are prepared for volatile oil/non volatile oil containing crude drugs. The volatile oil containing drugs include clove, fennel, dill, caraway,, etc., whereas non volatile oil containing drugs are mainly fixed oil and resin and colouring matter found in capsicum, cocoa, linseed, etc.

9. **Spectroscopic Analysis** : Certain molecule of a drug has capacity to absorb vibration at a specific wave length. It is a very useful parameter for evaluation of drugs. Various phytochemical groups are determined by the spectroscopic analysis (U.V, I.R., N.M.R, Mass, etc.) such as alkaloids of solanaceous drugs, glycoside of cardiotonic drugs, etc.

10. **Microbial Contamination** : The crude drugs are also contaminated by attack of certain microbes like bacteria, fungi or mold. The contamination's cause certain toxicity that is not actually desirable to the crude drugs. In these circumstances the drugs should be sterilized in a special equipment by treatment with ethylene oxide.

11. **Ash Value** : For determination of total ash content, a known quantity of air dried vegetable drug is incinerated in a silica crucible and the residual ash is weighed to calculate the percentage of ash on the basis of initial dry weight of the drug sample. Total ash of peeled drug is less than the unpeeled drug. Although total ash value are

of little significance in drug evaluation, but still very high ash values are indicative of contamination, adulteration or carelessness, in preparing the drug for the market. In the determination of total ash values, the carbon must be removed at as low a temperature (450°C) as possible. Since alkali chlorides, which may be volatile at high temperatures, would otherwise be lost. The total ash usually consists of phosphates, silicates, carbonates & silica. Sulphated ash is prepared by treating the drug with dilute sulphuric acid before ignition. In this all oxidies & carbonates are converted to sulphates and the ignition is carried out at a higher temperature (600 °C). Acid insoluble ash may be determined by treating the total ash with dilute hydrochloric acid, which usually consists mainly of silica and high acid-insoluble ash, in drug such as senna, clove, liquorice and tragacanth indicates contamination with earthy metals. Pharmacopoeial limits for acid insoluble ashes vary from 0.5% (Agar) to 12% (Hyoscyamus). If no limit of acid insoluble ash is given for a crude drug in the pharmacopoeial monograph, then this value should not exceed 2%.

CHEMICAL EVALUATION

It is very useful for determining the purity of crude drugs. Isolation, Purification, different chemical assays of active constituents is performed for evaluation of crude drugs. Chemical evaluation also comprises various quantitative chemical tests like acid value, saponfication value, ester value, acetyl value, peroxide value and hydroxyl value. *Vitali morin* reaction is performed for the determination of tropane alkaloid in Datura, Belladonna, etc. Gums are identified by using lead acetate or lead subacetate solution. Emetine in ipecac is estimated by potassium chlorate and hydrochloric acid. Borntrager's test is performed for anthraquinones. *Murexide* test is performed for purine bases for example caffeine. In nux-vomica, strychnine is detected by ammonium vandate and sulphuric acid and brucine is detected by concentrated nitric acid. Five member lactone ring present at c-17 (steroidal glycoside) in digitalis is detected by *Keller-Killiani* test, *Legal* test and *Baljet* test, protein and free amino acids are detected by *Millon's, Biuret* and *Ninhydrin* tests. *Molisch's* test is used for the detection of carbohydrate.

Crude drugs contain primary and secondary metabolites. Generally secondary metabolites are physiologically active. Phytochemical screening is performed for chemical evaluation of crude drugs which give a clear cut picture of chemical constituents present in a plant. Generally successive solvent extraction for crude drugs performed with petroleum ether, benzene, chloroform, acetone, ethanol and water in succession. Bioactive molecules are estimated and evaluated by chemical evaluation e.g. Sennosides in senna, eugenol in clove oil, morphine in opium, reserpine in rauwolfia, emetine in ipecac, etc. Sometimes titrimetric and gravimetric methods are used for chemical assay of crude drugs.

BIOLOGICAL EVALUATION

When physical or chemical means are not able to produce satisfactory result in crude drugs then the drugs are evaluated by biological method. In this evaluation, the tests are performed on living animals, animal preparations, isolated living tissues, micro-organisms and intact or excised organs. Since living organisms are used these tests are called bioassays or biological assays. In this method pharmacological activity or biological effect of a certain drug is measured and compared with that of standard drug in same conditions for evaluation of certain drugs. Drugs containing hepatoprotective activity can be biologically evaluated on albino rats. Anthelmintic drugs are evaluated on earth worms. Cardiac glycoside containing drugs are evaluated on cats, frogs or pigeons. Antiseptic property of certain drugs is evaluated on bacteria such as *Salmonella typhi, Staphylococcus aureus*. Antibiotics and vitamins are microbiologically evaluated on yeast, mold and the living bacteria. Bitter principle is evaluated for chirata, gentian and quassia where as pungency principle is evaluated for capsicum and ginger. Biological evaluation is expensive, time consuming and less precise than chemical evaluation. Quantitative accuracy is also less as compared to chemical analysis.

CHAPTER 6

DIFFERENT CHEMICAL GROUPS OF NATURAL DRUGS

INTRODUCTION

In the struggle for health promotion, the role of crude drugs is very important. Most of the active constituents are of plant origin. Plants are the major source of natural products used as pharmaceuticals, flavour and fragrance, ingredients, agrochemicals, food additives, etc. Several crude drugs are the sources of pharmacologically potent chemical substances, also known as active constituent of drugs and have a definite mode of action. On the other hand, some of the constituents present in the crude drugs are therapeutically inert but are used in the preparation of various pharmaceutical formulations as pharmaceutical aid.

Table 6.1 : Active chemical constituent of some natural drugs and their use

CRUDE DRUG	CHEMICAL CONSTITUENT	USES
Cinchona bark (Alkaloid)	Quinine	Antimalarial
Opium (Alkaloid)	Morphine	Analgesic
Vinca (Alkaloid)	Vincristine Vinblastine	Anticancer
Senna (Glycoside)	Sennosides	Purgative
Aloe (Glycoside)	Aloin	Laxative

Contd.

CRUDE DRUG	CHEMICAL CONSTITUENT	USES
Agar (Carbohydrate)	Agarose	Gelling and thickening agent
Honey (Carbohydrate)	Saccharine	Sweetener, Pharmaceutical aid
Starch (Carbohydrate)	Polysaccharides (Amylose, Amylopectin)	Disintegrating agent Diluent.
Pale Catechu (Tannin)	Catechin	Astringent
Tolu balsam (Resin)	Benzyl cinnamate	Scabicide,rubefacient, protectant
Turmeric (Resin)	Curcumin	Antimicrobial Antiinflammatory
Cinnamon bark (Volatile oil)	Cinnamic aldehyde	Astringent, Carminative
Clove (Volatile oil)	Eugenol	Antiseptic, Carminative
Chaulmoogra oil (Fixed oil)	Hydnocarpic acid Chaulmoogric acid Gorlic acid	Antileprotic
Papaya (Protein)	Papain	Protein digestant
Beeswax (wax)	Myricin, Myricyl acetate	Ointment, Wax-paper

ALKALOIDS

Alkaloids are complex compounds generally produced from plant. They are basic in nature and contain one or more nitrogen atom (usually present in heterocyclic ring) and have pronounced pharmacological actions on man or animals.

Properties : Most of the alkaloids are solid crystalline substance but a few are liquid (Nicotine, coniine). Generally alkaloids are colourless (but berberine - Yellow and Salts of Sanguinorine - copper red). They are soluble in organic solvents but insoluble in water. Alkaloidal salts are soluble in water and insoluble in organic solvents. A number of alkaloids are degraded by exposure to light and air.

Distribution : Alkaloids are distributed in the various part of the Plant.

Leaves : Belladonna, Datura, Tobacco, Vinca, Hyoscyamus, Coca, etc.
Bark : Cinchona, Kurchi, etc.
Roots and Rhizomes : Rauwolfia, Ipecac, Aconite, etc.
Fruit : Black pepper, Opium, etc.
Seeds : Nuxvomica, Colchicum.
Whole areal plant : Ephedra, Lobelia, Tylophora, etc.

Many alkaloids are obtained from bacteria, fungi (Ergot) and algae.

Isolation of alkaloid : The isolation of alkaloid involves three stages. (a) Extraction (b) Preparation of crude alkaloid (c) Purification of crude alkaloid and separation of several alkaloids usually step (b) and (c) are not separated from one another. Alkaloid can be isolated by any one of the following method.

Method A

Powder Material

(a) Keep moisten with water
(b) Mixed with lime
(Acids, tannins and other phenolic compound combine with lime)
(c) Extrated with organic solvent such as ether or pet. Spirit

Powder (Discarded)

Organic phase (containing alkaloidal extract)

(a) Concentrated the above extract.
(b) Shake with aqueous acid
(c) Allow to stand

Organic phase discarded (containing impurities)

Aqueous phase containing alkaloidal salt

Method B

Power Material

(a) Extract with water and aqueous alcohol containing dilute acid.

Shake with chloroform and other organic solvent

Chloroform layer (Pigment and other unwanted material)

Aqueous layer (Alkaloidal salt present)

Added Excess of sodium bicarbonate or ammonia

Free alkaloid precipitated

(a) Extract with organic solvent
(b) Concentrate the solution

Concentrated organic solvent contain alkaloid

Alkaloid is purified by crystallization using suitable solvent.

Table 6.2 : General Chemical test for alkaloids.

Reagent	Observation
1. Mayer's reagent (Potassium mercuric iodide solution)	Creamy precipitate
2. Wagner's reagent (aqueous iodine solution)	Reddish brown precipitate
3. Tannic Acid test (freshly prepared tannic acid)	Precipitate which is soluble in dilute acid or ammonia solution.
4. Dragendorff's reagents (potassium bismuth iodide solution)	Reddish brown precipitate
5. Hager's reagents (saturated picric acid solution)	Yellow precipitate

Note : Caffeine and some other alkaloids do not give positive test with above mentioned tests.

Murexide test : Alkaloid is digested with potassium chlorate and a drop of hydrochloric acid and this is exposed to vapours of ammonia - purple colour is formed with **Caffeine** and **Purine** group of alkaloid.

Classification of Alkaloids : The alkaloids are classified according to basic ring present in them. A detailed chart of classification with their use and basic structure is given in Table 6.3.

Table 6.3 : Classification of alkaloids

Type of alkaloids	Structure	Source	Example	Use
(A) Non heterocyclic alkaloids				
(1) Phenyl ethyl amine	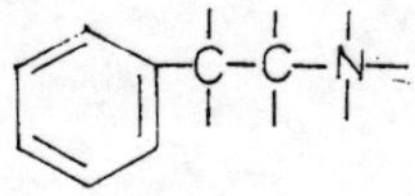	Ephedra	Ephedrine Pseudoephedrine	Asthma
(2) Tropolone	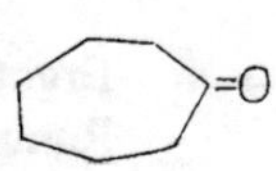	Colchicum	Colchicine	Gout & polyploidy
(3) Steroidal	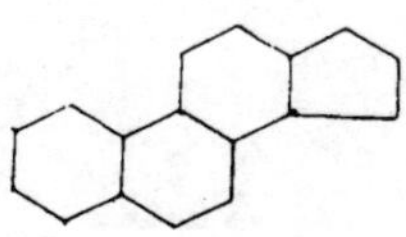	Kurchi Veratrum	Conessine Veratramine	Dysentry Hypotensive
(B) Heterocyclic Alkaloids				
(I) Monocyclic				
(1) Pyridine and	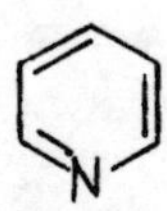	Lobelia	Lobeline	Spasmodic, Asthma
Piperidine	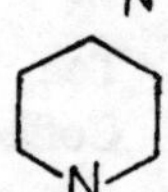	Hemlock Piper	Coniine Piperine	Gonorrhoea, Condiment
(2) Pyrrole and	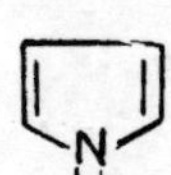	Coca	Hygrine	C.N.S
pyrrolidine	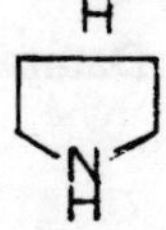	Tobacco	Nicotine	stimulant
(3) Imidazole	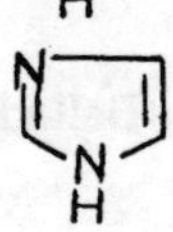	Pilocarpus	Pilocarpine	Atropine antagonist (Contraction of pupil)

Contd.

Type of alkaloids	Structure	Source	Example	Use
(II) Polynuclear Heterocyclics				
(1) Isoquinoline	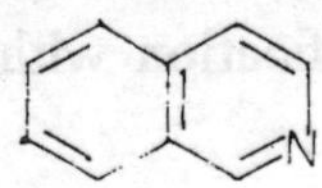	Opium	Papaverine Narcotine	Narcotic Analgesic
(2) Quinoline	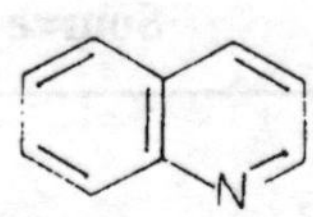	Cinchona	Quinine	Antimalarial
(3) Indole	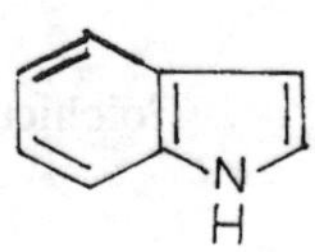	Ergot Rauwolfia	Ergotamine Reserpine	Oxytocic Hyper-tension
(4) Quinazolin	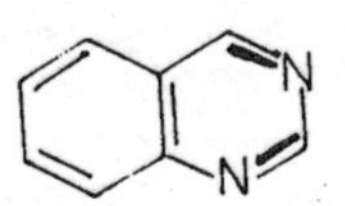	Vasaka	Vasicine	Antitussive
(5) Purine	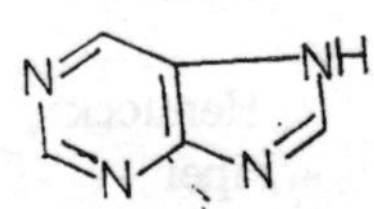	Tea, Coffee	Caffeine	C.N.S. stimulant
(6) Tropane	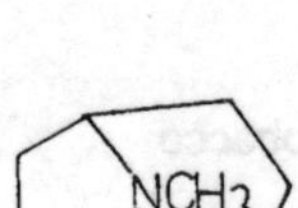	Datura	Atropine	Parasym-pathetic depressant
		Belladonna	Hyoscine	Parasym-pathetic depressant

TERPENOIDS

Terpenoids are polymers derived from two or more isoprene molecules (C_5H_8).As all the terenoids are derived from one monomeric structural unit, Isoprene and here they are sometimes referred as isoprenoid compounds.

$$
\begin{array}{c}
\quad CH_3 \\
\quad | \\
CH_2{=}C\text{-}CH{=}CH_2
\end{array}
$$

Isoprene or 2 methyl-1,3-butadiene

On the basis of number of isoprene units they are classified as

Class	Number of isoprene units	Molecular Formula
Hemiterpenes	1	C_5H_8
Monoterpenes or Terpenes	2	$C_{10}H_{16}$
Sesquiterpenes	3	$C_{15}H_{24}$
Diterpenes	4	$C_{20}H_{32}$
Triterpenes	6	$C_{30}H_{48}$
Tetraterpenes or Carotenoids	8	$C_{40}H_{64}$
Polyterpenes or Rubber	n	$(C_5H_8)n$

Each class of terpenoids except, hemiterpenes which is represented by a single member (isoprene), is further classified into subclasses on the basis of number of rings present in the molecular.

(a) Acyclic : That contains an open chain structure.

(b) Monocyclic: That contains one ring in their structure.

(c) Bicyclic : That having two rings in their structure.

(d) Tricyclic : That having three rings in their structure.

Table 6.4 : Classification of Terpenoids

Terpenoids	Consitituents	Drug
Monoterpenoids	Citral & Citronellal	Lemon, Orange
	Cannabinoids	Resin of cannabis
	Fenchone	Fennel
	Gentiopicroside	Gentian
	Limonene	Cardamom, Lemon, Caraway, Dill
	Pinene	Turpentine oil, Coriander, Chenopodium
Sesquiterpenoids	Caryophyllene	Clove, Copaiba
	Santaline	Sondalwood
	Bisaboline	Lemon oil.
	Cadinene	Lemon oil, Cubeb
	Gossypol	Cotton plant.
Diterpenoids	Aconitine alkaloid	Aconite root
	Forskolin	Coleus
	Gibberlins	Fungi and higher plants.
	Pimaric and abietic acids	Pine resins
Triterpenoids	Arjunollic acid	Arjuna bark.
	Asiatic & brahmic acids	Brahmi
	Glycyrrhitinic acid	Glycyrrhiza
	Quinovic acid	Cinchona bark
	Sterol	Wool fat, yeast, Rasna herb
	Squalene	Animals, Arachis and olive seeds.
Tetraterpenoids	Carotenoids (Color pigments)	
	Crocin	Saffron
Polyterpenoids	Solanesol	Tobacco

Isolation & identification tests

Different methods for isolation and identification tests of individual constituents are used on the basis of their chemical groups such as Alkaloids, Glycoside, Volatile oil, Saponin, Resin,, etc.

Therapeutic and Pharmaceutical uses

Terpenoids that exists in nature, may be used as medicinal agents for pharmaceutical purpose. For example.

(i) Arjunolic acid	: Diuretic
(ii) Asiatic & brahmic acids	: Antibacterial & in treatment of wound
(iii) Cannabinoid Δ^9 THC	: Anticancer activity.
(iv) Glycyrrhitinic acid	: In treatment of rheumatoid, arthritis and addision's disease.
(v) Gossypol	: As male antifertility agent.
(vi) Volatile constituents	: Flavouring agents.

GLYCOSIDES

Glycosides are compounds that contain aglycone and glycone molecule. These are widely present in plants and rarely in animals. In plant ß - D glucose sugar moiety is present. Glycosides on hydrolysis produce aglycone (genin) and glycone (sugar) molecules.

Chemically glycosides are considered as sugar ethers (acetals).

$$\text{Glycoside} \xrightarrow[\text{Acid/enzyme}]{\text{Hydrolysis}} \underset{\text{(genin)}}{\text{Aglycone}} + \underset{\text{(sugar)}}{\text{Glycone}}$$

Properties : Most of the glycosides are crystalline, colourless compounds (anthracene glycoside - red or orange; flavanoids - yellow in colour) and optically levo-rotatary. Glycosides are soluble in water and alcohol but insoluble in other organic solvent like chloroform, carbon tetrachloride, petroleum ether; while aglycone moiety is soluble in organic solvent but insoluble in aqueous solvent.

Classification : Glycosides are classified on the basis of linkage between glycone and aglycone moiety and also on the basis of chemical nature of aglycon (genin) molecule.

(A) Classification on the basis of linkage

" O " glycosides : These glycosides contain sugar molecule, attached to alcoholic or phenolic group of aglycone. e.g. Sennoside, glycyrrhizine, digitoxin, etc.

" C " glycosides : In these types of glycosides,. sugar molecule is directly attached to carbon atom of aglycone. e.g. Aloein, cascaroside, etc.

" N " glycosides : In these types of glycosides, sugar molecule is attached to nitrogen of aglycone molecule e.g. Adenosine, guannine, cytosine, etc.

" S " glycosides : In these types of glycosides, sugar molecule is attached to sulphur of aglycone molecule e.g. Sinigrin.

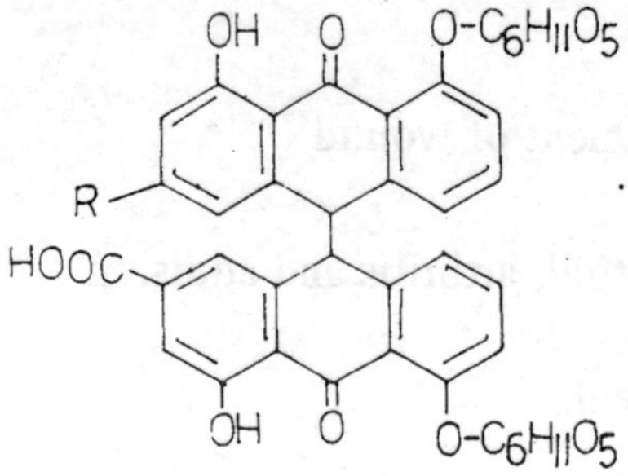

Sennoside

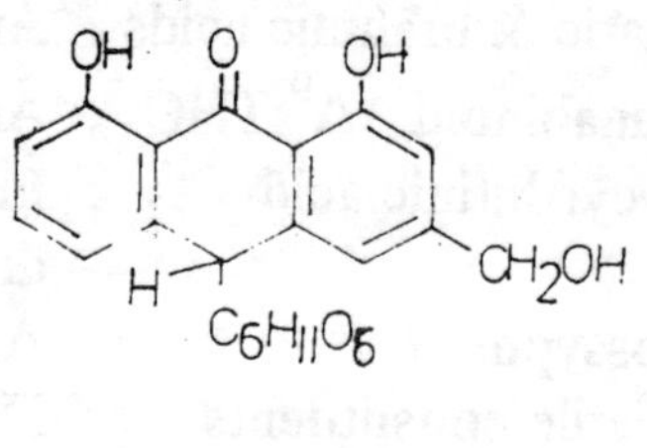

Aloin

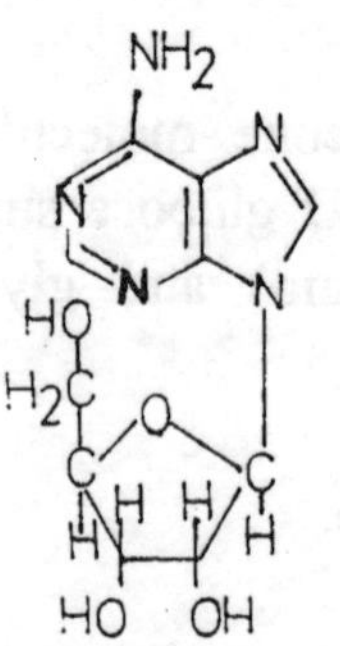

Adenosine

$$
\begin{array}{c}
C_3H_5\text{-}C\text{-}S\text{-}C_6H_{11}O_5 \\
\| \\
N\text{-}O\text{-}SO_3K
\end{array}
$$

Sinigrin

(B) Classification based on chemical nature of aglycone

(1) Alcoholic glycosides: Alcoholic glycosides are glycosides in which aglycone moiety is alcohol or its derivative i.e. salicin, in which aglycone part is O - hydroxy benzyl alcohol.

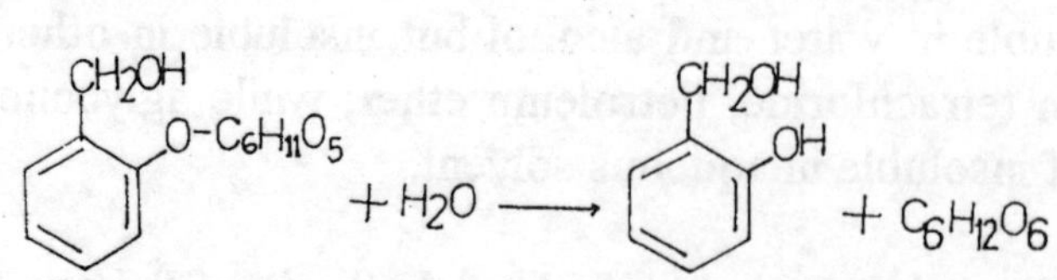

(2) Aldehyde glycosides : These glycosides contain aglycone molecule that is aldehydic compound. i.e. vanillin drug contains vanillin as aldehydic aglycone.

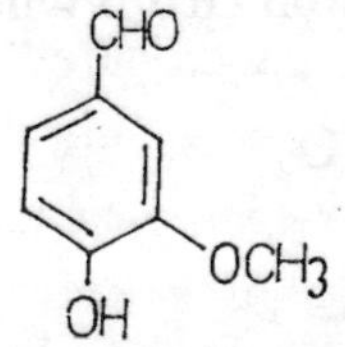

Vanillin (aglycon)

(3) Anthraquinone glycosides : These types of glycosides on hydrolysis give aglycone which is a derivative of di, tri, or tetra hydroxy anthraquinones. e.g. Sennoside, etc.

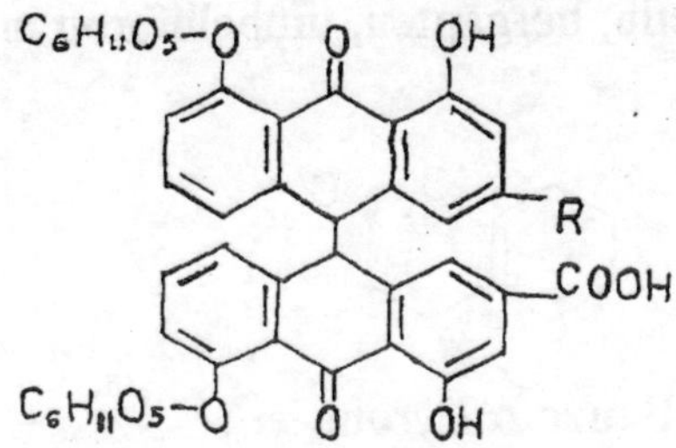

(4) Cyanophoric glycosides : These types of glycosides on hydrolysis give aglycone containing free cyanide group that breaks down to produce hydrocyanic acid. i.e. Amygdalin glycoside contains mandelonitrile aglycone that liberates hydrocyanic acid.

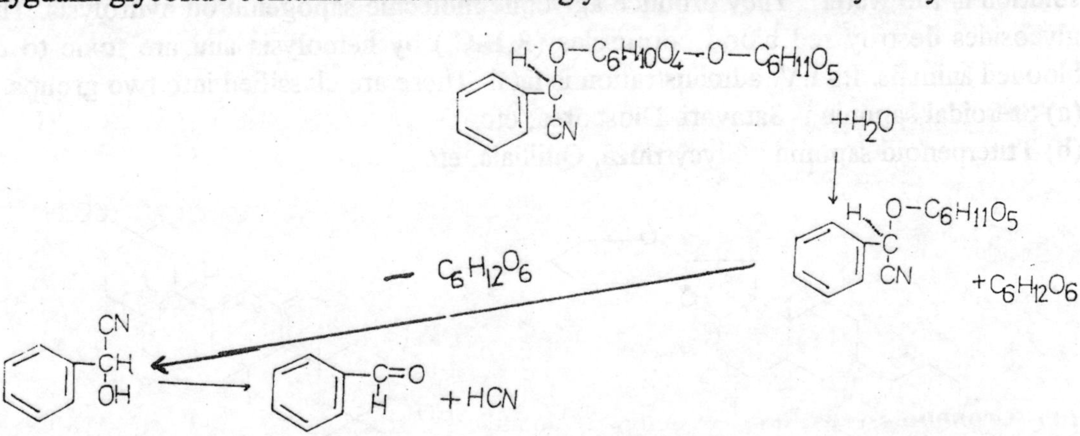

(5) Flavonol glycosides : Flavonol glycoside and its aglycone is termed as flavonoid. It occurs in plant as a yellow pigment [Latin-Flavous - yellow]. The basic moiety of flavonoide is Benzo γ pyrone type. e.g. Rutin, quercitin, biflavonoid, etc.

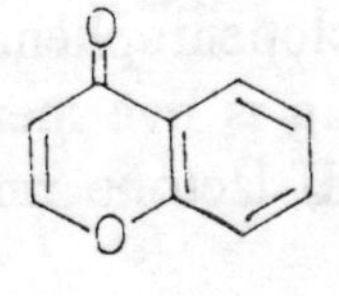

Benzo γ pyrone

(6) Isothiocynate glycosides : The aglycone moiety of this glycoside is isothiocynate. The aglycone may be aliphatic or aromatic. The examples of these glycosides are sinigrin (from black mustard) and sinalbin (from white mustard).

$$
\begin{array}{l}
C_3H_5\text{-}C\text{-}S\text{-}C_6H_{11}O_5 \\
\quad\quad\;\, \| \\
\quad\quad N\text{-}O\text{-}SO_3K
\end{array}
$$

Sinigrin

7) Lactone glycosides : These glycosides contain Benzo α Pyrone nucleus like aesculetin, coumarin, scopoletin, bergapten, umbelliferon in their aglycone moiety.

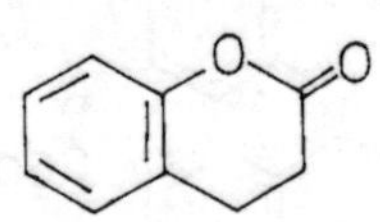

Benzo α Pyrone
(coumarin)

(8) Saponin glycosides : Saponin glycosides on shaking with water form colloidal solution in the water . They produce aglycone molecule sapogenin on hydrolysis. These glycosides destroy red blood corpuscles (R.B.C.) by hemolysis and are toxic to cold blooded animals. Its I.V. administration is fatal. These are classified into two groups.

(a) Steroidal saponin : Satavari, Dioscorea, etc.

(b) Triterpenoid saponin : Glycyrrhiza, Quilliaia, etc.

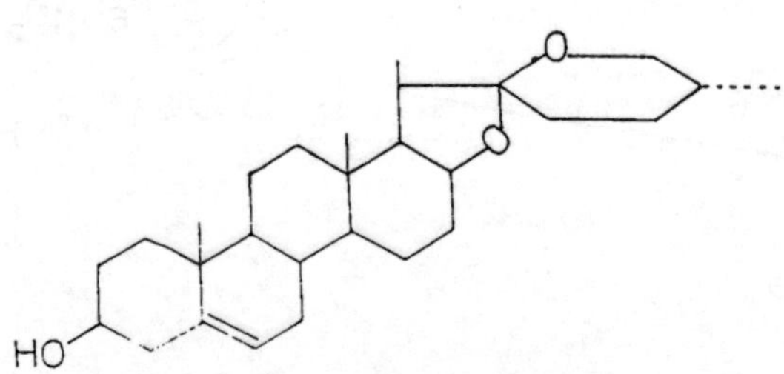

Diosgenin

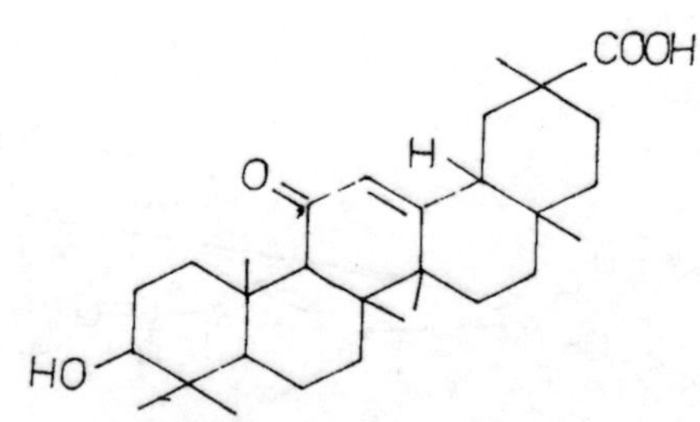

Glycyrrhetinic acid

(9) Steroidal glycosides : These glycosides are also called cardiac glycosides. Their aglycone moiety contains steroidal (cyclopentophenanthrene) nucleus. A lactone ring is attached to steroidal ring. If lactone ring is five members then it is called cardenolides e.g. digitoxgenin, strophanthidin, etc. If lactone ring is six members then it is called bufadienolide e.g. scillarenin.

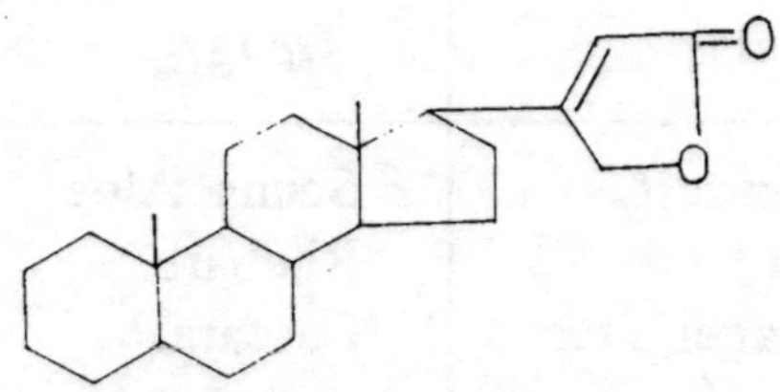

Cardenolide

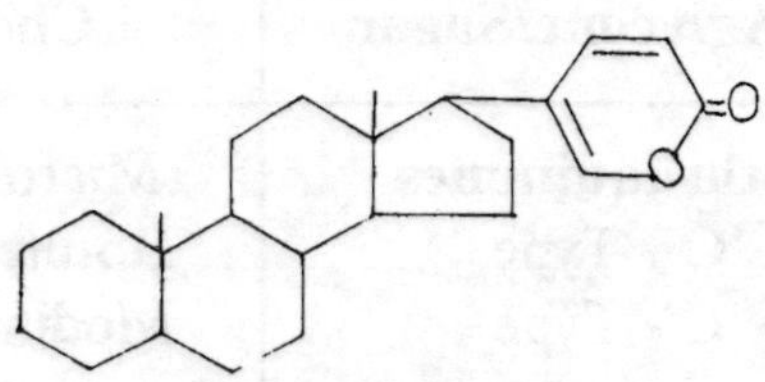

Bufadienolide

Distribution : Glycosides are distributed in almost every part of the plant.

Part of the Plant	Drug
Bark	Arjuna, quillaia
Whole aerial parts	Brahmi, Chirata
Fruits	Gokhru, Senna
Leaves	Aloe, Digitalis, Senna
Rhizomes	Dioscorea, Picrorrhiza
Roots	Satavari, Senega
Seeds	Musturd, Strophanthus

Isolation of glycosides : Generally glycosides are extracted with mixture of water and methanol (ethanol). Particular group of glycosides is efficiently extracted by a particular proportion of water and alcohol. Inactivation of enzyme is essential before or during extraction of particular glycoside from the fresh plant material. Fresh plant materials are heated at 100°C for 15-30 minutes. Inactivation of enzymes can also be carried out by any of the given methods.

(i) Boiling with acetone.
(ii) Acid treatment in cold condition. (pH 1.2)
(iii) Keeping in boiling water or boiling alcohol for 10-20 minutes.
(iv) Extraction at low temperature.

Identification of glycosides : There is no general test for the identification of glycosides. The glycosides are detected according to the nature of aglycone. Hydrolysis of glycoside liberates free aglycone.

Table 6.5 : Identification tests of some glycosides

Aglycone/Sugar	Chemical Test	Drugs
(1) **Anthraquinones**	Microsublimation test	Senna, Aloe
(a) 'O'- Type	Borntrager's test	Rhubarb.
(b) 'C'- Type	Modified Borntrager's test	Cascara.
(2) **Cardiac glycosides**		
(a) Deoxy sugars	Keller killiani test	Digitalis, Scilla
(b) Bufadienolides	Libermann Buchard's	Scilla
(c) Cardenolides	Baljet & Legal	Digitalis
(3) **Coumarins**	Fluorescence in alkali	Psoralea
(4) **Cyanogetic**	Sodium Picrate test	Linseed
(5) **Saponins**	Foam test	Liquorice
(6) **Reducing sugars**	Fehling solution	Acacia, Honey

VOLATILE OILS

Volatile oils are mixture of hydrodrocarbon terpenes, sesquiterpenes and polyterpenes and their oxygenated derivatives obtained from various parts of the plant. At ordinary temperature they evaporate and therefore are called etheral oils. They contain odourous or flavouring compounds hence known as essential oils because they produce essence. Fresh volatile oils are colourless. They oxidise and resinify on exposure to atmosphere for longer duration, so they should be stored in well closed amber coloured bottles in a cool and dry place.

Volatile oil may be present in particular secretory part they are

Glandular hair : Mint stem and leaves(Labiatae).
Mosophyll : Eucalyptus leaves
Modified : Piperaceae Parenchyma
Vittae : Anise (Umbelliferae)
Lysigenous or : Gossypium species
Schizogenous gland : Pinaceae, Rutaceae

All tissues	:	Conifers
Petels	:	Rose
Bark	:	Cinnamon
Rind	:	Orange
Heart wood	:	Sandal wood

Volatile oils are generally insoluble in water and soluble in organic solvents, their density is less than one and refractive index is very high. They are optically active.

Classification and Chemistry of Volatile oil : The out line of classification of volatile oils are given in following table:

Table 6.6 : Classification of Volatile oils

Class	Structure	Constituent	Drugs
1. Alcohol (a) Acyclic	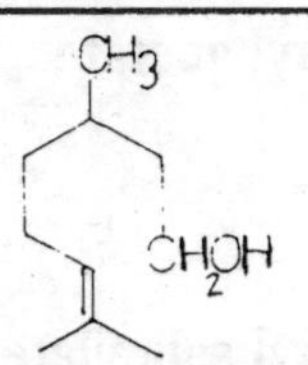	Citronellol	Lemon grass
(b) Monocyclic	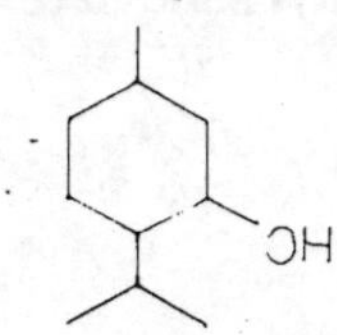	Menthol	Peppermint
(c) Bicyclic	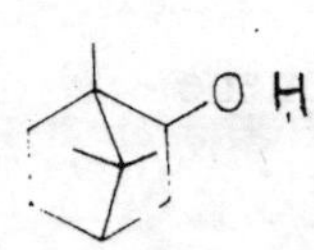	Borneol	Berneo camphor
2. Aldehyde	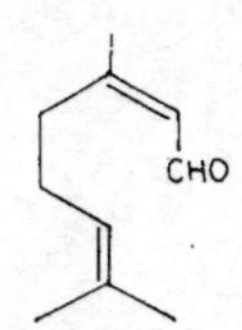	Citral	Lemon
	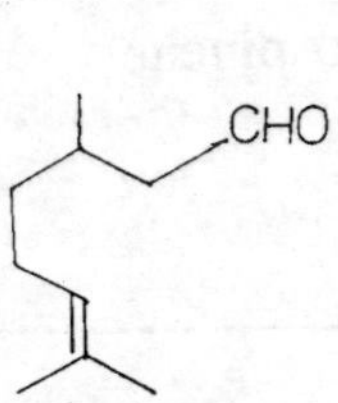	Citronellal	Lemon grass

Contd.

Class	Structure	Constituent	Drugs
3. Ether	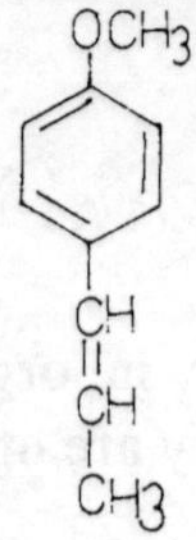	Anethol	Fennel ,Anise
	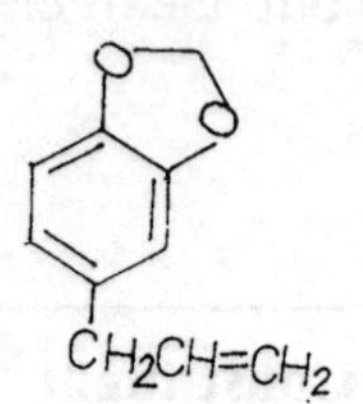	Safrole	Nutmeg
4. Esters	CH_3COOCH_3	Methyl acetate	Peppermint
	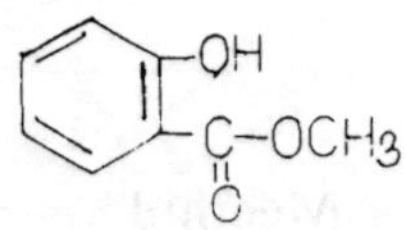	Methyl salicylate	Wintergreen oil
5. Hydrocarbon (a) Monocyclic	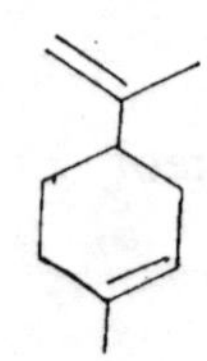	Limonene	Cardamom
(b) Bicyclic	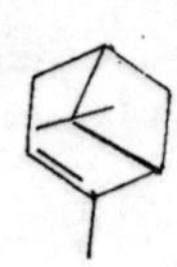	α pinene	Coriander oil

Contd..

Class	Structure	Constituent	Drugs
6. Ketons	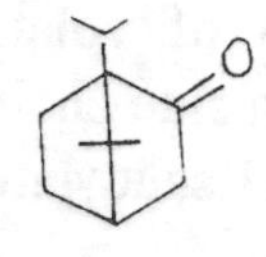	Camphor	Camphor
	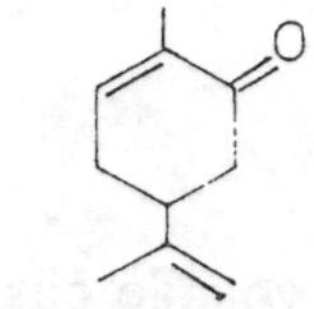	Carvone	Caraway oil
7. Nonterpenoid & derived from glycosidal	S=C=N-CH_2-CH=CH_2	Allyl isothiocynate	Musted oil
	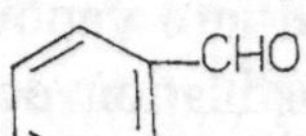	Benzaldehyde	Bitter almond
8. Oxides	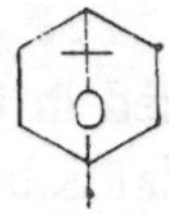	Cineole	Eucalyptus oil
9. Phenols	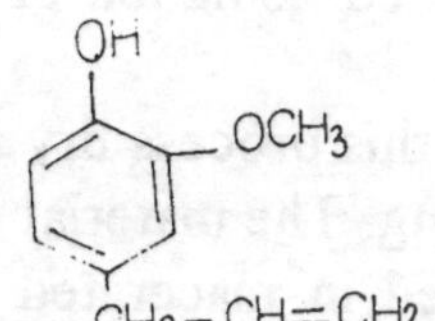	Eugenol	Clove
	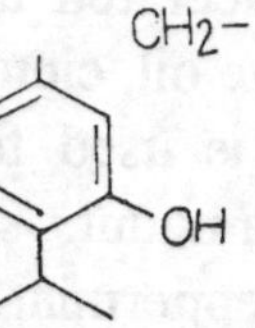	Thymol	Mint

Volatile oils mainly contain terpene. Terpene is a natural compound having isoprene (C_5H_8) unit. These isoprene units are linked by head to tail arrangement as per "special isoprene rule" in the terpene.

Monoterpenes	:	$(C_5H_8)_2$
Sesquiterpenes	:	$(C_5H_8)_3$
Diterpenes	:	$(C_5H_8)_4$
Triterpenes	:	$(C_5H_8)_6$
Polyterpenes	:	$[(C_5H_8)_2)]_n$

The monoterpenes are the major constituents of volatile oils. They may be acyclic, monocyclic or bicyclic, either as hydrocarbons(terpene) or their oxygenated derivatives

(terpenoids) i.e. aldehyde, ester, alcohol, phenol, etc. The terpenoids are responsible for odour and taste. The terpeneless volatile oils are possessing better fragrance.

Phenyl propanoids are also an important group of volatile oils. These compounds contain a phenylic nucleus attached to three carbon side chains (propane, allyl, etc.). The examples of such volatile oils are eugenol, methyl salicylate, anethol, cinnamaldehyde, etc,.

ISOLATION OF VOLATILE OILS

The following methods are used for isolation of volatile oils, first method (distillation) is widely applicable.

(1) **Distillation** : The process of converting liquid into vapour and again condensing to liquid is called distillation. The method of distillation depends on the condition of plant material. There are three methods used for oil distillation.

   a) **Water distillation** : This process is used in those plant materials which can not be destroyed by boiling. The material is boiled with water and vapours are condensed, volatile oil is separated. Isolation of turpentine oil is the main example of this method.
   b) **Water and steam distillation** : In this process dry and fresh plant material is used, which may be injured by boiling. The material is grounded and dipped in water. A stream of steam is passed in macerated material. The oily layers condense and distillate is separated e.g. clove oil, cinnamon oil.
   c) **Direct steam distillation** : This process is used for fresh plant materials which contain moisture in considerable amount, so there is no need of maceration. The fresh plant materials like peppermint, spearmint are placed in perforated basket or tray. The steam under pressure is passed through fresh plant material and volatile oil is collected with condensed vapours.

(2) **Expression** : Some volatile oils are obtained by expression because they can't be obtained by distillation process without decomposition.

   (a) **Sponge method** : The fruit is cut and pulp is removed with a sharp knife. The peel is soaked in water for few hours and peel curvature is reversed and oil gland present on peel is ruptured. Ejected oil is absorbed on sponge and is squeezed. The oil is separated and filtered.
   (b) **Ecuelle a Piquer method** : Ecuelle a piquer means "a bowl for pricking". In this process oil gland present over peel is ruptured with the help of pin (about 0.5 cm long). Lemon peel is rotated with hand and oil is sucked.

(3) **Extraction** : The volatile oil is obtained by solvent - solvent extraction with the help of organic liquid like petroleum ether and benzene. This process is performed at 50°C so that maximum volatile oil is collected. It is a significant process for perfumery industry because it contains more natural odour than the oil obtained by distillation. This process is economical as compared to distillation process in perfumery industry.

(4) **Enfleurage** : The fixed oil or fat is smeared on the glass sheet and fresh flowers containing volatile oil are spread. The flowers are removed from smeared fat with hand. Volatile oil is absorbed by fat or fixed oil. The volatile oil is extracted using alcohol. This process is used in perfumery industry e.g. rose oil from rose petals.

RESINS

Definition : Resins are solid or semisolid amorphous plant exudates of complex chemical nature. They are formed in schizogenous or schizolysigenous duct or cavities. They are the end products of metabolism.

Properties : Resins are hard translucent or transparent substance which on heating soften, melt and forms adhesive fluid. Their specific gravity is more than water. They are insoluble in water but soluble in organic solvents like chloroform, solution of chloral hydrate, volatile oil, etc.

Resins are chemically complex mixture of (i) Resin alcohol (resinols) (ii) resin phenols (resinotannols) (iii) resin acids (iv) resenes.

(i) **Resinols** : They give negative test with ferric chloride. They may be present in free or in combination with resin acids to form esters. These acids may be benzoic acids, salicylic acid, etc. The examples of resinols are benzoresinol (in benzoin), storesinol (in storax).

(ii) **Resino-tannols** : They contain tannins and give positive test for phenol with ferric chloride. They have high molecular weight and occur as esters or free. e.g. Toluresinotannol (in Tolu Balsam), Aloeresinotannol (in Aloes).

(iii) **Resin acids** : Resin acids contain a large proportion of oxy-acids. They are found in free and esterified form. They are soluble in aqueous alkali solutions and form soap like froth on shaking or colloidal suspension. Their metallic salts are called resinates. The examples are abietic acid (in colophony), copaivic and oxycopaivic acid (in copaiba) and commiphoric acid (in myrrh).

(iv) **Resenes** : They are inert neutral complex and high molecular weight substances. They are very stable and not affected by any chemical reactions. They are insoluble in acid and alkali. e.g. asaresene (in Asafoetida), dracoresene (in Dragons blood), etc.

Classification of resins : Resins are classified as per occurrence in combination with other compounds.

(1) **Oleo - resin** : When resin is associated with volatile oil, mixture is called as oleo-resins. e.g. Turpentine, Copaiba, Ginger & Capsicum.

(2) **Oleo gum resin** : When oleo resin is associated with gum, the mixture is called oleo-gum-resin. e.g. Myrrh, Asafoetida, etc.

(3) **Balsams** : Balsams are resinous mixtures containing large proportion of free or combined benzoic or cinnamic acid. e.g. Tolu Balsam, Benzoin, Peru Balsam,, etc.

(4) **Glycoresin** : Glycoresins are mixtures of resin with glycosides. These on hydrolysis give aglycone (complex resin) and sugar. Glycoresins are present in Podophyllum & Jalap.

Resins are obtained from plants by various methods.

(1) The incision is made over plant and pathological exudate is collected e.g. Asafoetida, Myrrh, etc.

(2) Fossil resins are collected e.g. Copal, Kauri.

(3) Resins are collected by heating plant material, e.g. Guaiacum.

(4) Material is distilled for separation of volatile oil e.g. Colophony.

(5) Material is extracted with alcohol and is precipitated with water e.g. Podophyllum, Capsicum.

FIXED OILS, FATS AND WAXES (LIPIDS)

The lipids are long chain fatty acids and alcohols. The type of alcohol is the differentiating feature between fixed oil, fats and waxes. Fixed oils and fats are esters of fatty acid with glycerol while waxes are esters of higher molecular weight alcohols (cetyl alcohol).

FIXED OILS AND FATS : They are reserve food material of plants and animals. Fixed oils are liquid at 15 - 16.5°C, while fats are semisolid or solid.

Properties : Fixed oils are obtained from seeds of the plant. These are thick, viscous, yellow colour liquids bearing characteristic odour and are non volatile. These can not be saponified. These are lighter than water and are soluble in organic solvents and insoluble in aqueous solvents. Fats and oils are greasy substances and produce permanent translucent stain on the paper. On exposure to air for longer duration causes rancidity (Acid liberated) and develop disagreeable odour. In moist condition these form free acids due to presence of enzyme lipase. These are emollient and demulcent in nature. Antioxidants, hydrocarbons, ketones, phospholipids, sterols and vitamins are present in oils and fats in traces, and are responsible for specific odour of oil. The fats contain more amount of saturated acids. The example of fixed oils and fats are Arachis oil, Castor oil, Codliver oil, Shark liver oil, etc.

Table 6.7 : Difference between Fixed oils and Volatile oils

Fixed oils	Volatile oils
1. These are non aromatic and does not volatalise at room temp.	These are aromatic and volatile at room temp. and produce essence.
2. These are ester of fatty acid with glycerol(glycerides of higher fatty acids).	Chemically these are terpenes and their oxygenated compounds (terpenoids)
3. They produces permanent, translucent stain on paper.	They don't produce permanent stain on paper
4. On prolong storage, they become rancid and give disagreeable odour.	On prolong storage they may resinify, oxidise & colour turns dark.
5. These are obtained by expression method	They are obtained by distillation, expression & extraction.
6. These have food value.	These do not contain food value.

WAXES : Waxes are esters of fatty acids with high molecular weight monohydric alcohols. In other way waxes are better defined as mixture of different molecular weight acids and alcohols. Waxes may contain paraffins. Waxes are similar to fats but difficult to saponify. Waxes are only saponified by alcoholic alkali where as fats are saponified by aqueous and alcoholic alkali both.

Wax is a viscous solid mass containing characteristic waxy lustre. Waxes are widely distributed in nature.

Animal : Bees wax, Wool fat.
Plant : Carnauba wax, Sesame wax, Bayberry wax.
Mineral : Paraffin.

Waxes are also present in the outer cell wall of epidermal tissues in fruits and leaves. It acts as a protective covering against penetration and water loss. Waxes are used in the preparation of ointments, creams & cerates,, etc.

TANNINS

Tannins are complex substances containing mixture of polyphenols and are widely distributed in plant kingdom. They give gold beater's skin test positive and absorb on standard hide powder. They combine with protein of animal hide to prevent putrefactions and convert hide and skin into leather. During growth of plant, tannins act as a protective. Most true tannins have molecular weight among 1000-5000. Low molecular weight substances are known as pseudotannins and they contain gallic acid (rhubarb), Catechins (Acacia & Catechu) and chlorogenic acid (nux vomica) are partly absorbed on standard hide powder and does not give gold beater's skin test. Tannins are non crystalline compounds that form colloidal and acidic solution with water. Tannins give precipitate with gelatin, alkaloids and heavy metals. Tannins may be hazardous due to their carcinogenic principles. Habitual chewing betel nut and drinking tea without milk is very harmful and produces cancer. Tannins have astringent property and are used as astringents, healing agents, gonorrhoea, burns, piles,, etc. These are also useful in alkaloidal poisoning due to formation of insoluble tannates.

Chemically tannins are classified into two groups

(i) **Hydrolysable tannins** (ii) **Condensed tannins.**

Hydrolysable tannins : These tannins are hydrolysed by acids, or enzyme (tannase) and produce gallic acid and ellagic acid. Chemically, these are esters of phenolic acid like gallic acid and ellagic acid. Tannins produced by gallic acid and ellagic acids are called gallic tannin and ellagic tannin respectively. The gallic tannins are found in clove, rhubarb and rose petals and ellagic tannins are found in eucalyptus leaves, rind and bark of pome granate. These tannins react with iron salts to give blue or black colour or precipitate which is used in the preparation of ink. These tannins on dry distillation produce pyrrogallol.

Condensed tannins : These tannins are resistant to hydrolysis and are formed by the condensation of many catechin, flavonols and flavon, 3,4 diols. These form red colour insoluble phlobaphenes after decomposition by treatment with acid or enzyme. The red colour of cinchona bark is due to presence of phlobaphenes. Catechol tannin on heating produces catechol. The condensed tannins give green colour with iron salts. These are widely distributed in plants and available in various parts of plant like bark (Cinchona,

Cinnamon), fruits(Amla, Harde, Bahera), leaves (Tea, Hemmanetis), rhizomes and roots (Male fern, Krameria), seed (Areca, Cocoa) and wood (Acacia)

Identification tests of tannins

(1) **Match stick test :** A match stick is dipped in aqueous extract containing tannin and dried . This stick on moistening with hydrochloric acid and subsequent heating turns pink. The stick woods contain lignin that turns pink due to formation of phlorogluci-nol.

(2) **Goldbeater's skin test :** A small membrane of ox intestine (Goldbeater's skin) is soaked in 2% hydrochloric acid for 5 minutes. Skin is washed with water and dipped in ferrous sulphate solution. A black brown colour is produced.

(3) **Phenazone test :** To the extract of tannin, sodium hydrogen phosphate and 2% phenazone is added. This solution is heated and bulky precipitate is formed.

(4) **Gelatin test :** A 10% sodium chloride and 1% gelatin solution is added to 1% tannin solution. A buff white coloured precipitate is obtained.

(5) **Chlorogenic acid test** : Tannins produce green colour on treating with aqueous ammonia solution. This is due to the presence of chlorogenic acid.

(6) **Vanillin hydrochloric acid test** : Tannins give red precipitate with vanillin hydrochloric acid reagent (Vanillin hydrochloric acid reagent is prepared by mixing 1gm Vanillin + 10ml hydrochloric acid + 10ml alcohol).

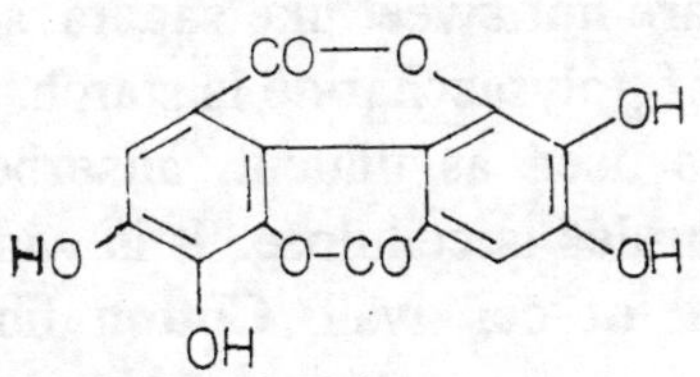

Ellagic acid

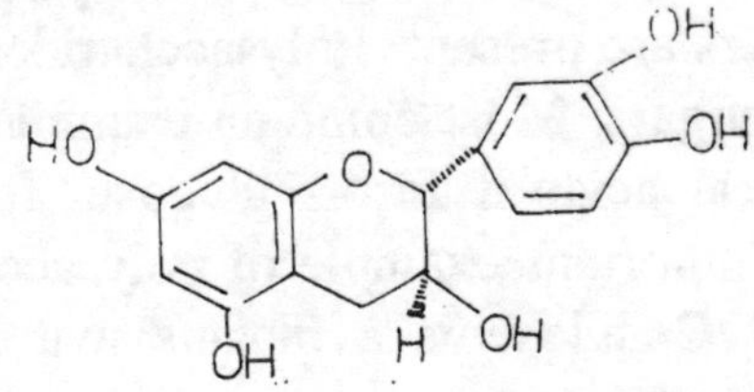

Catechin

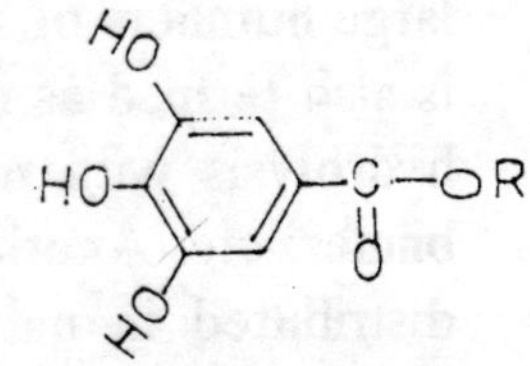

R=H = Gallic acid
$R=C_6H_{11}O_5$ = Glucogallin

CARBOHYDRATES : Carbohydrates are plant and animal product which contain carbon, hydrogen and oxygen, where hydrogen and oxygen are in the same ratio as in water. Carbohydrates are the first products of photosynthesis.

Carbohydrates are classified into two groups

(i) Saccharides or simple sugars
(ii) Polysaccharides (non sugars)

I. **Saccharides or Simple sugars** : Sugars are monosaccharides, containing only one sugar unit. It can not be hydrolyzed into simpler sugars.

$$\text{Disaccharides} \xrightarrow{\text{hydrolysis}} \text{2 monosaccharide units}$$

$$\text{Trisaccharides} \xrightarrow{\text{hydrolysis}} \text{monosaccharide units}$$

$$\text{Tetra saccharides} \xrightarrow{\text{hydrolysis}} \text{4 monosaccharide units}$$

Monosaccharides are classified on the basis of number of carbon atoms in the molecule

Trioses	:	3 carbon sugar
Tetroses	:	4 carbon sugar
Pentoses	:	5 carbon sugar
Hexoses	:	6 carbon sugar

Chemically simple sugar is a aldehydic or ketonic substitution product of poly hydroxy alcohol. Glucose contains aldehydic group so it is known as aldose where as fructose contains ketonic group and is known as ketose. It contains unbroken chain of carbon atoms. Sugars are soluble in water giving sweet taste. These are crystalline solids and optically active and are inert substances. These are used to mask the taste in various formulations. Honey is one of examples of saccharides.

II. **Polysaccharides** : Polysaccharides contain large number of sugars e.g. monosaccharides. They are joined together through oxygen. Polysaccharides on hydrolysis form hexoses or pentoses or their derivatives as final products. In oligosaccharides two to ten units of sugars are present, whereas in polysaccharides large numbers of sugars are present. Polysaccharides are not sweet like sugars, so it is also termed as nonsugars. Most common example of polysaccharide is starch. On hydrolysis with mineral acids it forms glucose. It is used as diluent, adsorbent, binder, etc. Another important example of polysaccharides is cellulose. It is widely distributed in nature. Cellulose is a fibrous material of cell wall. Cotton fibres contain about 98% of cellulose.

Chemical test for carbohydrates

1. **Reduction of Fehling's solution** : To the heated solution of carbohydrate, add equal parts of Fehling's solution A and B drop by drop, on heating, a brick red precipitate of cuprous oxide is formed. In case of non reducing carbohydrates, these are boiled with acid which converts them into reducing sugars, neutralised and then other tests are performed.
2. **Molisch's Test** : This is a common test for identification of all carbohydrates. Carbohydrate solution is prepared in water containing α-naphthol. Concentrated sulphuric acid is added along the side of test tube. A purple ring is formed below the aqueous solution. In case of insoluble carbohydrates such as cotton wool (i.e. cellulose) colour will be produced after shaking the reaction mixture.

CHAPTER 7

NATURAL DRUGS AND THEIR THERAPEUTIC EFFICACY

7 - A. LAXATIVE

The term laxative is derived from a latin word Laxare, meaning to loosen. The drugs that promote evacuation of feacal matter by loosening bowel are called laxative. Aperint, laxative,purgative and cathartic are similar terms but these are used to define the magnitude of laxative action.

Cathartic >	Purgative >	laxative >	Aperint
(strongest)			(mildest)

The laxatives are classified into four categories according to their mode of action.

(1) **Stimulants** : They act by local irritation on the intestinal tract and increase peristaltic activity e.g. Cascara, Rhubarb, Senna, Castor oil, etc.

(2) **Bulk forming** : These drugs absorb water and swell. This increases the bulk of intestinal content that stimulates peristalsis. e.g. Ispaghula, Psyllum, Agar-agar, etc.

(3) **Emollient** : These drugs act either as stool softners or as lubricants to facilitate evacuation of compact stool. e.g. Liquid paraffin.

(4) **Cathartic** : These agents act intensively by violent irritation of gut. e.g. Croton oil, Podophyllum resin, Jalap resin, etc.

ALOES

Vernacular name : Sans. - Ghrit-Kumari.

Biological source : Aloe is the dried juice of the leaves of various species of Aloe. It is a member of *Liliaceae* family. There are various species of aloe (i) *Aloe perryi* Baker (Socotrine aloes) (ii) *Aloe barbadensis* Miller (Curacao aloes) and (iii) *Aloe ferox* and its hybrids (Cape aloes).

Geographical source : Various species of aloe are indigineous to Africa but the plant is available also in West-Indies and Europe. In India, it is cultivated mainly in the north west Himalayan region. Cape aloe is found in South Africa, Kenya, etc. Curacao aloe is found in West-Indian islands of Curacao, Aruba and Bonaire. Indian aloe is *Aloe vera*.

Cultivation, collection and preparation : Aloe is a xerophytic plant containing thick fleshy leaves, spines at the margin. The leaves are in the rosette form, the parenchymatous cells of pericycle contain juice which is surrounded by mucilaginous cells. The fleshy leaves are cut at the base and juice exudes out. The juice is collected in a V shaped vessel, or in goat skin or in canvas. Commercial varieties of aloe vary, depending on the various methods of collection, concentration and cooling of juice either by gradual heating or by boiling.

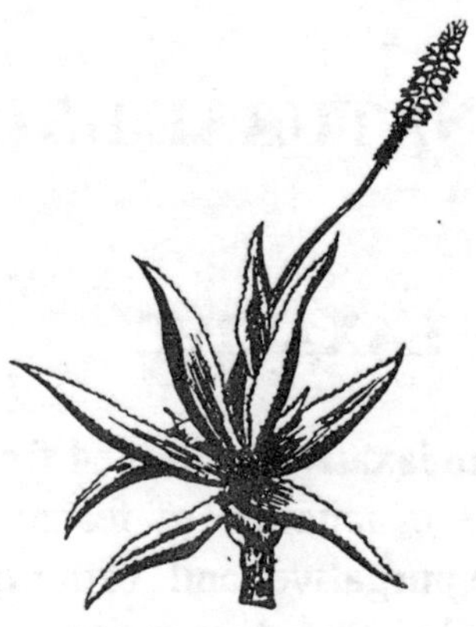

Fig. 7. 1: Aloe: A mature plant of *Aloe vera*.

Socotorine Aloe : This is also known as *Zangibar Aloe*. Juice is collected in goat or sheep skin and is allowed to evaporate naturally.

Curacao aloe : This is also known as Barbados aloe. The cut leaves of aloe plant are placed one above the other. V shaped structure is formed in this way. The juice draining out from the V shaped structure is collected in a tin vessel and evaporated into a semi-solid mass. This mass is cooled slowly to give crystalline Barbaloin. It is allowed to solidify to obtain an opaque mass. This is known as hepatic aloe or livery aloe.

Cape aloe : The juice of aloe is collected in canvas or goat skin from fleshy leaves. These are boiled for few hours till it attains solid consistency and quickly cooled to prevent crystallization of Barbaloin. This is also known as vitreous or shiny aloe.

Socotrine aloe is an opaque mass reddish black to brown in colour, fracture is porous. Curacao aloe is yellowish-brown to chocolate-brown in colour and fracture is waxy. Cape aloe is glassy dark brown in colour and fracture is glassy. All the forms of aloe have strong characteristic, unpleasant odour and a disagreeable, bitter and nauseous taste.

Chemical constituents : Aloe contains 10-30% aloin. It is a mixture of three substance, barbaloin, ß-barbaloin and iso-barbaloin. The proportion of these isomers differs in the different commercial varieties. Barbaloin is a pale yellow, crystalline glycoside, soluble in water, present in all the varieties of aloe whereas the amorphous ß-barbaloin which is obtained from barbaloin on heating is present only in the cape aloe. Isobarbaloin is present in curacao aloe and trace of isobarbaloin is also present in cape aloe but it is not present in socotrine aloe. Barbaloin is a C-glycoside and is not hydrolysed easily as compared to the O-glycoside present in aloe. It also contains emodine-8-glucoside and emodine oxanthrone glucoside. These are O-glycoside present in aloe. On hydrolysis it produces aloe-emodin and arabinose. Aloe also contains a resin ester formed from ferulic acid, para coumaric acid and cinnamic acid. Polysaccharides aloeferon and aloeulcin are also present in aloe. It also containsglycoprotein, alocutin A & B.

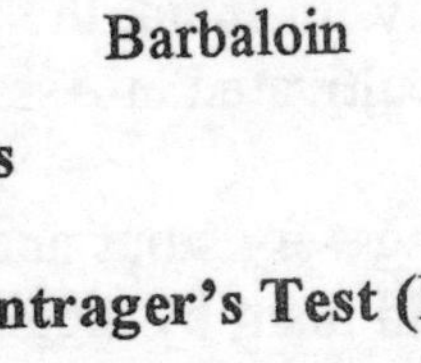

Barbaloin

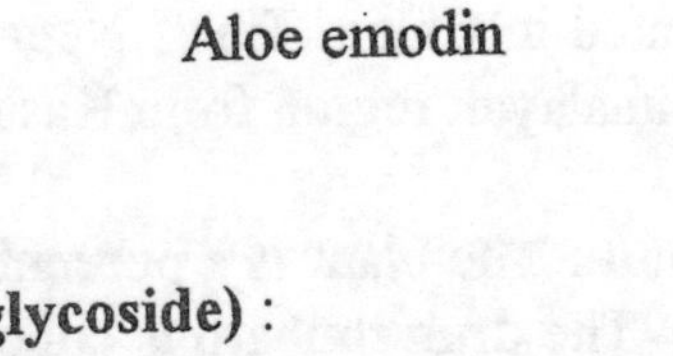

Aloe emodin

Chemical tests

Modified Borntrager's Test (For anthraquinone glycoside) :

1. Aloe is boiled with 5ml of dil. HCl and 5ml of 5% solution of ferric chloride for five minutes. The solution is cooled, filtered and filtrate is shaken with benzene. The benzene layer is made alkaline with ammonia, pink colour is formed.

2. **Bromine Test** : To the solution of aloe, add equal volume of bromine solution, yellow precipitate of tetrabromaloin is formed.

3. **Schouteten's Test (Borax test)** : To 5ml solution of aloe, add 0.2gm of borax. This is heated to dissolve completely. This is poured into water, green fluorescence is produced due to aloe -emodin anthranol.
4. **Klunge's Isobarbaloin Test (Praloin test)** : To an aqueous solution of aloe add 1 drop of copper sulphate, 1gm sodium chloride and (few ml) 90% alcohol, a purple colour is formed. This test is sensitive with curacao aloe but not with socotorine aloe.
5. **Nitrous Acid Test** : To an aqueous solution of aloe a small amount of sodium nitrite and few ml of acetic acid are added, pink colour is developed.
6. **Nitric Acid Test** : To aloe solution(aqueous), add nitric acid; cape aloe forms brownish colour, which changes rapidly to green; curacao gives deep brownish red; Socotrine a pale brownish - yellow; Zanzibar a yellowish - brown colour.

Uses : Aloe is used as irritant purgative. Its activity is increased when it is administered with small amounts of alkaline salt or soaps. Aloe gel is viscous viscid juice. It is mucilaginous and colourless, widely used in the cosmetic industry as a protective in the treatment of sun-burn. It is one of the ingredients of compound benzoin tincture.

RHUBARB (RHEUM)

Vernacular name: Sans.: Gandhini, Pitamulika; Hindi-Revendchini; Tam.-Nattuirevalchini; Eng.- Himalayan rhubarb.

Biological source : The drug rhubarb consists of dried rhizomes and roots of *Rheum officinale* Baillon, *Rheum palmatum* Linn. and other species of Rheum excluding *R. rhaponticum*. It is the member of *polygonaceae* family. Indian rhubarb consists of rhizomes of *R. emodi* Wall or *R. webbiannum* Royle.

Geographical source : The plant is grown at an altitude of over 3000 metres. The plant is cultivated in China, Tibet, Nepal, Europe and Germany. In India, the plant is available in the Himalayan region from Kashmir to Sikkim and is cultivated in Assam.

Collection : The plant is a perennial stout herb containing very stout and thick roots and rhizome. The drug rhubarb is collected from 6-8 years old plant by digging out rhizomes, during September to October. The roots and rhizomes are cut, the outer bark is separated by peeling. The big rhizomes are cut longitudinally into small pieces and drugs are dried in shade or by artificial heat. The quality of shade dried drug is superior.

Morphology : The drug occurs in round, flat or conical pieces. The outer surface of chinese drug is pale brown to reddish in colour, whereas Indian rhubarb is yellowish brown in colour. It is 2-15 cm in length and 3-8 cm in diameter. Surface is smooth, non-shrunken and light yellow showing white reticulations. These white tissues are phloem or xylem parenchyma filled with starch and calcium oxalate, reddish orange lines and medullary rays are seen in the tangential section of the rhizomes. Odour is faint, aromatic and characteristic. Taste is bitter and astringent.

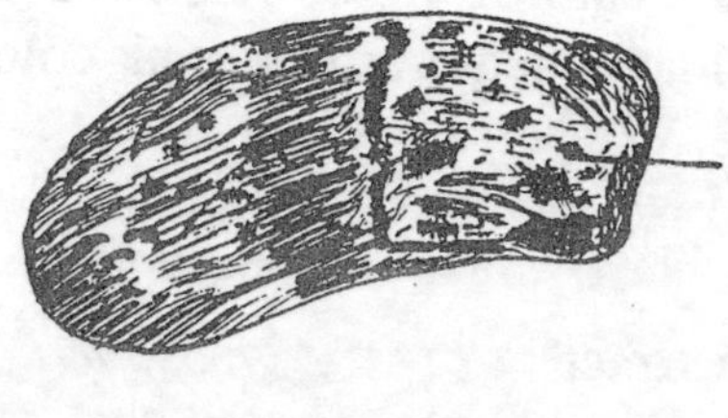

Fig. 7.2. : Rhubarb : Rhizome of *Rheum officinale.*

Chemical constituents : It contains four type of anthraquinone derivatives.

(I) Anthraquinone with carboxylic group : ex- Rhein and its glycoside, glucorhein.
(II) Anthraquinonewithout carboxylic group : ex-Chrysophanol, emodine, aloe emodine physcion and their glucosides.
(III)Anthrone & dianthrone of chrysophanol, aloe-emodin, emodine and physcion. The other dianthrone glucosides of rhein i.e., sennoside A & B.
(IV)Heterodianthrones obtained from two different anthrone molecules, e.g.

Palmidin A=(aloe-emodine+emodine) anthrone
Palmidin B=(aloe modine+chrysophanol) anthrone
Palmidin C = (emodine+chrysophanol) anthrone.

It also contains glucogallin, free gallic acid, epicatechin gallate and catechin as astringent compounds, starch and calcium oxalate.

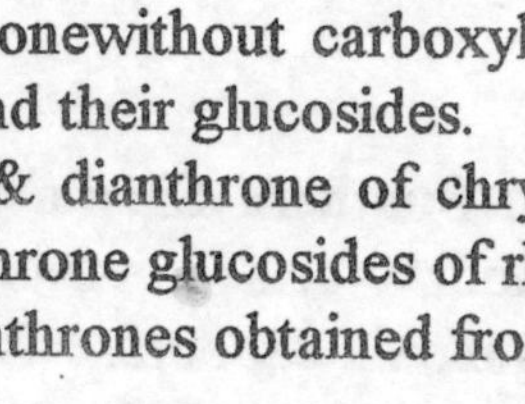

R	Compound
-H	emodin
-COOH	Rhein
$-CH_3$	Chrysophanol
$-CH_2OH$	Aloe-emodin

Chemical tests

(1) **With ammonia** : When powdered drug is kept with ammonia for 15 minutes, pink coloured crystals of rhaponticin are formed.

(2) **Borntrager's Test** : Boil the drug with dilute sulphuric acid, filter, cool the filtrate and add organic solvent like chloroform or benzene followed by ammonia solution to make alkaline. Ammonical layer acquires rose pink colour.

Standards

Acid insoluble ash	:	≤ 1%
45% Alcohol soluble extract	:	≤ 35%
Hydroxy quinone derivatives	:	≥ 3%

Uses : It is used as laxative and in larger dose as purgative, followed by an astringent effect due to the presence of tannoid. It is also used as bitter stomachic, powder root is applied externally in ulcer. It is an important ingredient in anumber of Ayurvedic formulations. It is contraindicated to patients suffering from rheumatism, gout, epilepsy and uric acid troubles.

Other rhubarb : Rhapontic rhubarb: It is found in Southern Siberia and regions of Volga river. It shows diffuse ring of star spots and hollow centre, it has sweet taste. It gives blue fluorescence that is further intensified by ammonia vapours.

CASTOR OIL

Vernacular names : Hind- Erandi; Sans.- shweteranda; Beng - Rehri; Tam.- Amanakku; Eng.- castor.

Biological source : Castor oil is a fixed oil obtained by cold expression of the seeds of *Ricinus communis* Linn. This is a member of *Euphorbiaceae* family.

Geographical source : The plant is native of India and cultivated throughout the country in gardens and fields and also grows wild in waste places. It is also cultivated in Brazil, China, USSR and Thialand.

Character of seeds : The seeds are oval, compressed 0.8-1.8 cm long and 0.4-1.2 cm broad. The tasta is smooth, brittle and thin. It is grey, brown or black in colour. There is a small yellowish caruncle present at one end, from which raphe extends on the flat or ventral side, to challaza at the opposite end of the seed. The testa is easily removed exposing the large white oily endosperm containing thin, flat foliaceous cotyledons and a radicle directed towards the caruncles.

(a) Fruit (b) Seed

Fig. 7.3 : Castor

Preparation of castor oil : The seed coats are removed and kernels are cold expressed with hydraulic presses to get 30% of oil using 1-2 atmospheric pressure per square inch. The cold expression yields medicinal oil (33%) and remaining quantity of oil is obtained by other methods. The medicinal oil is steamed at 80°C to destroy lipase and ricin (toxic protein). The medicinal castor oil is colorless or pale yellow liquid, possessing slightly nauseating odour and a faintly acrid taste. The acid value of çastor oil increases with time and poor storage conditions. But initially high acid value shows use of damaged seed sand careless extraction.

Standards

Density	:	0.945-0.965
Acid value	:	≤ 2
Acetyl value	:	≥ 143
Iodine value	:	82-90
Sap.value	:	177 to 185
Optical rotation	:	$\geq +3.5$
Refractive Index	:	1.475

Chemical constituents : The castor seeds contain 46-53% fixed oil, albumin, globulin, glycoprotein, ricin and crystalline alkaloid ricinine. Fixed oil contains glycerides of ricinolic acid, isoricinolic acid, stearic acid and dihydroxystearic acids. The free ricinolic acid and its stearic isomers are responsible for its purgative action. These are formed by the hydrolysis of tricinolein by the lipases in the duodenum.

$$CH_3(CH_2)_5\underset{\substack{|\\ OH}}{CH}\text{-}CH_2\ CH=CH(CH_2)_7COOH.$$

Ricinoleic acid

Uses : It is a well-known purgative and emollient. It is also useful in the preparation of flexible collodione (as ointment bases), hair fixers and perfumed hair oil. Ricinoleic acid is used in preparation of contraceptive creams and jellies.

ISPAGHULA [psyllium seed]

Biological source: It is a dried seed of *Plantago ovata* Forskal. It is a member of *Plantaginaceae* family.

Geographical source : Plant is cultivated largely in Gujarat, Punjab, Southern Rajasthan, Maharastra and Karnataka. The variety *P. psyllium* Linn is cultivated in Spain, Cuba and France.

Cultivation and collection : The plant is stem-less, containing soft hair and is an annual herb. The piant is cultivated by spreading the seeds in the month of November. The field is irrigated about 7-8 times at the interval of 8-10 days. Ammonium sulphate is a suitable fertilizer for the satisfactory growth of the plant. The crop is harvested after 4 months, i.e., in the month of March and April and the average yield of seed per hectare is 750 Kg. The plants are collected by cutting just above the ground and dried. The seeds are separated by thrashing and are cleaned by winnowing and sieving.

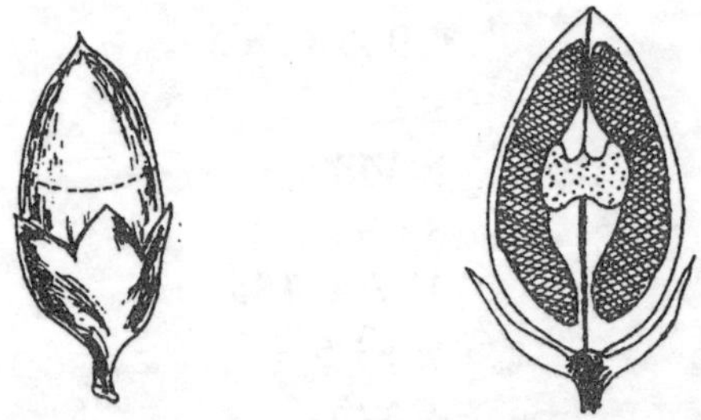

(a) Fruit (b) Longitudinal section of fruit.

Fig. 7.4 : Ispaghula

Characters : The seeds of *P. ovata* are 2-3 mm long and 1-1.6 mm in breadth, pinkish-grey to brown in colour. They are boat shaped with shinning and glossy surface. The dorsal surface is convex containing a small elliptical or elongated reddish-brown spot. The ventral surface is concave containing a deep furrow with a hilum covered by a thin membrane that appears as a red spot in the centre. The seeds are odourless, mucilaginous and containing blaňd taste.

Chemical constituents : Ispaghula seed and husk contains 10-30% of hydrocolloid as mucilage. Chemically, it contains pentosan and aldobionic acid. D-xylose, rhamnose, arabinose and galactouronic acids are hydrolysed products of mucilage. Fixed oils and proteinsare also present in the drug.

Standards

		Seed	Husk
Ash	:	≤ 3%	2. 9%
Acid insoluble ash	:	≤ 0.6%	0.45%
Foreign organic matter	:	≤ 2%	2.00%
Swelling factor	:	≥ 10ml	20ml

Chemical tests

1. **Swelling factor** : Swelling factor should be in between 10-14.
2. **Mucilage test** : With rethunium red, it gives pink colour.

Uses : It is used as demulcent, bulk laxative, in amoebic and in bacillary dysentery, duodenal ulcer, diarrhoea, constipation and piles. It contains indigestible mucilage hence intestinal flora and enzymes cannot react with it and it comes out unchanged.
It is also used as a stabilizer in ice cream industry.

Adulterants :

1. The seeds of *P.lanceolata* Linn. are oblong, elliptical in shape, yellowish brown in colour and swelling factor is 4.75. It is widely available in India.
2. The seeds of *P. asiatica* (syn.*P.major* Linn.) are available in Andra Pradesh and Tamil Nadu and used as substitute of ispaghula.

SENNA

Vernacular name : Sans.- Kalyani; Hindi-Sona-Ka-Pat; Beng.Sona-Mukhi; Tam.-Nila virai; Eng.-Senna.

Biological source : Senna consist of dried leaflets of *Cassia acutifola* Delile, known as **Alexandrian senna**, and *Cassia angustifolia* vahal, known as **Tinnevelly senna** (Indian senna). These are commonly known as *Cassia senna.* These plants are the members of *Leguminosae* family.

Geographical source: *Cassia acutifolia* is indigenous to tropical Africa and cultivated in Sudan. *Cassia angustifolia* is indigenous to Somaliland, Sind, Arabia, Punjab and cultivated in South India (Tinnevelly).

Cultivation and collection : The plant is a small shrub about half to one metre height, containing paripinnate leaves. Leaf-lets are 7-8 in pairs, glabrous,yellowish-green in colour. The cultivation of senna plant is done by sowing the seeds. Generally it is cultivated twice in a year, i.e, in March or April and November or December. Generally well drained irrigated land is preferred for cultivation but it can also be cultivated in dry area. In the dry area, collection of leaves is inferior than that of irrigated area. The plant is allowed to grow for 4-5 months and is harvested by cutting the stem above the ground. These stems containing leaves and pods are dried in the sun. The pods and large stalks are separated with the help of sieve, leaves are then graded by means of sieves and hand picking method into following groups.

(a) Whole leaves
(b) Whole and half leaves mix
(c) Siftings

Morphology : The drug senna occurs in leaflets, lamina has an entire margin containing an acute apex and asymmetric base. Leaves are lanceolate 2-4 cm long and 1 cm wide, surface is pubescent and venation is pinnate. It has a slight characteristic odour, mucilaginous, bitter and unpleasant taste.

(a) Indian senna (leaf) (b) Alexandrian senna (leaf)

Fig. 7. 5 :

Chemical constituents: Senna contains anthraquinone glycosides as sennoside A, sennoside B, sennoside C, sennoside D, emodine, chrysophanol, aloe emodine, rhein, and two naphthalene glycoside,i.e. 6-hydroxy musizin glycoside and Tinnevellin glycoside. It also contains yellow flavinol, colouring matter kaempferol and its glucosides kaempfrin, sterol and its glucoside, mucilage, resin and calcium oxalate.

Table : 7.1 Difference between Alexandrian Senna and Indian Senna.

Character	Alexandrian Senna	Indian Senna
Leaf length	upto 40 mm	upto 50 mm
Colour	Greyish-green	Yellowish-green
Leaf base	More asymmetric	Less asymmetric
Leaf edge	More curled and more broken	Rarely broken & flat
Vein-islet number	25 to 29.5	19.5 to 22.5
Stomatal index	11.4 to 13.3	17 to 20
Palisade ratio	9.5 (upper epidermis) 7.0 (lower epidermis)	7.5 5.1

Anthraquinone glycoside —> Anthraquinone (aglycone) + Sugar (glycone)
Sennoside A —> Sennidine A +2 glucose)

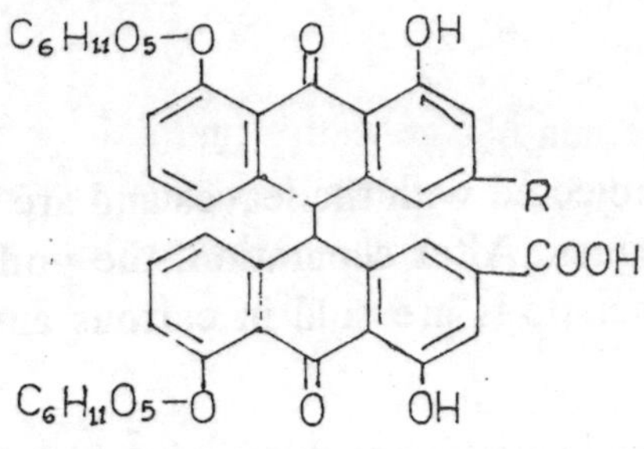

Compound	R	10-10'
Sennoside A	-COOH	trans
Sennoside B	-COOH	meso
Sennoside C	$-CH_2OH$	trans
Sennoside D	$-CH_2OH$	meso

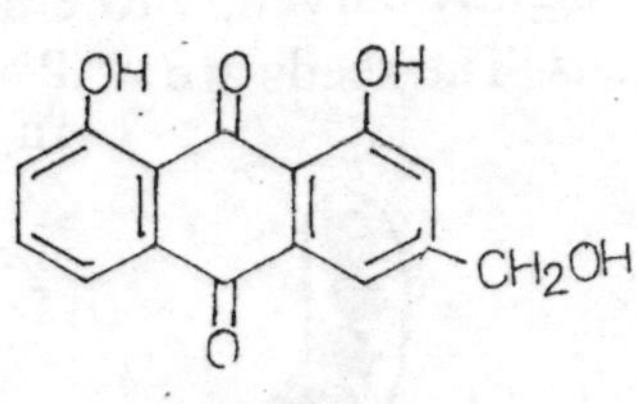

Aloe - emodin

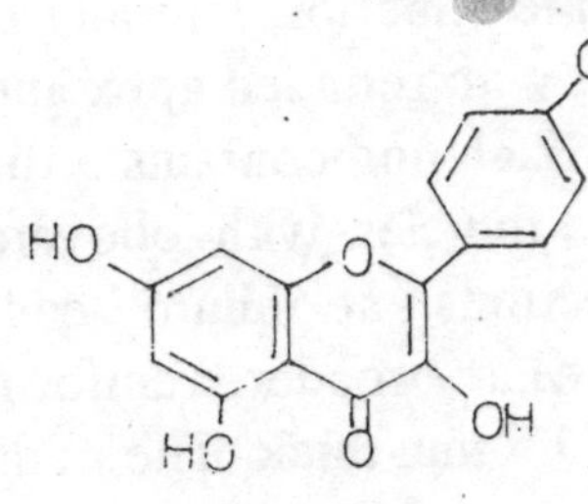

Kaempferol

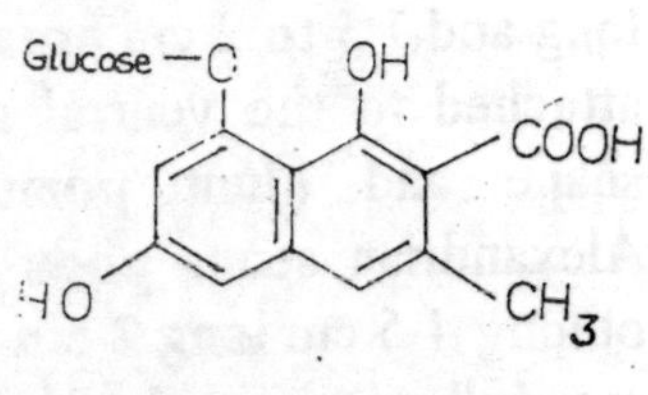

6-hydroxy musizin glycoside

Chemical test

1. **Due to presence of anthraquinone derivative. Senna give positive Borntrager's test. Powdered leaves of senna are boiled with dilute sulphuric acid, filtered and cooled. The filtrate is extracted with chloroform or benzene and dilute ammonia is added to it. The ammoniacal layer becomes pink to red due to the presence of anthraquinone derivative.**

Uses : Senna leaves are used as laxative and cathartic. It acts as an irritant purgative due to the presence of anthraquinone derivative. Senna is mixed with carminative drugs due to its gripping action. Powdered Senna is mixed with vinegar and applied externally to cure skin diseases.

Allied drugs

1. **Arabian Senna** : This is the wild plant of *Cassia angustifolia* available in Arabia and is used as a substitute.
2. **Palthe Senna** : This is the dried plant of *Cassia auriculata* Leaves are used as substitute for senna.
3. **Dog Senna** : It is obtained from the leaves of *Cassia obovata.* The leaves are ovate in shape.

SENNA POD

Synonyms : Senna legumes; senna fruit; seena fructus.

Biological source : Senna pods are the dried ripe fruit of *C. angustifolia* Vahal (Indian senna) and *C. acutifolia* Delile (Alexandrian senna). It is a member of leguminosea family.

Geographical source : See senna leaf.

Collection and preparation : The senna pods are collected with the leaves and are dried in sunlight then the pods are separated from the leaves. After separation, the pods are hand picked into various qualities. The best and finer pods are sold in cartons and the inferior ones are used for making galenicals.

Morphology : Indian senna pods are superior, laterally flattened, thin and dehiscing by both sutures. Their shape is oblong, with rounded apex and are slightly curved, 5 to 6 cm long and 1.5 to 2 cm broad in size. Each pod contains 5 to 8 seeds. The seeds are attached to the ventral surface by funicles with obovate shape and blunt pointed projections at hilum end. Alexandrian senna pods are somewhat broader, reniform oblong 4-5 cm long 2 cm wide and 0.5 mm thick. The pods are dull green or brownish green in colour. The dorsal sutures of senna pod have a larger convex curvature and the ventral sutures are slightly concave or may be straight with a small point like scar at the distal end.

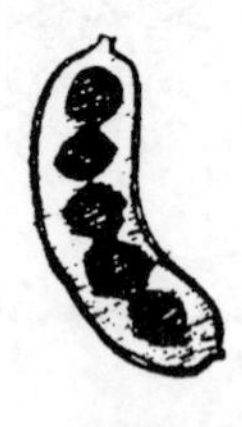

Fig. 7.6 : Senna pod

Chemical constituents : In senna pod, maximum active constituents are found in pericarp. Seena pods contain sennoside A and sennoside B. The anthraquinone derivatives and other constituents of senna pods are similar to senna leaves but mucilage is absent in senna pod.

Uses : Senna pods are used as laxative.

7 - B. CARDIOTONICS

Cardiotonic drugs are used to increase the heart contraction. (Cardiotonic, Prefix cardiac-meaning heart and suffix tonic -means strength or energy). They provide energy and strength to cardiac muscles, which increase the activity of heart. Certain plant glycosides directly act on the heart muscles. Digitalis, Squill, Strophanthus, Arjuna bark, etc. are examples of natural cardiotonic drugs.

DIGITALIS (FOX GLOVE LEAVES)

Biological source : Digitalis consists of dried leaves of *Digitalis purpurea* Linn. It is a member of *Scrophulariaceae* family. The dried leaves should not contain less than 0.3% of total cardenolides calculated as digitoxin.

Geographical source : It is cultivated in England, U.S.A, Holland, other European countries and in India. In India, it is cultivated in Kashmir & Nilgiri hills.

Cultivation & collection : Digitalis is a biennial or perennial herb. It is about 1 to 2 metre in height. The seeds of digitalis are small in size, so they are mixed with sand for sowing. Leaves are collected in both the years but the leaves collected in the first year have highest glycoside content. Leaves are collected when 2/3 of the flowers are fully developed. The seedlings are then transplanted into the field. Generally the leaves are collected in the early afternoon, with a belief that maximum cardio-active glycosides are present at that time. The leaves are immediately dried after collection below 60°C and dried leaves are stored in air tight containers. The dried leaves should not contain more than 5% moisture, since it promotes hydrolysis of cardiac glycosides resulting in loss of cardiac activity.

Morphology : Digitalis leaves are ovate-lanceolate to broadly ovate in shape. It is about 10-30 cm long and 4-10 cm wide having subacute apex. It is dark greyish-green in colour. The margin of the leaf is crenate or dentate, containing water pores. Both surfaces are hairy but lower surface contains more hairs than upper surface. The leaves are borne on a 2.5-10 cm long winged petiole. Leaf is bitter in taste and contains slight odour.

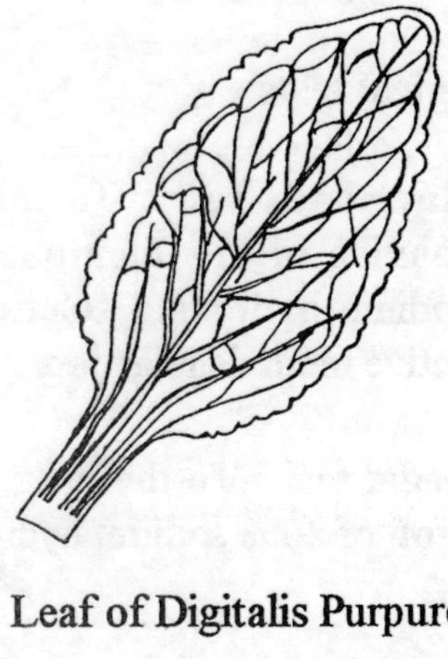

Fig 7.7 Leaf of Digitalis Purpurea

Chemical constituents : *Digitalis purpurea* contains 35 glycosides. The carderiolides are 0.2-0.4%. The primary glycosides are purpurea glycosides A & B. It also contains odoroside H, glucogitaloxin, gitaloxin, verodoxin and glucoverodoxin.

Purpurea glycoside A (Primary glucoside) $\xrightarrow[\text{enzymatic hydrolysis}]{\text{-glucose}}$ Digitoxin $\longrightarrow$ Digitoxigenin + 2Digitose (Secondary glycoside)

Purpurea glycoside B (primary glycoside) $\xrightarrow[\text{enzymatic hydrolysis}]{\text{-glucose}}$ Gitoxin $\longrightarrow$ Gitoxigenin + 2Digitose (Secondary glycoside)

Odoroside H $\xrightarrow[\text{enzymatic hydrolysis}]{}$ Digitoxigenin + Digitalose

The digitoxigenin, Digitoxin, gitoxigenin, gitaloxin are important medicinal compounds. They are also called secondary glycosides. They contain anthraquinone derivatives like digitolutin, methoxy-2 methyl anthraquinone, etc. It also contains saponin, flavonoid, tannin and pectin.

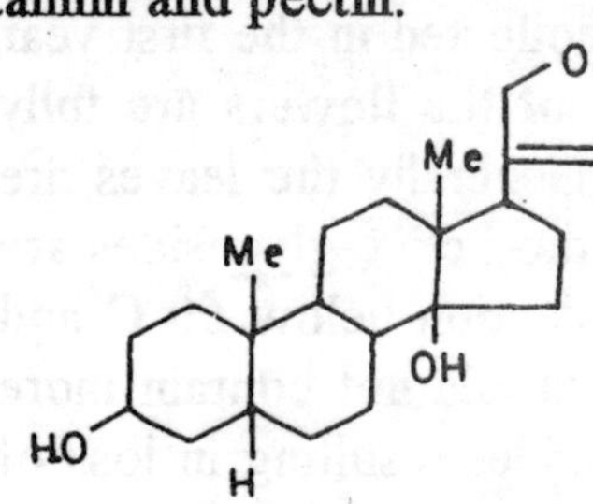

Digitoxigenin

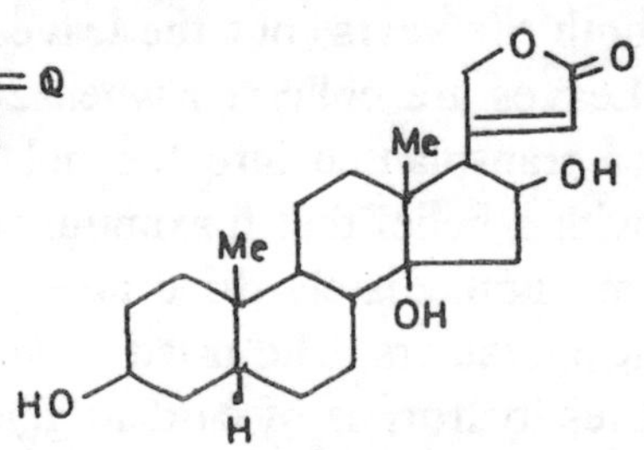

Gitoxigenin

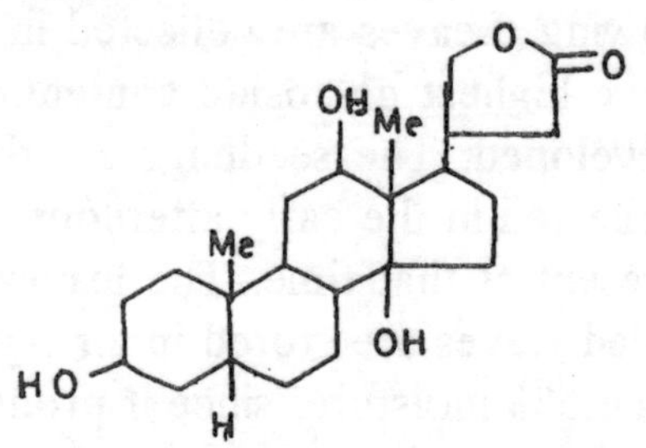

Digoxigenin

Chemical tests

(1) **Raymonds test** : To the drug, add a few ml of 50% ethanol and 0.1 ml of 1% solution of m - dinitrobenzene in ethanol. To this solution, add 2-3 drops of 20% sodium hydroxide solution. Violet colour appears, this is due to the presence of active methylene group.

(2) **Legal test** : To the drug, add few ml of pyridine and 2 drops of nitroprusside and a drop of 20% sodium hydroxide solution. A deep red colour is produced.

(3) **Keller Kiliani test** : Glycoside is dissolved in a mixture of 1% ferric sulphate solution in (5%) glacial acetic acid. Add one or two drops of concentrated sulphuric acid. A blue colour develops due to the presence of deoxy sugar.

(4) **Xanthydrol test** : The crude drug is heated with 0.1 to 5% solution of Xanthydrol in glacial acetic acid containing 1% hydrochloric acid. A red colour is produced due to the presence of 2-deoxysugar.

Uses : It is a cardiac stimulant and tonic. The drug directly stimulates the cardiac muscles. It is used in various forms, like tablets or capsule in the treatment of congestive cardiac failure, atrial flutter, atrial fibrillation and peroxysmal atrial tachycardia. The preparation of digitalis produce cumulative effect on cardic muscles due to digoxin hence, it should be administered under strict medical supervision. It is also used as diuretic.

Adulterants

(1) **Primrose leaves** : Leaves of *Primula vulgaris* Huds. (family - *Pimulaceae*).
(2) **Comfrey leaves** : Leaves of *Symphytum officinale* Linn. (family *Boraginaceae*).
(3) **Mullein leaves** : Leaves of *Verbascum thapsus* Linn. (family - *Scrophulariceae*).

These leaves are used as adulterant for digitalis due to similar appearance.

DIGITALIS LANATA (WOOLLY FOX GLOVE)

Biological source : The drug consists of dried leaves of *Digitalis lanata*. It is a member of *scrophulariaceae* family.

Geographical source : The drug is indigenous to Central and South Europe and cultivated in Holland, Eucador and U.S.A.

Description : It is biennial or perennial herb, about 1 metre in height. The leaves are sessile, linear, lanceolate, about 30 cm in length, 4 cm broad bearing acuminate apex and entire margin. Veins leave the midrib at a very acute angle.

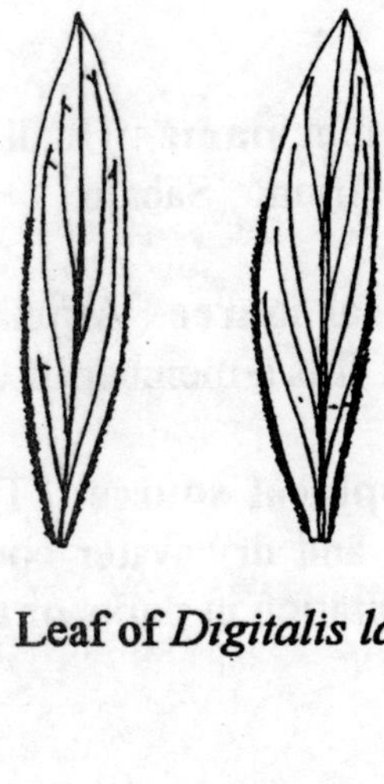

Fig. 7.8 : Leaf of *Digitalis lanata*

Chemical constituents : Leave contains digitoxin, gitoxin, digoxin, lanatoside A,B,C,D & E. It also contains flavone derivatives like scutellarein, dinatin, etc. These lanatosides are acetylated products of purpurea glycosides.

Lanatoside A	Lanatoside B	Lanatoside C	Lanatoside D	Lanatoside E
↓ alkaline hydrolysis $-CH_3COOH$	↓ alkaline hydrolysis $-CH_3COOH$	↓ alkaline hydrolysis $-CH_3COOH$	↓ alkaline hydrolysis $-CH_3COOH$	↓ alkaline hydrolysis $-CH_3COOH$
Purpurea glycoside A	Purpurea glycoside B	Deacetyl lanatoside C	Deacetyl lanatoside D	Deacetyl lanatoside E
↓ enzymatic hydrolysis -glucose	↓ enzymatic hydrolysis -glucose	↓ enzymatic hydrolysis -glucose	↓ enzymatic hydrolysis -glucose	↓ enzymatic hydrolysis -glucose
Digitoxin	Gitoxin	Digoxin	Diginatin	Gitaloxin
↓ -2 digitose	↓	↓	↓	↓
Digitoxigenin	Gitoxigenin	Digoxigenin	Diginatigenin	Gitaloxigenin

Uses : *D. lanata* is used commercially in the preparation of digoxin and lantoside. Digoxin is rapidly absorbed from G.I.T. than other glycoside are used in atrial fibrillation and congestive heart failure. Lanatoside C is preferred for long term therapy because of less cumulative effect.

ARJUNA

Vernacular name : Hindi, Sanskrit & Beng.-Arjun; Tamil- Vellamatta; English - Arjun; Oriya - Arjuno, Sahajo.

Biological source : Arjuna consist of dried stem and bark of *Terminalia arjuna* (Roxb) W.&.A. It is a member of *Combretaceae* family.

Geographical source : The plant is found throughout India, on the banks of rivers, streams and dry water courses in sub Himalayan tract. It is also planted for shade or ornamentation in parks or avenues.

Cultivation & collection : It is a large tree 20-25 metre high containing smooth grey bark. It is raised by sowing seeds or stumps. It grows satisfactorily at about 45°C temperature. Bark is collected from the plant.

Characters : The Arjuna bark occurs in flat pieces of various sizes. The outer surface of the bark is smooth and grey in colour while the inner surface is striated and reddish. The fracture of bark is short and fibrous. It is odourless and has an astringent taste.

Chemical constituents : Arjuna bark contains tannins (about 12-15%) and triterpenoid saponins. It also contains ß sitosterol, ellagic acid, arjunolic acid, tomentosic acid, arjunine, arjunetine, arjunoside 1 to 4 and Ca, Al & Mg salts are also reported.

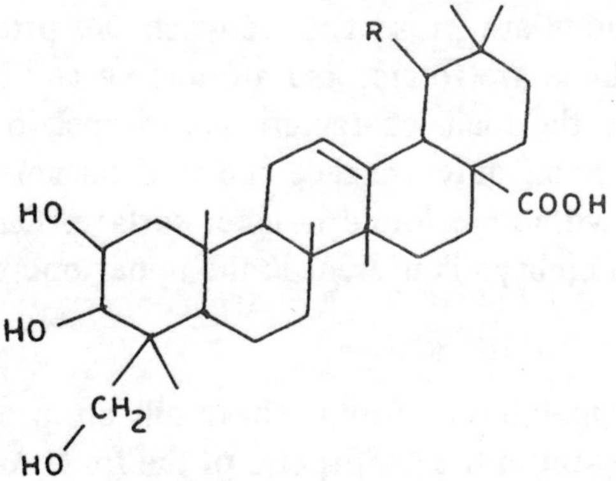

R = H = Arjunolic acid
R = ß - OH = Tomentosic acid

Uses : Arjuna bark is used in heart diseases as a cardiotonic due to presence of triterpenoid. It is also used in cirrhosis of liver, in ulcers and as a diuretic too. The presence of tannins exerts an astringent action. Arjuna bark is useful in the treatment of diarrhoea, dysentery and acts as an antidote to poisons.

7 - C. CARMINATIVES AND GASTRO-INTESTINAL REGULATORS

Carminatives (Latin : carminare - to cleanse; Eng. carminat-relieve flatulence) are the drugs that relieve flatulence and gas from gastro intestinal tract used in the treatment of gastric colic and discomfort. This is due to peristaltic movement of gas from the stomach. The natural carminative drugs discussed in this chapter are Coriander, Fennel, Ajowan, Cardamom, Ginger, Black pepper, Asafoetida, Nut-meg, Cinnamon, Clove, etc. These crude drugs are generally used as stomachic, aromatic, appetizers, stimulants, etc.

UMBELLIFEROUS FRUITS

The umbelliferous plants are annual, biennial or perennial herbs. Pinnate type leaves are found in this family, which are alternate in arrangement. The fruits belonging to this family are known as umbelliferous fruits. The fruits are schizocarp or splitting fruits known as cremocarp. The cremocarp splits into two, dry, partial fruits that are known as mericarps. These mericarps are attached by a stalk like structure known as carpophore. There are two surfaces of mericarp, outer or dorsal surface and inner or ventral or commissural surface. Five longitudinal primary ridges are found in dorsal surface which run from apex to base. These ridges are straight or wavy prominent or obscure. These ridges are called primary ridges, which contain vascular bundles. The coriander fruit has primary ridges and secondary ridge's that are arranged alternatively. The two mericarps are separated by a line known as commissure. In Dill, the lateral primary ridges extend to form wing like structure. Furrows or depressions are present in between the primary ridges, below which the volatile oil secreting ducts are found, and are known as vittae. The number and arrangement of the vittae are the main characteristics of such fruits; Fennel, Dill, Caraway, etc., have six vittae, four on outer surface and two on inner or commissural surface but in coriander only two vittae are found in inner surface. On the inner surface, a single seed is found and a small embryo is present in the upper one third part of seed.

The volatile oils are the main constituents of umbelliferous fruits. These oils are present in the vittae. Fixed oils and proteins are also present in the endosperm of the fruit. Anise, Ajowan, Coriander, Caraway, Cumin, Dill and Fennel are the important drugs of this family. Umbelliferous fruits are very useful in medicine and as flavouring agents, condiments and spices.

CORIANDER

Vernacular names : Hindi-Dhania; Sanskrit - Dhanyaka; Beng.-Dhane; Tam-Kottamalli; English-Coriander.

Biological source : It is the dried ripe fruit of *Coriandrum sativum*. This is a member of *umbelliferae (Apiaceae)* family.

Geographical source : The plant coriander is indigenous to Italy. The plant is widely cultivated in India, Egypt, Morocco, Holland, Argentina, Eastern Europe, China, Russia and Bangladesh. In India, the plant is cultivated throughout the country.

Collection & preparation : The plant is an annual herb, about 0.7 to 1 metre hight containing small white and pinkish flowers. The green plant and unripe fruits give unpleasant odour like bug but odour disappears during ripening and changes to an aromatic odour. Plants are cut and collected when the fruits are ripen. After drying, fruits are separated.

Morphology : The drug consists of the whole cremocarps and is about 2.3 to 4.3 mm in diametre, subglobose in shape and straw yellow in colour. The fruit consists of two hemispherical mericarps united at their margin. The apex of the fruit bears two divergent styles. Each fruit surface contains ten wavy and inconspicuous primary ridges, Alternating with primary ridges, there are eight more prominent straight, secondary ridges. Fruit bears aromatic odour and spicy taste.

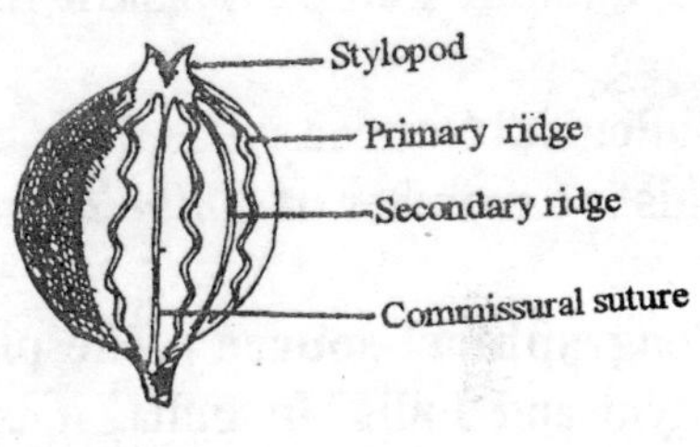

Fig. 7.9 : Coriander fruit, entire cremocarp

Constituents : Coriander fruits contain volatile oil (about 1%). The main constituent of volatile oil are (+) linalol (coriandrol) and α pinene. It also contains limonene, α and γ terpinene, p- cymene, camphor, geraniol,borneol, fixed oils, malic acid, tannin, etc. Coriander leaves also contain vitamin A.

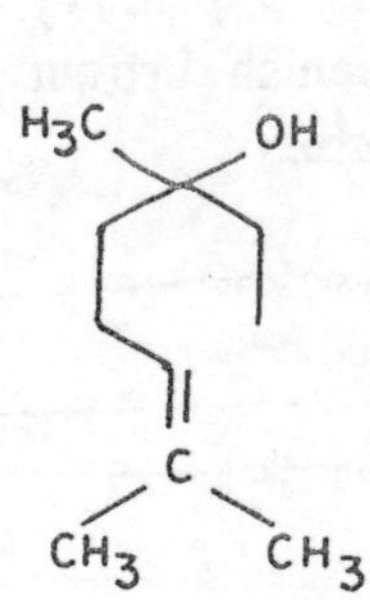

Coriandrol

Standards

Acid insoluble ash : $\leq$ 1.5%
Foreign organic matter : $\leq$ 2%.

Uses : Coriander fruits and volatile oils are used as a carminative and flavouring agent. It is also useful as anthelmintic, aromatic, diuretic, stimulant stomachic and aphrodisiac. It is one of the important ingredient for cooking.

FENNEL

Synonyms : *Foeniculum capillaceum* Gilib., *F. officinale* All.

Vernacular name : Sanskrit-Misreya; Hindi-Saunf; Beng.-Panmauri; English-Fennel.

Biological Source : The drug consists of the dried ripe fruit of *Foeniculum vulgare* Mill. This is a member of *Umbelliferae (Apiaceae)* family.

Geographical source : The plant is widely cultivated in many parts of Europe, China, Egypt and India. In India, it is commonly cultivated throughout the country and often grows wild.

Collection and preparation : The plant is a glabrous, biennial or perennial tall herb. Seeds are sown in spring, Ripen fruits with stem are collected in autumn. They are dried in sun and thrashing is done for separation of fruits.

Morphology : The drug consists partly of whole cremocarp and partly of mericarps with pedicel. The fruit is straight or slightly curved 5 to 10 mm long and 2-4 mm broad. The surface of fruit is glabrous containing 5 primary straight prominent ridges and bifid stylopod at the apex. Colour is greenish brown to yellowish brown. The drug has aromatic odour and sweet aromatic taste.

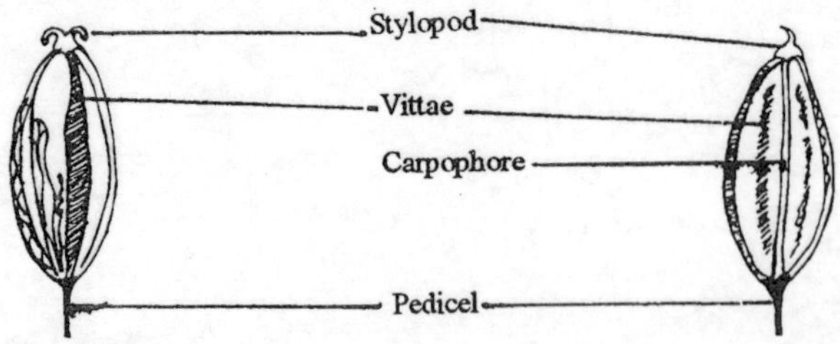

(a) Lateral view (b) Commissural surface

Fig. 7.10 : Fennel fruit, entire cremocarp

Chemical constituents : Fennel contains volatile oil (1-4%), fixed oil (9-12%) and proteins (20%). The chief constituents of volatile oils are a phenolic ether anethole (50-60%) and the ketone fenchone (18-20%). Anethole has an aromatic odour and sweet taste whereas fenchone has a camphoraceous odour and taste. Volatile oil also contains methyl chavicol, anisic aldehyde, α and ß-Pinene, citral, ascorbic acid, niacin, riboflavin, etc.

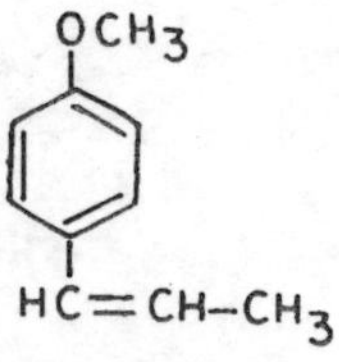

Anethole

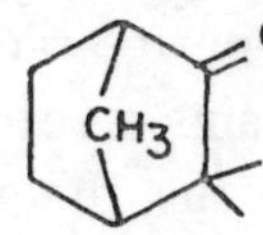

Fenchone

Standards : Similar to coriander.

Uses : Fennel and its volatile oil are used as a flavouring agent carminative, expectorant, stimulant, stomachic and anthelmintic. It is also useful in dental and mouth wash preparations due to pleasant taste of anethole. Fennel water is useful in colic and flatulence in children.

Adulterants : The drug is adulterated with exhausted fennel from which volatile oil has been extracted out by steam distillation or volatile oil has been removed by treating with alcohol.

AJOWAN

Synonyms: *Carum copticum* (L) Hiern., *Ammi copticum* L., *Sison ammi* L.

Vernacular names : Hindi - Ajown; Beng.- Jowan; Sans.- Javani; Tamil-Omum; English-Ajowan.

Biological source : The drug consists of dried ripe fruits of the plant *Trachyspermum ammi* (L) Sprague. It is a member of the *umbelliferae* family.

Geographical source : The plant Ajowan is native of Egypt. It is cultivated in Afghanistan, Iran, Iraq, Pakistan and India. In India, it is widely cultivated in Punjab, Madhya Pradesh, Uttar Pradesh, Gujarat, Rajasthan, Maharastra, Bihar and West Bengal.

Morphology : The drug consists of cremocarps or separate mericarp with bifid stylopod. It is yellowish brown in colour 2 to 3 mm long, 1.5 to 2.4 mm broad and 0.5 to 1.5 mm thick. The fruits are ovoid, muricate subhispid in shape. The drugs contain agreeable odour and aromatic (thymol like) taste.

Chemical constituents : Ajowan fruit consists of 2-4% of volatile oil. The main constituents of volatile oil are thymol, (35-60%) p-cymene, terpinene, etc. Due to high content of thymol in volatile oil, it imparts characteristic odour. It also contains nicotinic acid, riboflavin, thiamine, protein, sugars, tannins, flavone and sterols.

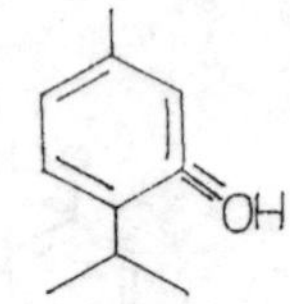

Thymol

Uses : Ajowan is used as antiseptic, antidiarrhoeal, antispasmodic and carminative. Its aqueous extract (Ajwan Ka arak) is useful in diarrhoea. It is one of the popular ingredients in the preparation of Ayurvedic formulations for cough, digestive disorders and infections. It is useful in preparation of various pharmaceutical formulations like lotions, ointments, mouth washes and gargles.

CARAWAY

Vernacular name : Sans.- sushavi; Hindi-shiajira; zira, Beng.-jira; Tam.- shimai-shembn; Tel.- shimaisapu; Bombay-wilayati-zirah.

Biological source : Caraway consists of dried, ripe fruits of *Carum carvi*. Linn. It is a member of *umbelliferae* family.

Geographical source : Caraway grows wildly and also cultivated in Holland, Denmark, Germany, England,Morocco, Russia, Norway, Sweden and China. In India, wild caraway is found in Northern Himalayan region. The plant is cultivated in the hills of Kashmir, Kumaon and Garhwal.

Collection and preparation : Caraway is a biennial herb about 1 metre in height. The cutting of the plants is done when fruits ripen, they are dried in the sun and fruits are separated by thrashing.

Morphology : The drug caraway is present in mericarps that are free from pedicel. The mericarps are about 4 to 7 mm long, 1 to 2.3 mm wide, 1 mm thick and tapered at both ends. It is slightly curved, glabrous and brown in colour. Each mericarp has five narrow primary ridges. It has characteristic aromatic odour and spicy taste.

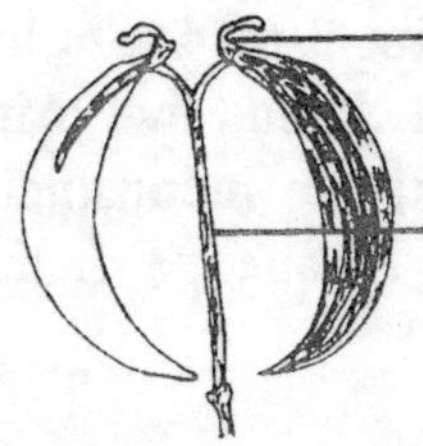

Fig. 7.11 : Caraway fruit

Chemical constituents : Caraway contains volatile oil (3 to 7%). The main constituents of volatile oil are carvone (50 to 60%) and limonene. It also contains α- pinene, α-phellandrene, carveol, etc. Caraway also contains fixed oils (8-20%) resins, proteins, colouring matters and calcium oxalate crystal.

Carvone Limonene

Standards

Ash value	: ≤ 8%
Acid insoluble ash	: ≤ 1.5%
Foreign organic substance	: ≤ 2%
Ketone content (calculated as carvone)	: 53-63% w/w

Uses : Caraway is used as a carminative, flavouring agent, stomachic and spice. Its oil is used in the preparation of mouth washes, tooth pastes, chewing gums, soaps, cosmetics, etc.

DILL

Vernacular name: Sans-Satapushpi; Hindi & Beng.- Sowa; Guj.-surva, Tam.-Sata Kuppi.

Biological source : Dill consists of dried ripe fruits of *Anethum graveolens* Linn. A. Sowa Kurr. This is a member of *umbelliferae* family. *A. sowa* is known as Indian Diii.

Geographical source : Dill is an annual herb and indigenous to southern Europe. It is cultivated in England, Germany, Romania, U.S.S.R., U.S.A. and India.

Morphology : Dill usually consists of separated mericarps generally free from pedicels. Mericarps are broadly oval in shape, about 3 to 4 mm long, 2 to 3 mm wide and 1 mm thick. The fruits are dorsally compressed. It has five primary yellows coloured ridges in which three of them (i.e., dorsal ridges) are inconspicuous (not clearly seen) but the lateral two ridges are extended as wings. At apex, a distinct stylopod is found. The fruits have an aromatic odour and spicy taste.

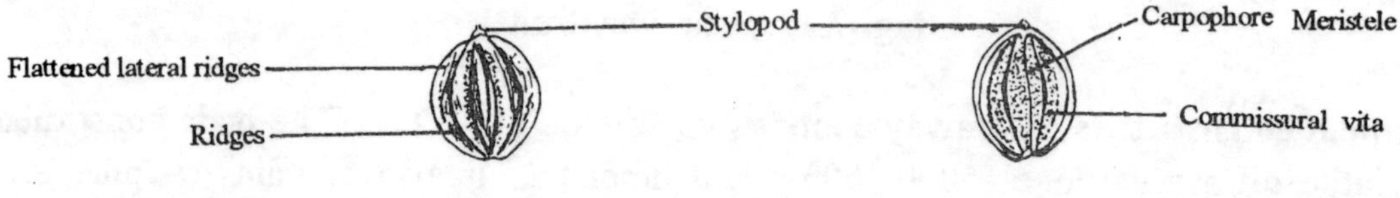

(a) Dorsal view of mericarp (b) Commissural view of mericarp

Fig. 7.12 : Dill fruit

Chemical constituents : Dill contains volatile oil (3 to 4%) which is known as oleum Anethi. The main constituents of volatile oil is carvone (50-60%) along with other components like limonene, phellandrene, α- thujene dihydrocarbon. The Indian Dill oil contains low carvone (i.e. 22-46%) and high dillapiole which is not present in European dill. Dill apiole is poisonous in character that can be separated by fractional distillation. The European Dill contains only one flavonoid, i.e., kaempferol while Indian Dill contains three flavonoids, quercetin, Kaempferol and isorhamnetin.

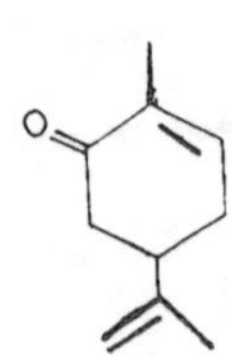

Carvone

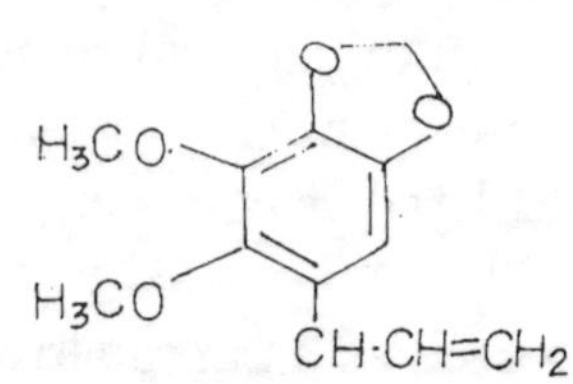

Dill apiole

Uses : Dill fruit is used as carminative, diuretic, stimulant and aromatic. It is used in the preparation of gripe water and Dill-water which is useful in flatulence, colic pain, vomiting and gastric disturbance of infants and children.

CUMIN

Vernacular name : Sans.-Jiraka, Jira; Hindi-Jira, Zeera; Beng.-Jira; Tam.-Siragam; Tel.-Jilakara, Jiraka, Kan.-Jeerige.

Biological source : Cumin consists of dried ripe fruits of *Cuminum cyminum* Linn. It is a member of *umbelliferae* family.

Geographical source : Cumin is a small annual plant, which is indigenous to Egypt. It is widely cultivated in Morocco, Sicily, Malta, Syria, China and India. In India, it is widely cultivated in Rajasthan and Gujarat.

Morphology : Cumin fruits resemble caraway fruit at first glance. It is about 4 to 6 mm long and 2 mm wide. The mericarps and cremocarp have pedicels which are ellipsoidal in shape. The mericarps have five primary and four secondary ridges and are densely covered with short bristly hairs. Four dorsal vittae and two commissural vittae are found in each mericarp. It is brown in colour. It has characteristic odour and aromatic taste.

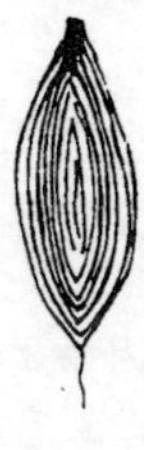

Fig. 7.13 : Cumin fruit

Chemical constituents : Cumin contains 2.5 to 4.5% of volatile oil. The volatile oil is mainly composed of cuminaldehyde. (25to 35%). It also contains α and ß pinene, limonene, p-cymene, cuminic acid, anisaldehyde, etc. The other reported constituents are fixed oil, protein and flavonoids.

Uses : Cumin is mainly used as stimulant, stomachic, astringent, carminative and as spices. The cumin oil is useful as an antispasmodic. Currently cumin is chiefly used in veterinary practice.

ANISE OR ANISEED

Biological source : Anise consists of dried ripe fruits of *Pimpinella anisum* Linn. It is a member of *umbelliferae* family.

Geographical source : Anise is an annual plant and indigenous to Levant. It is widely cultivated in Germany, Spain, Russia, Italy, Egypt, America, Bulgaria and India. In India, the plant is cultivated in Orissa, Punjab and U.P.

Morphology : The drug consists of greyish-brown pear shaped, entire compressed cremocarps with pedicels 2 to 12 mm in length. The cremocarps are 3 to 6 mm long and 2 to 3 mm wide. The mesocarps have five wavy ridges and are slightly pubescent on the outer surface. The fruits have an aromatic odour and a sweet aromatic taste.

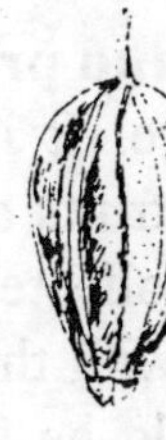

Fig. 7.14 : Aniseed fruit

Chemical constituents : Anise fruit contains volatile oil (2 to 3%). The main constituent of volatile oil is anethole (90%) and others are chavicol and anisaldehyde. Proteins, fixed oil, starch and mucilages are also present in anise fruit.

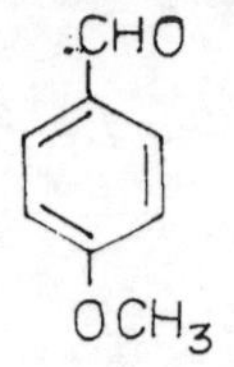

Anisaldehyde

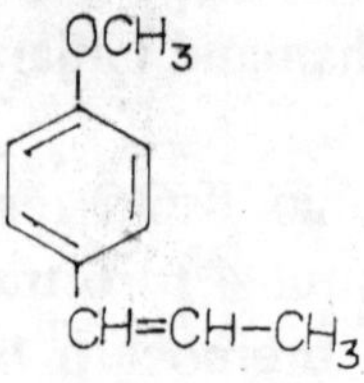

Anethole

Standards

Acid insoluble ash	: ≤ 1.5%
Foreign organic matter	: ≤ 1.0%

Uses : Anise fruit is used as carminative, stimulant, diuretic, diaphoretic and expectorant. It is also used to prevent flatulence and colic. Various mouths and dental preparations, asthma powders and veterinary medicine are also prepared from anise fruits.

CARDAMOM

Vernacular name : Hindi & Beng.-choti elachi; Sans.-Upakunchika, ela; Mar.-Veldode; Tam.-Yelakkai; Tel.-Yelakkayalu.

Biological source : Cardamom consists of the dried nearly ripe fruits of *Elettaria cardamomum* Var. minuscula. It is a member of the *Zingiberaceae* family. The seeds of cardamom contain about 2.8 to 6.2% of volatile oil. Seeds are used in medicine and as spices. These are removed from fruits as and when required.

Geographical source : Cardamom is grown in Ceylon, Srilanka, Mayanmar (Burma), Malaysia and India. In India, the plant is widely cultivated in Mysore and Kerala.

Collection and preparation : The plant of cardamom is a perennial herb containing reed like structure. It is 3-4 metre in height and three to four years old plant bears fruits. Cardamom fruits are in racemes. Flowering and fruiting continue through out the year. Crops are collected when the fruits are nearly ripe. It is better to cut off each fruit, at right stage with the help of a pair of short blade scissors. Fruits are dried slowly. Rapid drying should be avoided because it may split the fruit to shed their seeds. Sometimes fruits are bleached in the sunlight or by placing fruits tray over the burning sulphur. Calyx, stalk and split fruits are removed. The fruits are graded by means of sieves into long, medium and short sizes and also by means of quality.

Morphology : Cardamom fruit is an inferior, ovoid or oblong capsule. Fruit is about 1 to 2 cm long. Naturally it is green to pale buff in colour but sulphur dioxide bleached cardamom turns to white. Apex of the fruit is beak shaped and base is rounded with remains of stalk and surface is longitudinally striated. Internally the fruit contains three chambers. Each chamber contains a double row of seeds about 5 to 10 in number attached to axial placenta. The seeds are about 4 mm in length and 3 mm breadth, irregularly angular in shape, dark reddish-brown in colour and wrinkled surface. Cardamom seed possesses aromatic odour and a pleasant, aromatic and Pungent taste.

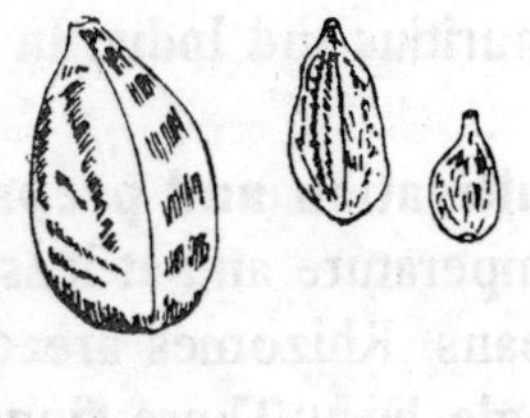

Fig. 7.15 : Cardamom fruits

Chemical constituents : Cardamom Seeds contain about 2.8 to 6.2% of volatile oils. The main constituent of volatile oil is cineole (50%). Volatile oil also contains borneol; terpinene, terpinyl acetate, limonene, geraniol, etc. Cardamom seeds also contain fixed oils starch, calcium oxalate and resins.

Stardards

Ash	:	≤ 6%
Acid insoluble ash	:	≤3.5%
Foreign organic matter	:	≤ 1% (fruits)

Uses : Principally Cardamom is used as flavouring agent. It is aromatic, stimulant and carminative. It is used in the preparation of compound cardamom tincture.

Allied Drugs

(i) ***Elettaria cardamomum*** var. major. This Species is along, wild native of Sri lanka. The fruits are much elongated, upto 4 cm in length. The pericarp of fruits are dark brown in colour and coarsely striated.

(ii) ***Amomum aromaticum*** or ***A. subulatum*** :*A. aromaticum* is found in Bengal and Assam. It is commonly known as Bengal cardamom (Bari elachi). *A. subulatum* is obtained from Nepal, Bengal, Sikkim and Assam. It is commonly known as Nepal or Greater cardamom.

GINGER

Vernacular name : Hindi - Adrak, ada; Sanskrit-Ardraka; Beng. -Ada, Tam.-Allam, inji; Mal.- Andrakam.

Biological Source : Ginger consists of either the scraped or unscraped rhizomes of *Zingiber officinale* Roscoe. This is a member of *Zingiberaceae* family.

Geographical source : The plant is native of South-eastern Asia. It is cultivated in the many parts of the world including Jamaica, West Africa, Nigeria, China, Australia, Mauritius and India. In India, it is cultivated throughout the country.

Cultivation and preparation : For good growth of ginger, the plant needs subtropical temperature and at least 80 mm rainfall annually. The plants are cultivated by vegetative means. Rhizomes are cut into peices called "fingers", each piece containing at least a single bud. These fingers are planted in March and April. In December and January rhizomes are dug out and soil is removed. For the scraped drug, rhizomes are boiled with water, peeled, washed and dried in the sun for 5 to 6 days and turned several times daily. It should be protected from damp weather.

Morphology : The dried rhizomes are thick, laterally compressed containing short, flatly ovate and oblique branches on the upper side with undeveloped bud at the apex. Rhizomes are 5-15 cm long, 3-4 cm wide and 1 to 1.5 cm thick. Externally rhizomes are buff coloured, showing longitudinal striations and fibres. The fracture of the drug is short, projecting numerous fibres from the broken surface.

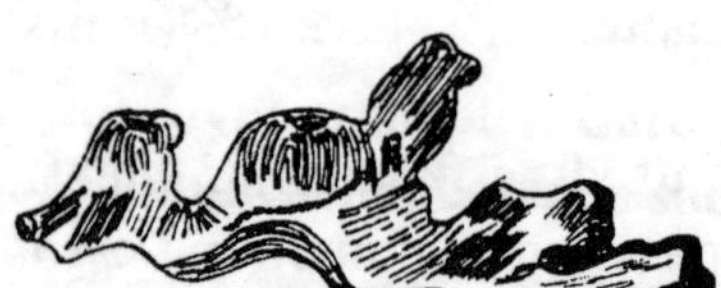

Fig. 7.16 : Ginger (*Zingiber officinale)* rhizome

Chemical Constituents : Ginger contains about 0.25 to 3 % of volatile oil, 5 to 8% resinous matter, 56% starch and Proteins. Volatile oil contains a mixture of more than 25 constituents containing monoterpene and sesquiterpenes. The pungent taste of ginger is due to the presence of gingerol. The pungency of gingerol is destroyed by boiling in 2% solution of KOH. Zingerone, a pungent compound also occurs in the rhizome but possesses a sweet odour, shogaol is a component of oil but is not present in fresh rhizomes, it is formed by dehydration of gingerol.

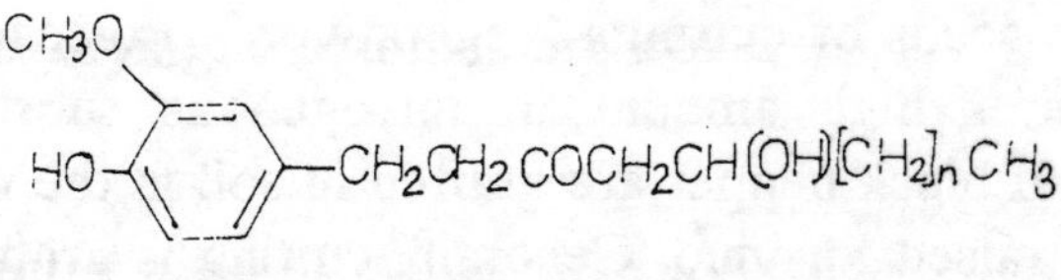

Gingerol (where n= 3,4 or 5)

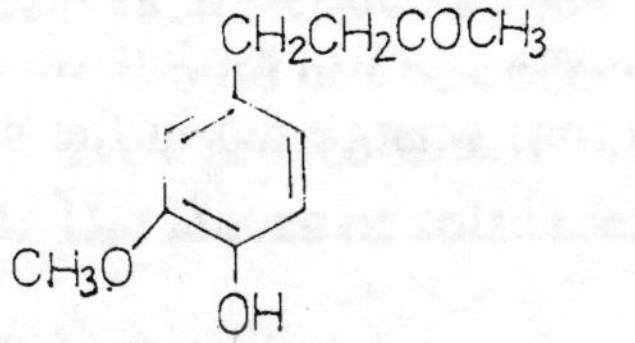

Zingerone

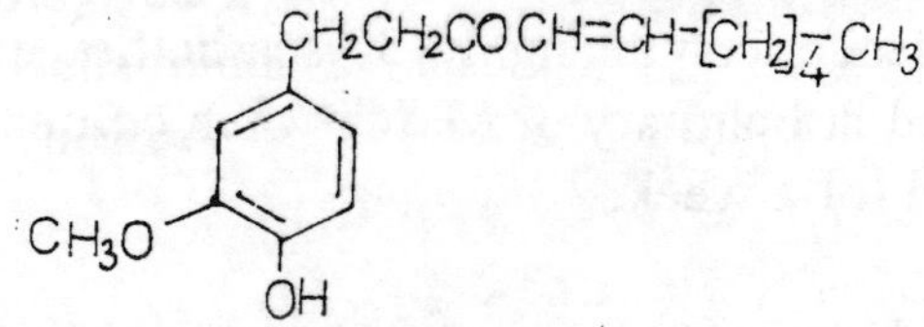

Shogaol

Standards

Total ash	: ≤ 6.0%
Water soluble ash	: ≥ 1.7%
Water soluble extractive value	: ≥ 10 %
Alcohol (90%) soluble extractive value	: ≥ 4.5%

Uses : Ginger is used as condiment. Medicinally it is used as aromatic, carminative, flavourant, stimulant and stomachic. The oil of ginger is used in mouth washes and beverages (as flavouring agent).

BLACK PEPPER

Vernacular name : Hindi- Kalimirch; Bengali -Golmarich; Tamil- Milagu; English- Black Pepper; Tel.- Miriyala tige.

Biological source : Black pepper consists of dried, unripe fruits of *Piper nigrum* Linn. This is a member of *Piperaceae* family.

Geographical source : Black Pepper is indigenous to India and widely cultivated in Assam, Kerala, Karnataka and Maharastra. This plant is wildly available from North Kanara to Kanyakumari. It is also cultivated in Malayasia, Indonesia, Brazil, Srilanka, South America and West Indies.

Cultivation and collections : The well distributed annual rainfall and altitude up to 1500 metre are ideal conditions for good cultivation of the Black Pepper. The plant is a perennial climbing vine. Supports and stands are provided for every vine. Fast growing tree is used as stands for vine. It provides support and shade to the plant. Generally plant is cultivated as mixed crop with coconut, arecanut, tea and coffee. Plant is generally cultivated by sowing the seeds or cuttings (vegetatively). For economical cultivation of black pepper soil requires high amount of nitrogenous substances (Fertilizers and Manures). The cuttings of black pepper are grafted in soil in the month of April to May, support or stand is also raised for vine. Generally cutting is grafted in north and north east side from stands, in this way severe western sun light is avoided, The plant starts fruiting from third year and onwards. The inflorescence of black pepper has a spike inflorescence, containing 20-30 sessile flowers, that develop into sessile fruits. Fruits are harvested in February or March when colour of fruits turn orange red in the spike. Fruits are dried for a week.

Morphology : Its fruits are globular in shape, 3.5 - 6 mm in diametre. The external surface is dark brown or greyish -black. The surface is strongly reticulated wrinkled with remains of stigma at apex. The pericarp is thin and encloses a single white kernel with hollow centre. This kernel contains perisperm, a small endosperm and embryo. Perisperm is horny in outer part.

Constituents : The Black pepper contains piperidine group of alkaloids like piperine, piperidine, piperettine, chavicine, 1-2.5% volatile oil, phellandrene, caryophyllene, piperonal, camphene, α pinene & ß pinene, citronellol, resin and starch (30%). It also contains arginine, ascorbic acid, carotene, thiamine and riboflavin. The pungency is due to alkaloid piperine and resins.

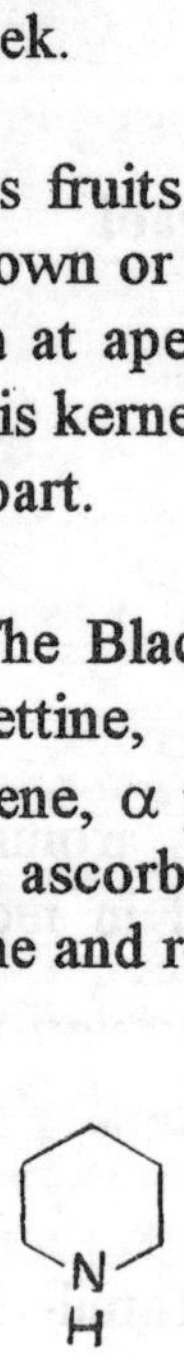

Piperidine

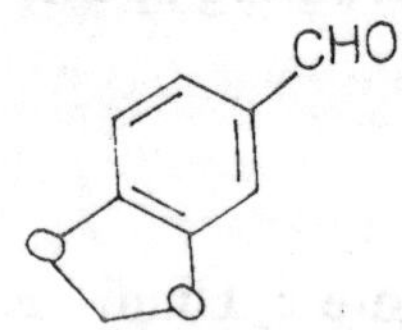

Piperonal

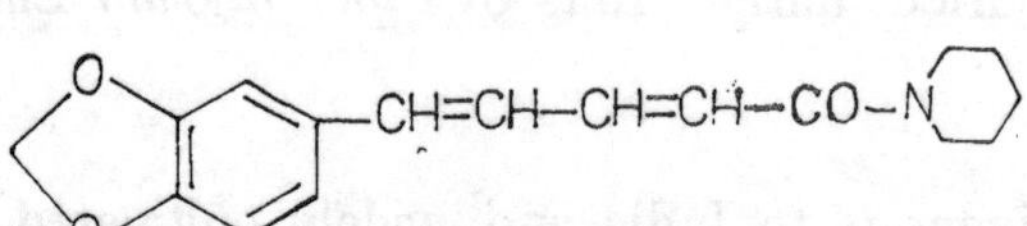

Piperine

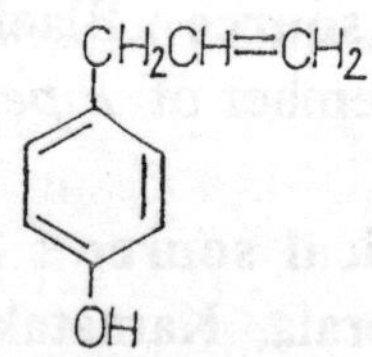

Chavicol

Standards

Ash	:	≤ 6.0%
Acid insoluble ash	:	≤ 1.0%
Foreign organic matter	:	≤ 2.0%
Crude fibres	:	≤ 15%

Uses : Black Pepper is used as carminative, stomachic, stimulant, flatulent, antimalarial and antiarthritic. It is also useful in sore throat, piles, dyspepsia and in skin diseases. It is also useful for the treatment of gonorrhoea and chronic bronchitis.

ASAFOETIDA

Vernacular name : Hindi & Bengali- Hing; Sans.- Hingu; Tam.-Perungayam; Eng.- Asafoetida.

Biological source : Asafoetida is an oleo gum resin obtained as exudation by incision from living rhizomes and roots of *Ferula foetida* Regel, *Ferula rubricaulis* Boiss and other species of Ferula. It is a member of *Umbelliferae* family.

Geographical source : The plant is distributed in eastern Persia, western Afghanistan, Iran, Turkistan and Pakistan. It is cultivated in the North Western part of India.

Collection : The plant is a perennial tree, 2-4 metre high containing schizogenous ducts and lysogenous cavity filled with whitish gum-resinous emulsion. Four to five years old plant's root contains sufficient oleo gum resin. Just before the flowering, upper part of the stem, close to crown is cut off. The exudation flows from cut surface and starts coagulating. The cut surface is protected by dome like covering made of leaves and branches to avoid contamination from foreign matter. After a few weeks, the hard and coagulated gum resin is scraped off. The process of successive incision is repeated at an interval of 10 days till complete collection of oleo gum resin is achieved. The average yield of oleo gum resin from each plant is about 1 kg. The product is packed in tin containers.

Morphology : Asafoetida occurs as soft and solid mass. There are two principle forms of asafoetida : (i) Tears form (ii) Mass form

(1) **Tears form** : Tears are rounded flattened 5-30 mm in diameter. These are solid, semi-solid, greyish-white, whitish yellow or reddish brown in colour. They are translucent or opaque in appearance.
(2) **Mass form** : It is similar to tears but agglutinated mas and usually mixed with fruits, root fragments and other foreign materials. It is the common commercial form of asafoetida.

Asafoetida has a bitter taste, strong alliaceous (garlic) odour and alliaceous taste. It should not contain more than 50% of matter insoluble in alcohol (90%) soluble matter, and the ash should not be more than 15%.

Constituents : Asafoetida contains 10-17% volatile oils, 25% gums and 40-64% resins. The alliaceous odour of drug is due to the presence of sulphur compound of the formula $C_7H_{14}S_2$, $C_8H_{16}S_2$, $C_{10}H_{18}S_2$, $C_7H_{14}S_3$, $C_8H_{16}S_3$ and $C_{16}H_{20}S_2$, The oil is obtained by steam distillation of oleo gum resin. The main constituent of oil is isobutyl propanyldisulphide ($C_8H_{16}S_2$). It also contains α pinene, phellendrine, gummosin, etc. The resin consists of asaresinotannol in combination with free or combined ferulic acid. Free umbelliferone is not present in the drug but after boiling the drug with HCl and filtering in ammonia will give positive test for umbelliferone e.g., blue fluorescence in ultra-violet (U.V) light.

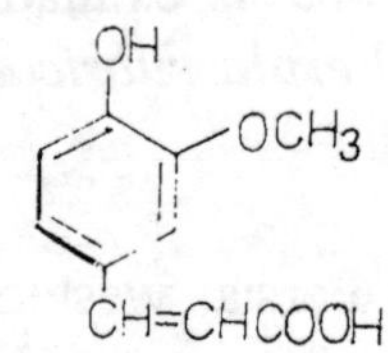

Ferulic acid

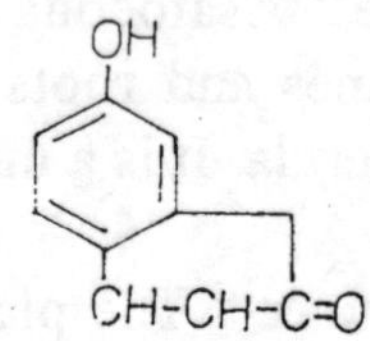

Umbelliferone

Standards

Ash	: ≤ 15%;
Alcohol soluble matter	: ≥ 50%

Chemical tests

1. If the fractured surface of drug is treated with 50% nitric acid, green colour is produced.
2. To the fractured surface of drug, add sulphuric acid. Red or reddish brown colour is produced.
3. The drug produces a yellow-orange emulsion when triturated with water.
4. It also gives above mentioned umbelliferone test

Uses : The drug is used as carminative, diuretic, expectorant, antispasmodic, anthelmintic and applied externally to ring worms. It is also used in veterinary practice.

NUTMEG

Vernacular name : Hindi- Jaiphal, Javitri; Beng.- Jaipal, Jaitri; Sans.- Jatiphala (Nutmeg); Tam. - Jadikai; Eng.- Nutmeg tree.

Biological source : Nutmeg is the dried kernels of the seeds of *Myristica fragrans* Houtt. This is a member of *Myristicaceae* family.

Geographical source : The nutmeg is indigenous to Molucca Island. The plant is widely cultivated in Malaysia, Indonesia, Zava, Ceylon and West-Indies. In India, nutmeg is found as specimen tree in Kerala, Karnataka, Nilgiri and West Bengal.

Cultivation, collection and preparation : Nutmeg is a dioecious or occasionally monoecious, ever green tree, usually 9-12 metre in height and often attains its height upto 20 metre. The plant requires a hot, moist climate, well drain rich loam soil and shelter from high wind. The plant is grown from fresh seed. The seed germinates within 5-6 weeks, then the plants are transplanted in the field. Banana trees are grown between the nutmeg plants to provide shelter. The male female plant ratio should be 1:7 or 1:8 and for this purpose, excess of male plants are removed from the field at their flowering stage, e.g. after 5-8 years. The plant starts bearing fruits from 8-9th year and continue upto 20-30 years, Every year two crops are taken one in November to December and other in April to June.

The female plant can also be propagated by vegetative means, i.e., from the branches of female tree. It saves time and loss due to growth of male tree.
The fruits are peach like, ovoid and dehisce longitudinally when ripe; 5-7 cm long, 4-5 cm wide and light yellow in colour. The fleshy pericarp splits and the brown seeds are surrounded by arillus (mace). The arillus is striped off from the seeds. Seeds are dried in the shade. Drying usually takes 2-3 weeks . Testa is separated with the help of wooden mallet and nutmeg is extracted out. Nutmeg is separated for commercial value as per their size and external appearance.

Morphology : Kernels are ovoid 2-3 cm long and about 2 cm wide. They are greyish brown in colour with reticulate furrows. There is a small projection at one end. Micropyle and hilum are present near the projection. Hilum is surrounded by a raised ring. From the hilum, ill defined furrow runs to a chalaza, that indicates the position of raphe. The cut surface of nutmeg yields oil easily. The nutmeg has strong aromatic odour and a bitter and aromatic taste.

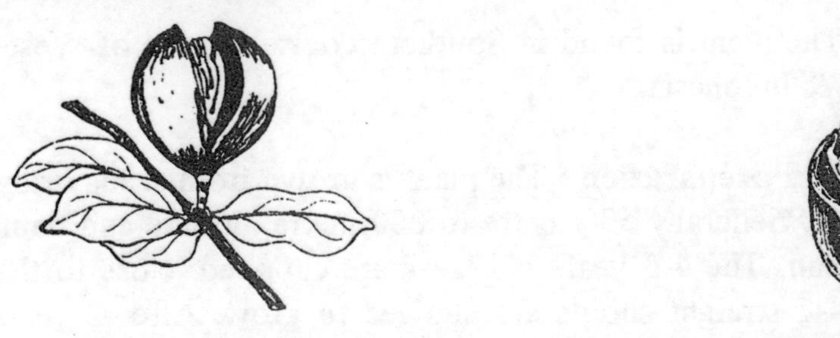

(a) fruiting branch (b) surrounded by mace

Fig. 7.17 : Nutmeg

Chemical constituents : Nutmeg contains 5-15% of volatile oils,30-40% fats(Nutmeg butter), proteins, phytosterin, colouring matter, starch, amylodextrin and saponin. Volatile oil contains myristicin (4-8%), trimyristicin, elemicin, safrol, apiole, methyl euginol,α terpinene, ß-pinene,, etc. Myristicin is responsible for hallucinogenic property. It also contains myrstic acid, polyphenols, tannins, thiamine, riboflavin, epicatechin, etc.

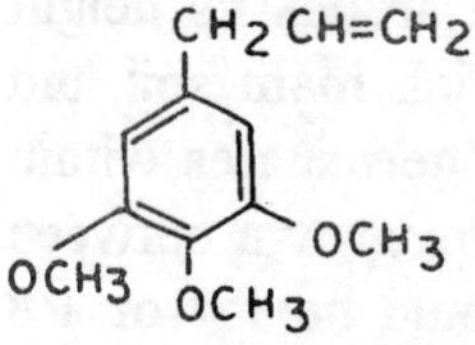

Elemicin

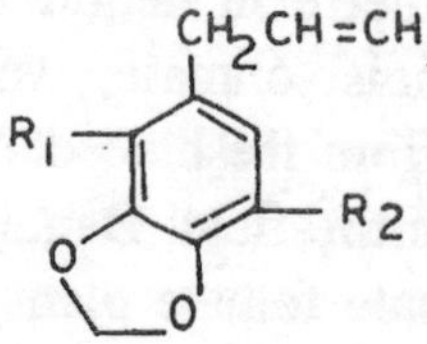

R1	R2	Compound
H	H	Safrol
H	$-OCH_3$	Myristicin
$-OCH_3$	$-OCH_3$	Apiole

Standards

Total ash	: ≤ 3.0%
Acid insoluble ash	: ≤0.2%

Uses : Nutmeg is used as carminative, stomachic, astringent, flatulent, nausea, vomiting, aphorodisiac. Nutmeg infusion is useful for cholera patients. The nutmeg oil and mace are useful in paralysis, sprain and rheumatism. It is also used as a flavouring agent.

CINNAMON

Synonym : *Cinnamomum verum.*

Vernacular name : Hindi- Tvakh; Sans. - Tvacha; Beng. - Dalchini; Tam. - Ilayangam; Eng. - Cinnamon.

Biological source : Cinnamon consists of dried bark of *Cinnamomum zeylanicum*. It is a member of *lauraceae* family.

Geographical source : The plant is found in Southern coastal region of Western India, Srilanka, Jamaica, Brazil & Indonesia.

Cultivation, collection and preparation : The plant is grown from seeds or by planting the cuttings (vegetatively). Generally 500 metre to 800 metre altitude and damp climate are preferred for cultivation. The 4-5 years old trees are chopped, close to the ground. From each plant about 4-7 straight shoots are allowed to grow. After 2 years straight branch is lobed off and bark is stripped off from the shoot with the help of copper or brass knife. Iron knives are avoided because they react with tannin present in bark. These barks are collected in the month of April to July after heavy rain fall. These are dried.in shade for 24 hours in open air. The dried bark is graded according to quality and appearance and tied in the bundle of 15 Kg.

Morphology : Cinnamon barks are found in single and double coils about one metre in length; 6-10 mm in diameter and about 0.5 mm in thickness. The fracture of bark is splintery, yellowish-brown and internal surface is dark brown. External surface shows longitudinal wavy lines of pericyclic fibres whereas internal surface is longitudinally striated. External surface also contains scars and holes. The bark has aromatic odour and sweet taste followed by warm sensation.

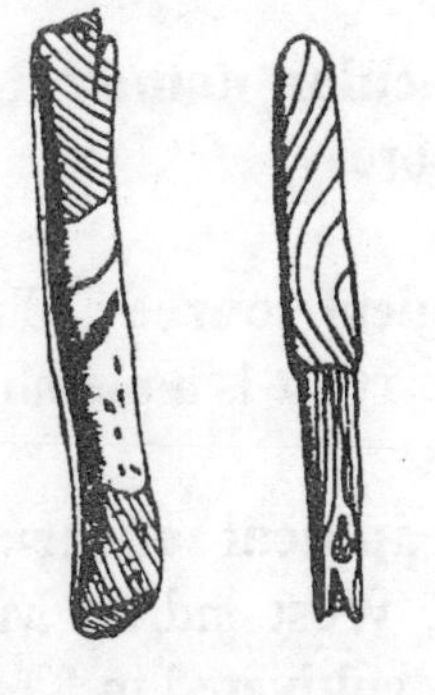

Fig. 7.18 : Compound quill of cinnamon bark

Chemical constituents : Cinnamon bark contains volatile oil, phlobatannin, mucilage, calcium oxalate, mannitol and starch. The constituents of volatile oil are cinnamic aldehyde $C_6H_5CH=CH-CHO$ (60-75%), eugenol, benzaldehyde, phellandrine, pinene, cymene, linalool, safrol, methyl eugenol, borneol, gerineol, etc.

Chemical tests

(1) Test for phenol : Volatile oil is dissolved in 5ml alcohol and a drop of ferric chloride is added. The pale green colour is produced due to presence of phenolic compound eugenol.

(2) Test for aldehyde : To the alcoholic extract of bark, add phenylhydrazine hydrochloride, a red coloured ppt. of phenyl hydrazone is formed.

Standards

Foreign organic matter	: $\leq$ 2%
Acid insoluble ash	: $\leq$ 2%
Crude fibres	: $\leq$ 26-36%
Alcohol (90%) soluble extract	: 14-16%

Uses : Cinnamon bark is used as carminative, astringent, flavouring agent, antiseptic and antidiarrhoeal. Cinnamon oil is used in the treatment of rheumatism, headache and toothache. It is also used as spices, condiments and perfumes.

CLOVE

Synonym : *Eugenia caryophyllata* Thunb; *E. aromatica* Kuntze.

Vernacular name : Hindi- Laung; Eng. - clove; Sans. & Bengali -Lavanga; Tamil - Kirambre.

Biological source : Clove is a dried flower bud of *Syzygium aromaticum* (Linn.) Merry and Perry. It is a member of the *Myrtaceae* family.

Geographical source : The clove tree is indigenous to Molucca Island. It is cultivated in Brazil, West indies, Madagascar, Mauritius, Pemba, Srilanka and India. In India, it is mainly cultivated in Kerala and Tamil-Nadu.

Cultivation, collection & preparation : Clove is a 9-12 metre evergreen tree. Plants are generally raised from seeds. Initially seedlings are protected from direct sunlight for a period of about 9 months, after that period, plant is exposed to gradual sun light for the period of 2-3 years. After that it can be exposed to full sun light. The plant begins to bear clove buds from 6th years and yields 3-4 Kg buds per tree annually till 70 years of age. Flower buds are collected when their lower part changes from green to crimson red in colour. Generally buds are collected twice in a year between August to December in dry weather. The cloves are dried in the open air and clove stalks are separated. If buds are not collected then buds open, blown clove is formed and finally converted into fruits, i.e., mother clove; which contain lesser amount of volatile oil in comparison to clove buds. Collected clove buds are dried in the sun light. During drying 60-70% water is evaporated. It is graded & packed into bales and exported.

Morphology : Cloves are about 1.6-2.1 cm long, reddish-brown in colour. The upper portion is known as crown or cap and lower flattened, cylindrical solid stalk is known as hypanthium. The lower stalk is about 10-13 mm long, 4 mm wide and 2 mm thick and tapers towards lower end. A bilocular ovary containing numerous ovules attached to axial placenta is present on the upper portion of the stalk. The head consists of four

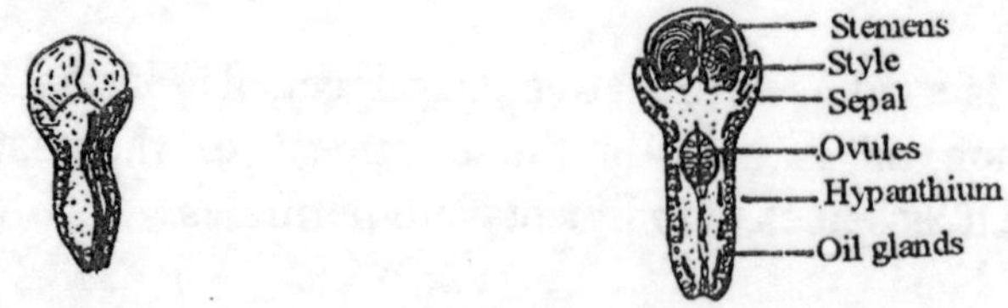

(a) Clove bud (b) Longitudinally cut clove

Fig. 7.19 :

projecting calyx teeth, four pale yellow dome shaped imbricated membranous petals, numerous incurved stamens surrounding a large style. Clove possesses strong fragrance, spicy odour and pungent aromatic taste.

Chemical constituents : Clove contains volatile oil 15-20%, tannin 10-13% and a colourless crystalline substance caryophyllene. The volatile oil contains Eugenol 85-90%, eugenyl acetate, α and ß caryophyllenes, methyl salicylate and α - humulene. It also contains resin, vanillin, glucose, fructose, rhamnose, sucrose, carvone and furfural.

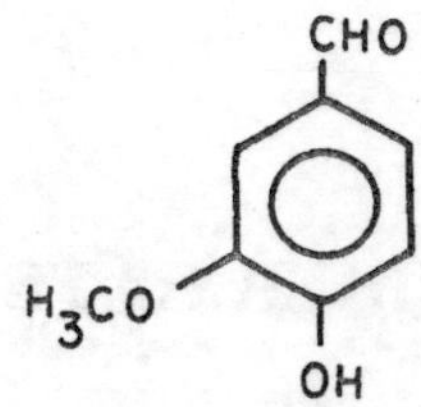

Vanillin

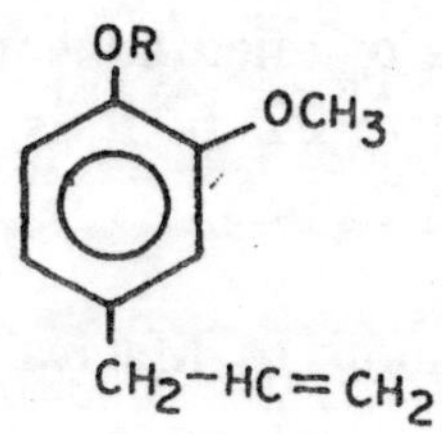

R=H = Eugenol
R= $-COCH_3$ = Acetyl eugenol

Standards

Density at 25°C	: 1.038 to 1.06
Refractive Index	: -1.53 to 1.531
Optical Rotation	: 0 to - 1.5°

Uses : Clove is used as carminative, antispasmodic, stimulant, flatulant, antiseptic, counter irritant, rubifacient, local anesthetic, flavouring agent, etc. Clove oil is used in various dental products. Externally it is applied in rheumatic pain.

Chemical tests

(1) Test for eugenol : When hypanthium of clove or clove oil is treated with 50% potassium hydroxide solution, needle shaped crystals of potasium eugenate are formed.

(2) Test for phenolic groups : When ferric chloride is added to clove extract, a blue black colour is formed.

7 - D ASTRINGENTS

Astringents are the agents in which cells shrink by precipitation of surface proteins. It is used in lotions to harden and protect the skin, and to reduce exudative secretions & bleeding from minor abrassions. They are also used in glossitis, mouth washes, antipesrpirants, throat lozenges, eye drops, piles and internally used for diarrhoea. The important natural astringents are

(I) Tannic acid	(II) Myrobalan
(III) Bahera	(IV) Amla
(V) Arnica	(VI) Catechu

PALE CATECHU/ GAMBIER CATECHU

Vernacular name : Hindi- Kath-Kutha; Beng.-Khayer; Tel.- Ankudukurra.

Biological source : The pale catechu consists of dried aqueous extract, prepared from leaves and twigs of *Uncaria gambier* (Hunter) Roxb. It is a member of *Rubiaceae* family.

Geographical source : The plant is indigenous to Malaya and largely cultivated in Indonesia and Malaya.

Preparation : The leaves and twigs of 2-10 years old plants are collected at an interval of 3-6 months. These leaves are boiled with water in a large container. The extract is filtered and concentrated till yellowish paste is formed. It is then transferred in a wooden tray and cut into cubes, which are then dried in sun.

Characters : Catechu cubes are dark reddish- brown in colour while internal surface is pale brown and dull. The cubes are friable, odourless and possess astringent taste.

Chemical constituents : It contains 7-33% of catechins, 22-50% catechutannic acid, catechu red, quercitin, pyrogallol and gambir fluorescin. It also contains fixed oil, starch, sugar, etc.

Standards

Ash	: $\leq 5\%$
Water insoluble matter	: $\leq 33\%$
Loss on drying	: $\leq 15\%$

Uses : It is used as astringent but its major use lies in dyeing and tanning industry. It is also used in diarrhoea and in preparation of lozenges.

Chemical tests : Gambier fluorescin test - Positive (see Black Catechu)
Chlorophyll test : Substance is heated with 5 ml chloroform and extract is evaporated in evaporating disc, green residue is observed.

BLACK CATECHU

Vernacular name : Sans. - Khadira; Hindi & Beng.- Khayir; Tamil - Karangalli; English - Cutch tree; Guj.- Kher.

Biological source : The black catechu consists of dried aqueous extract, prepared from the heart wood of the plant *Acacia catechu* (L.F) wild. This is a member of *Mimosoideae* (*Leguminosae*) family.

Geographical source : The tree is indigenous to India & distributed in the dry regions of Sub Himalayan tract from Punjab to north eastern state, Madya Pradesh, Gujarat, Andra Pradesh, Tamil Nadu, & Konkan region.

Preparation : The whole tree is fallen by cutting. Bark & heart wood are separated and cut into small chips and boiled with water in an earthen-ware or stainless-steel vessel for decoction. It is filtered and concentrated till thick syrupy mass is obtained. It is solidified in a wooden frame, covered with leaves.

Characters : Black catechu occurs as brown to black irregular mass, hard and brittle externally and soft and porous internally. Freshly broken surface is dull, glossy and brittle. The drug is completely soluble in hot water and partially soluble in cold water and alcohol. Taste is astringent and it is odourless.

Standards

Ash	: $\leq 6\%$
Loose on drying	: $\leq 12\%$
Alcohol insoluble residue	: $\leq 40\%$
Water insoluble residue	: $\leq 25\%$

Chemical constituents : Black Catechu contains isomeric mixture of catechin, acacatechin, catechutannic acid or phlobatannin, l-epicatechin, quercitrin, quercitin gum and catchu red. The acid hydrolysis of the gum gives L-arabinose, D-galactose, D-

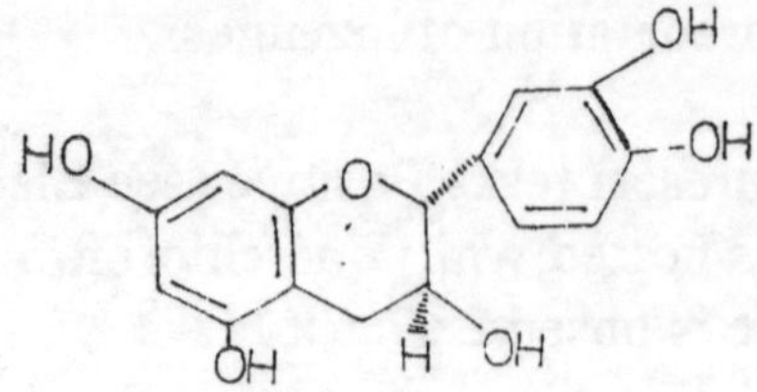

(+) - Catechin

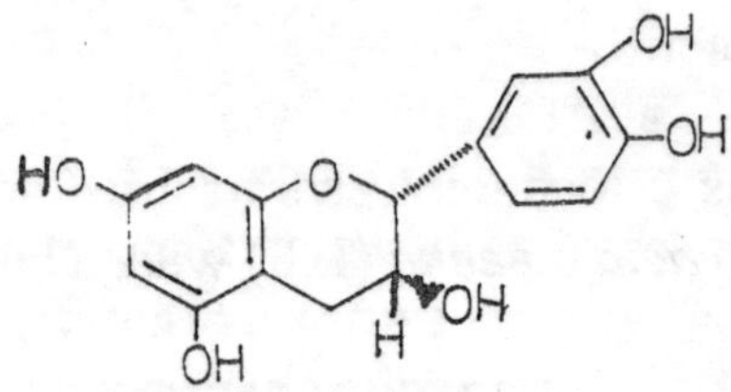

(+) - Epicatechin

Chemical tests

(1) **Vanillin hydrochloride test : The solution of catechu is treated with vanillin hydrochloric acid (vanillin : alcohol : hydrochloric acid : 1:10 : 10) a pink or red colour produces due to the formation of phloroglucinol.**

(2) **Match stick test : Paste of black catechu in water is smeared on the rear end of match stick and a drop of hydrochloric acid is put on it and warmed, purple colour is produced due to the formation of phloroglucinol which reacts with lignin present in the wood of stick.**

(3) **Gambier fluorescin test : This test is negative for Black catechu but positive for Gambier or pale catechu. The drug is extracted with alcohol, filtered and a solution of sodium hydroxide is added, followed by shaking with the addition of a few drops of light petroleum. The petroleum layer acquires green fluorescence due to pale catechu.**

Uses : It is used as astringent, passive antidiarrhoeatic either alone or in combination with cinnamon or opium. Also used as a colic anthelmintic, apetizer, antidysentric, anti-pyretic and indigestion, leprosy, leucoderma, elephantiasis, piles,, etc. It is mainly used as an important constituent of *pan-masala*. It is used as masticatory together with betle leaves, areca nut and lime.

7 - E. DRUGS ACTING ON NERVOUS SYSTEM

1. AUTONOMIC NERVOUS SYSTEM (Autonomous - self goverining)

Autonomic nervous system, is involuntary part of nervous system, which controls the functions of the body going automatically. The autonomic nervous system is also called the visceral; vegetative, or involuntary nervous system. A.N.S. control the vital functions of the body such as blood circulation, blood pressure, body temperature, water balance, respiration, digestion, urination, etc.

Autonomic nervous system is divided into two parts
1. Parasympathetic
2.. Sympathetic

Usually, sympathetic system is inhibitory in nature and parasympathetic is excitatory in nature. These two systems are always in a state of dynamic equilibrium. The two important neurotransmitters of ANS are acetyl choline and noradrenaline and it's derivative. Drugs by mimicking or antagonising the actions of either of these two produce a remarkable physiological response and are divided into four groups on basis of its action.

DRUGS ACTING ON A.N.S.

A) **Parasympathomimetic (cholinergic agents)** : These drugs stimulate the parasympathetic system and mimic the action of acetyl choline.

e.g. : (i) Pilocarpine (*Pilocarpus microphyllus*)
(ii) Physostigmine (*Physostigma venenosum*)
(iii) Muscarine (*Amanita* spp.)
(iv) Arecholine (*Areca catechu*)

(B) **Parasympatholytic (Cholinergic blocking agents)** : These agents antagonise the action of acetyl choline.

(i) Tropane alkaloids (Hyoscine, Atropine, etc.) : Datura, Belladonna, Stramonium, etc.
(ii) Tubocurarine : (Chondodrendon spp.)

(C) **Sympathomimetic (Adrenergic agents)** : These agents mimic the action of Adr.
Ephedrine : Ephedra spp.

(D) Sympatholytic (adrenergic blocking agents) : Drugs which antagonise the action of adrenaline and noradrenaline, comes under this. e.g. : Ergot alkaloids (*Claviceps purpurea*)

2. CENTRAL NERVOUS SYSTEM

The central nervous systems consist of the brain and the spinal cord. This system mainly co-ordinates the voluntary functionsof the body. The proper interaction and co-ordination between A.N.S. & C.N.S. produces many responses.

Drugs acting on C.N.S. : On the basis of action (either excitatory or inhibitory) these drugs are classified as below

1. **Drugs affecting mental activity**		
(I) Depressant	Reserpine	*Rauwolfia serpentina*
(II) Hallucinogens	Lysergic acid	Ergot
	Cannabinoids	*Cannabis sativa*
(III) Stimulants	Caffeine	Coffee,Tea.
	Cocaine	*Erythroxylum coca*
2. **Analeptics**	Strychnine	*Strychnos nuxvomica*
	Camphor	*Cinnamomum camphora*
3. **Analgesics**	Morphine & Codeine	*Papaver somniferum*
4. **Depressant**	Tropane alkaloid- atropine, hyoscine.	*Solanaceous* plant (Datura, Belladonna)

HYOSCYAMUS [HENBANE]

Vernacular Name : Hindi - Khurasaniajvayan; Beng. - Khorasaniajowan; Tam. - Kurasaniyomam; Kashmir - Bazarbang & English - Black Henbane.

Biological source : It consists of dried leaves and flowering tops of plant *Hyoscyamus niger* Linn. This is a member of *solanaceae* family. It contains not less than 0.05% total alkaloids, calculated as hyoscyamine.

Geographical source : In India, it is found in temperate Western Himalayan from Kashmir to Garhwal. It is also cultivated in certain part of western Himalaya. World wide it is distributed in England, Germany and Russia.

Collection and cultivation : The drug is cultivated in commercial scale in Europe. In India, it is cultivated in western region of Himalayan. It is annual or biennial plant. The drug is propagated from seed. These take two weeks for germination, then seedlings are transplanted in the field in the month of May and June. The plant is sprayed by derris or pyrethrum (as insecticide) to protect the plant from the "potato beetle".
The biennial plant flowers in May and June and annual plant flowers in July or August. In European countries drug is collected before fruiting and dried rapidly by artificial heat at 40-50°c temperature.

Morphology : The leaves of Henbane are more or less broken, crumpled and sessile. It is characterized by greyish green colour; Midrib is very broad with numerous hairs. The stems are hairy and about 5 mm in diametre. Flowers are subsessile, unilateral, lower axillary, solitary, upper forming a dense racemose or subscorpioid cyme. Calyx is softly hairy and teeth is mucronate, persistent of five lobes, corolla lurid yellow or greenish deep purple, funnel shaped, limb oblique, lobes more or less unequal. Dry flowers are compressed and broken, its yellowish corollas with purple vein are visible in the drug. The ovary is bilocular. Seeds are flat and reniform, dark grey coloured. The taste of Henbane plant is bitter. It has unpleasant and characteristic heavy odour. The first year biennial plant stem is very short, leaves are rossette form near the ground, normally not flowering in first year but in second year leaves are sessile, 10-20 cm. long, margin is dentate, it is very hairy and flowering in May and June. In the annual plant, leaves are also sessile but smaller than biennial plant, contains lesser hairs and flowering in July and August.

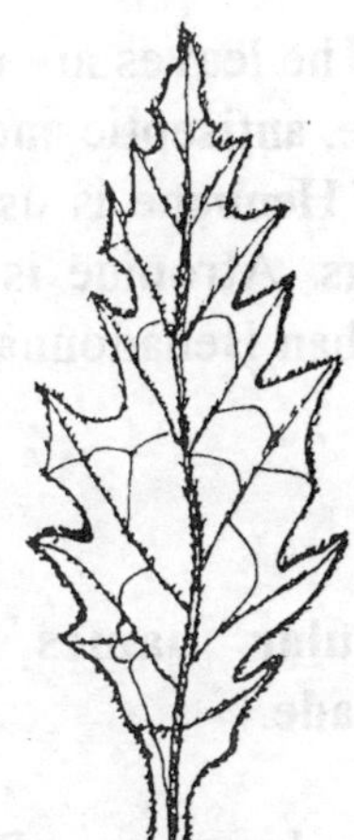

Fig. 7.20 : *Hyoscymus niger* leaf

Chemical constituents : Hyoscyamus leaves contain tropane alkaloids 0.05% to 0.15%. L-Hyoscyamine (atropine) is main active constituent of leaves. It also contains hyoscine (scopolamine). The petioles contain more alkaloid than that lamina and stem. In seed the percentage of alkaloid is less than leaf. It also contains apohyoscine, α and ß belladonine, ascorbic acid and other amino acids like alanine, arginine, aspartic acid, glutamic acid, glycine, etc. Apoatropine, cuscohygrine, daturamine, tropine. hyoscypicrin, hyoscine N-oxide and choline are also isolated from the plant.

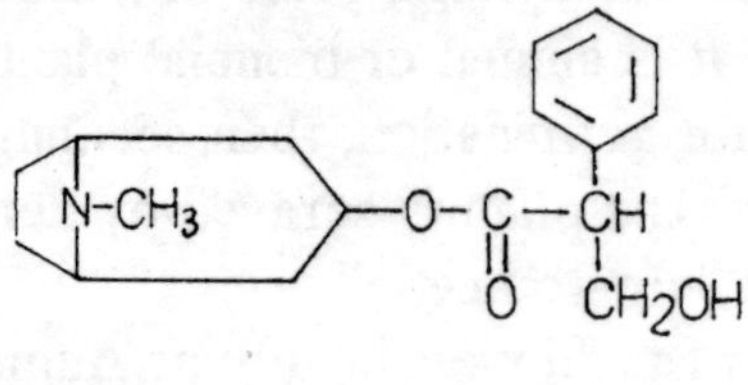

Hyoscyamus or Atropin.

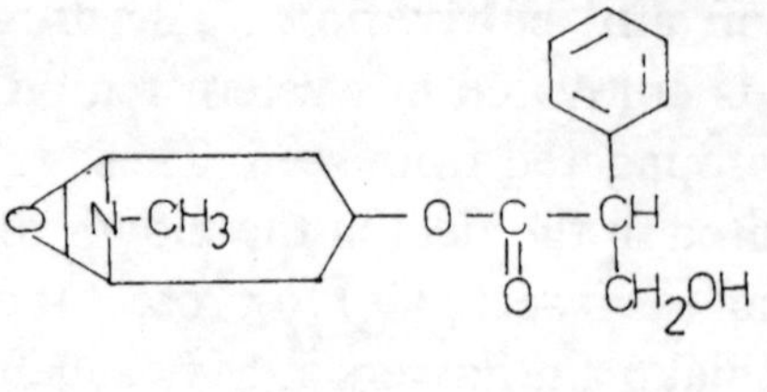

Hyoscine or Scopolamine

Standards

Ash	: ≤ 20%
Acid insoluble ash	: ≤ 12%
Total alkaloid	: ≥ 0.05%
Foreign organic matter	: ≤ 2%

Uses : The leaves are used as mydriatic (atropine and hyoscine), antispasmodic, laxative, anodyne, antiseptic and in asthma and whooping cough. The oil prepared from leaves and seed of Henbane is useful as anthelmintic, narcotic, stomachic and in inflammation and swellings. Atropine is a C.N.S. stimulant. Hyoscyamus has weaker parasympatholytic action than Belladonna and Stramonium; prevent gripping pain when added to cathartics.

BELLADONNA

Vernacular names : Hindi-Sag-angur; Sans.-Suchi; Beng.-Yebruj; Eng.-Deadly Nightshade.

Biological source : Belladonna consist of dried leaves and flowering tops of *Atropa belladonna* Linn. and *Atropa acuminata* Royle (Indian belladonna). It is a member of family *solanaceae* Atropa is a greek word; Atropose means cuts the thread of life, i.e., poisionous nature of plant. Belladonna is an Italian word; bella means beautiful and donna means lady. Here by means that by putting its fruit juice in eye makes more sparking due to dilation effect on pupil. This is a member of *solanaceae* family. It contains not less than 0.3% of alkaloids, calculated as hyoscyamine.

Geographical source : The drugs is indigenous to England and cultivated in England and other European countries like Italy, Yugoslavia, Russia, Rumania, etc. It is also cultivated in Germany, U.S.A. and India. In India, it is found in western Himalayan from Kashmir to Simla.

Collection and cultivation : Belladonna plant is grown by seed. Three years old plant gives maximum yield. Two or more crops of leaves are collected annually. The leaves are collected at the end of June or July when it contains maximum content of alkaloid. The leaves are collected in peak sun light because in shady period leaves contain low percentage of active constituents. The collected leaves are dried immediately at about 60°C and stored. If moisture is present in leaf, it is detoriated and ammonia is liberated.

Morphology : The belladonna consists of leaves, smaller stem having diameter about 5 mm; flowers and fruits. The leaves are dull green or yellowish green in colour. The upper side of leaf is darker than lower side. It is 5-20 cm long and 2.5-12 cm wide. Apex is acuminate, margin is entire and is broadly ovate, or lanciolate and slightly decurrent lamina. Petiole is 0.5 to 4 cm long.

The stems are green or purple green in colour. The flowers are purple to yellowish brown in colour. Corolla bell shaped 2.5 cm long and 1.5 cm wide. Fruits are green to brown in colour, it is globose berries. Due to presence of sandy crystals of calcium oxalate in mesophyll cell, it gives minute points on the surface of dried leaf, because all other cells are contracted on drying except these crystals.

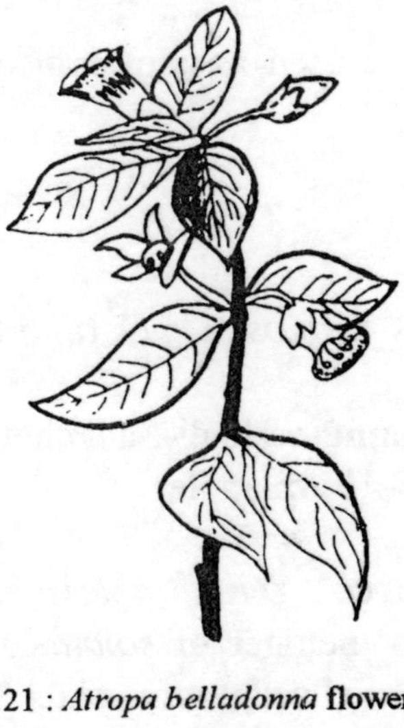

Fig. 7.21 : *Atropa belladonna* flowering shoot

Chemical constituents : Belladona contains 0.3% to 0.6% of tropane alkaloid. The chief alakloids are hyoscyamine, atropine and scopolamin (hyoscine). The other components are apoatropine, asparagine and choline. It also contains small quantity of bases like pyridine, N-methylpyrroline. The leaves also contain florescence substance ß-methyl aesculetin (scopoletin) and calcium oxalate.

Standards

Ash (acid insoluble)	: ≤ 3%
Foreign organic matter	: ≤ 2%

Uses : It is used as anticholinergic, narcotic, sedative, and diuretic. It is used for the spasm of gut and respiratory tract. Herb is used to reduce secretion of salivary, gastric and sweat gland and in bronchal asthma, G.I.T. Hyper motility, peptic ulcer, motion sickness. The aqueous extract of atropine is applied as sulphate for the dilation of pupil of the eyes. It is important antidote for opium, muscarine and chloral hydrate poisoning. *A. belladonna* leaves are used in internal preparations whereas roots are mainly used externally.

Adulterants

(1) Leaves of *Phytolacca decandra*
(2) Leaves of *Ailanthus glandulosa*
(3) Leaves of *Scopolia carniolica*
(4) Leaves of *Datura stramonium*
(5) Leaves of *Solanum nigrum*

These plants are used as adulterant due to some what similar morphological feature to genuine drugs.

DATURA

Synonyms : *D. fastuosa* L.; *D. alba* Nees; *D. fastuosa* L. Var.-alba (Nees) Cl.

Vernacular name : Hindi-Sadadhatura; Sans.-Dhastura; Beng.-Dhutura; Tam.-Vellum mattai; English-Thorn apple.

Biological source : Datura consist of dried leaves and flowering tops of *Datura metel* Linn. This is a member of *solanaceae* family. It contains not less than 0.5% of total alkaloid, calculated as hyoscyamine.

Geographical source : The drug is commonly found in waste places along road side and railway line, scrub jungles throughout the tropical part of country.

Collection and cultivation : The drug is usually cultivated by seeds. The germination rate of seeds is poor. The germination rate can be increased by soaking seeds in water for 24 hours, to soften the seed coat. The seed takes about 2-3 weeks for germination. The leaves and flowering tops are collected after 3-4 months after cultivation. The crude drug is dried in sun and stored in air tight containers.

Morphology : The plant contains cylindrical, glabrous, stem and leaves. Leaves are green, unequal at the base, acute apex, ovate, triangular, 8-12 cm long and 6-7 cm broad; an entire sinuate or tooth head margin. The flowers are whitish to reddish purple in colour, 6-7 cm in length and funnel shaped. The stem and branches of the Datura are purple in colour; capsule is globose or ellipsoid, nodding, spinous, 4-valved or irregular breaking up near the apex. Seeds are compressed, brown and rugose.

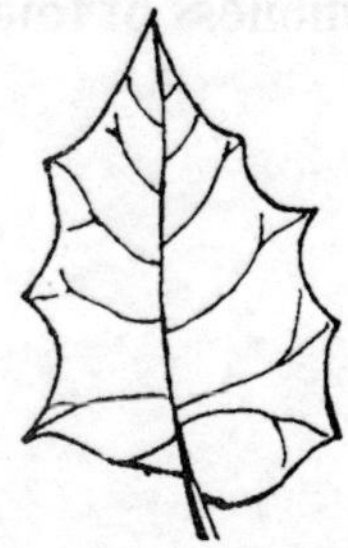

Fig. 7.22 : *Datura metal* leaf

Chemical constituents : Datura contains tropane alkaloid. The drug contains hyoscine (scopolamine) and hyoscyamine (atropine). It also contains fastudine, fastunine, fastusic acid, alantoin, ascorbic acid, etc.

Uses : Datura is an anticholinergic and parasympatholytic drug. It is used similar to belladonna.

Chemical test

1. **Vitali - Morin reaction** : The drug is treated with concentrated nitric acid, filtered and solution is evaporated to dryness. To the residue, add acetone and methanolic potassium hydroxide solution, violet colour is produced due to tropane derivative.

ACONITE (Wolfsbane root)

Vernacular name : Hindi- Dudhi-bish; Sans.- Visha; Beng. - Katbish.

Biological source : It consist of the dried tuberous roots of *Aconitum napellus* Linn. This is the member of *ranunculaceae* family.

Geographical source: It is wildly distributed in Southern Europe, Spain, England, Hungary, Germany and Switzerland. In India, it is found in alpine and sub alpine belt of Himalayan.

Cultivation and collection : It is a perennial herb. The plant is cultivated from the daughter roots due to poor rate of germination by seeds. The roots are collected from flowering plants in autumn, washed, dried and stored in well closed containers.

Morphology : The crude drugs consist, parent and daughter roots. They are dark brown in colour, obconical and tapering below in shape. The drug is 4-10 cm in length and 1-3 cm in diameter at the crown. The drug has slight odour and taste is slightly sweet followed by numbness of tounge.

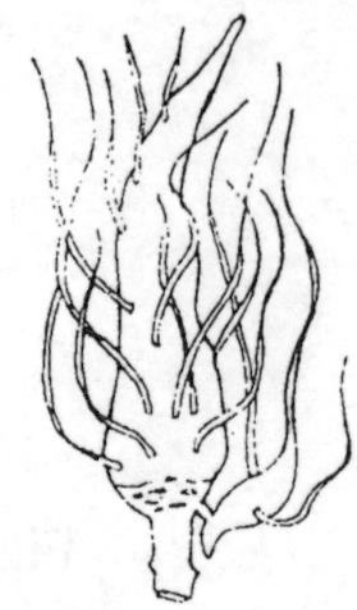

Fig. 7.23 : *Aconitum napellus* root, showing parent and daughter root.

Chemical constituents : The drug contain 0.3-1.2% of total terpene ester alkaloids. The most important alkaloids are aconitine, aconine and benzyl aconine. Aconitine on hydrolysis produce benzoyl aconine and acetic acid. It also contains aconitic acid and abundance of starch. A traces of ephedrine, spartein, neoline, napelline, ascorbic acid, etc. are also present.

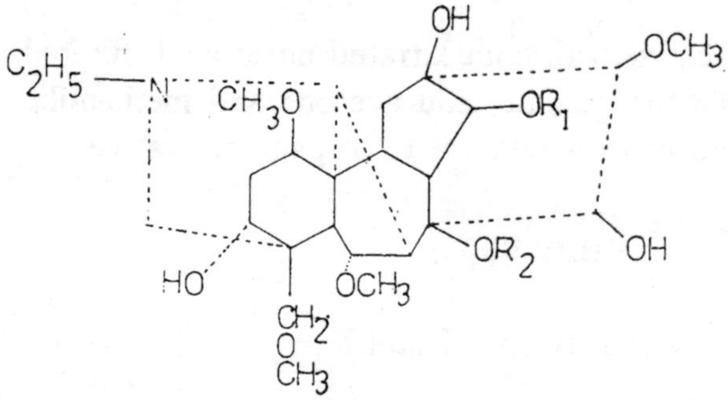

Compound	R_1	R_2
Aconine	-H	-H
Benzoyl aconine	$-COC_6H_5$	-H
Aconitine	$-COC_6H_5$	$-COCH_3$

Standards

Ash	: ≤ 5%
Acid insoluble ash	: ≤ 1%
Foreign organic matter	: ≤ 2%

Uses : It is a cardiac drug as C.V.S. depressant. It is used in respiratory failure, gout, rheumatism, neuralgia and nervous debility and as antipyretic,. In Ayurveda, it is used after mitigation (boiling roots in cow's urine) so that poisonous effect is lost. It is extremely toxic in large dose and milk is given as anti dote in aconite poisoning.

ASHWAGANDHA

Vernacular name : Beng., Hindi and Sans.- Ashwagandha; Tam.-Achuvgandi; Tel.-Panneru; Rajasthan-Chirpotan.

Biological source : Ashwagandha is dried roots and stem bases of *Withania somnifera* Dunal. This is a member of *solanaceae* family.

Geographical source : It is found throughout the drier and sub tropical parts of country like Rajasthan, Madhya Pradesh, Maharastra, etc. It is also available in Africa, Israel and Srilanka.

Cultivation and collection : The plant is cultivated by sowing the seeds in rainy season, plant flowers in the month of December. The whole plant is uprooted from February. Roots are separated, cut into small pieces (transversely) cleaned, dried and stored in a suitable airtight container.

Characters : The plant of Aswagandha is perennial, branched and erects under shrub. It attains 0.5 to 2 meter height. The plants contain tuberous root and used as crude drug. It is straight unbranched and conical in shape, 5 to 12 mm in diameter. The outer surface is buff to grey-yellow or dark brown coloured, longitudinally wrinkled and internally cream coloured. Fracture of drug is short and uneven. Taste is acrid, bitter and mucilaginous.

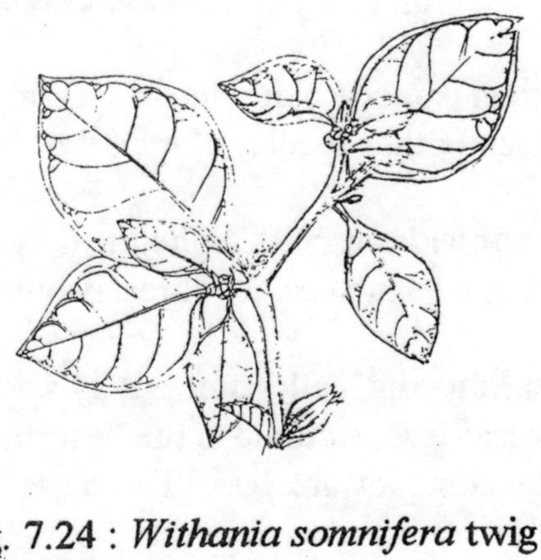

Fig. 7.24 : *Withania somnifera* twig

Chemical constituents : Withania contains mainly alkaloids and steroidal lactones (withanolides). The important alkaloids are tropine, pseudotropine, hygrine, cuscohygrine, anaferine anahygrine, withasomine, visamine, etc. The most important steroidal lactone is withaferin A. It also contain starch, reducing sugar, protein and amino acids.

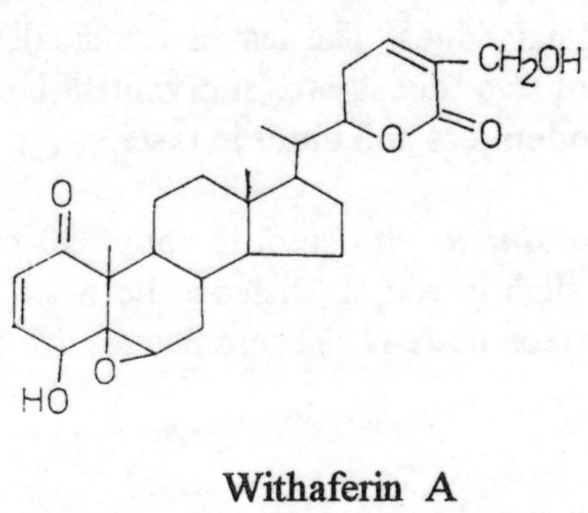

Withaferin A

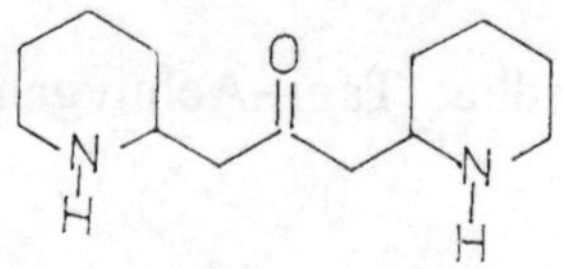

Anaferine

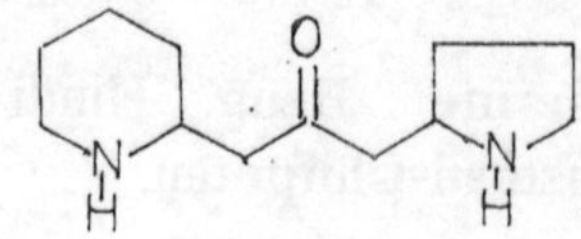

Anahygrine

Uses : Drug is used as hypotensive and depressant. It is adaptogenic, alterative, aphrodisac, diuretic and tonic. It is also useful in cough, dropsy, menstrual trouble and restores loss of memory. In Ayurveda, it is used as tonic. *Withania somnifera* along with *Asparagus racemosus* (Satavari) and *Ocimum sanctum* (Tulsi) come under the classifications of Rasayana plants that are supposed to increase the quality of life. These drugs are immunostimulants,therefore might be good in the battle against various diseases including AIDS.

EPHEDRA (Ma-huang)

Biological source : It consists entire plant of *Ephedra sinica* Stapf., *E. equisetina* Bunge. and other species of *ephedra*. It is a member of family *ephedraceae*.

Geographical source : Ephedra is widely distributed in China, India and Pakistan. In India, it grows in Western Himalayan region.

Cultivation and collection : It is a low dioecious shurb and 60-90 cm in height. It is usually leaf-less. Autumn is the best period for collection of drugs and in other season its alkaloid contents are less. The aerial part of plant is dried, compressed in bale and packed.

Characters : Ephedra stem is a cylindrical piece, containing numerous fine and longitudinal ridges. The leaves are small about 4 mm long connate at the base, usually whorls of two, decussate, and whitish lamina. Fresh drug is aromatic in odour but dried drug is odourless and bitter in taste.

Ephedra sinica : Its stem is about 30 cm in length, cylindrical, ashy greyish green in colour, slightly rough; distance between internodes are about 3-6 cm and diameter of lowest green node is 1-2 mm, leaves are 4 mm long, opposite, recurved; Base is reddish brown.

(ii) *Ephedra equisetina* : The stem are usually woody and much branched 25-200 cm long; ashy yellowish-green in colour. Internodes are shorter than *Ephedra sinica* (1-2.5 cm). The apex of leaf is shorter and not recurved. The leaves are brownish purple in colour.

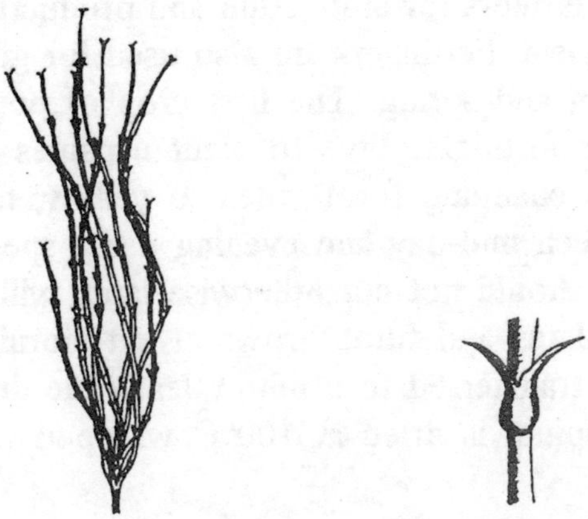

(a) Plant (b) Leaf

Fig. : 7.25 : *Ephedra sinica*

Chemical constituents : Ephedra contains about 0.5-2% of phenylethyl amine type of alkaloids in which ephedrine is a main constituent, i.e., about 30-90% of total alkaloids. The other alkaloids are pseudoephedrine; 1-methyl ephedrine; dimethyl ephedrine; norephedrine and ephedroxane. It also contains glucaric acid and leucodelphidine.

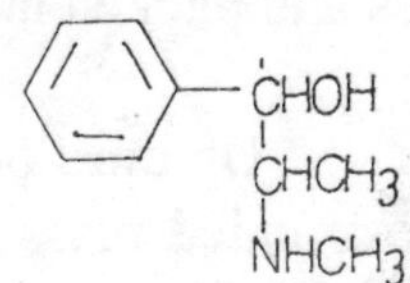

Ephedrine

Uses : Ephedrine is used in asthma, bronchitis, hay fever and whooping cough. It is an adrenergic drug having bronchiodilatory action and is slower and more prolong acting than adrenaline, it may be administered by mouth. Epherda is also used as anti-inflammatory drug due to presence of oxazolidone.

OPIUM

Vernacular names : Sans.- Aphuka; Hindi- Afim; Beng.- Posto; Tam.-Postaka. Eng.- Opium poppy.

Biological source : Opium is the air dried latex obtained by incision of unripe capsule of *Papaver somniferum* Linn. This is a member of *papaveraceae* family. 9.5% of morphine is present in raw opium.

Geographical source : Plant is a native of West Asia. It is cultivated and collected mainly in India, Iran, Yugoslavia; Pakistan, Afghanistan, Burma, Thailand, etc. In India, plants are mainly grown in Uttar Pradesh (Gazipur), Hoshiarpur and Jallandhar in Punjab and Neemuch in Madhya Pradesh.

Cultivation and collection : It is an annual herb. Opium is cultivated under strict government control. *Papaver somniferum* var. glabrum cultivated in Turkey, *Papaver somniferum* var. album cultivated in India, *Papaver somniferum* var. nigrum cultivated in Europe, opium has a strong export potential for India. India produces largest amount of opium in the world. Government issue licence to farmers for cultivation and production. Rich alluvial soil is generally preferred for good yield. Fertilizers are also used for good productions. Generally seeds are sown in autumn and spring. The first crop of poppy flowers in May and June and second crop after fortnight. Five to eight capsules are present in each plant, when colour of capsule is changing form green to yellow, then incision are made vertically or horizontally between mid-day and evening using special knife containing 4-7 blades. Endocarp of poppy should not cut otherwise latex will be lost. Latex is white in colour but rapidly coagulates and turns brown. Next-morning, dried latex is scraped off with help of knife and transferred to a poppy leaf. The dried latex is collected and it is kneaded into balls. Opium is dried at 100°C wrapped with poppy leaves and packed in air tight container.

Characters : Opium occurs in flattened or rounded mass weighing from 0.3 to 2 kg. External colour is pale or chocolate brown. Opium is plastic like when fresh, but becomes hard and brittle after some time. Internal surface is reddish brown in colour. It has characteristic odour and bitter taste.

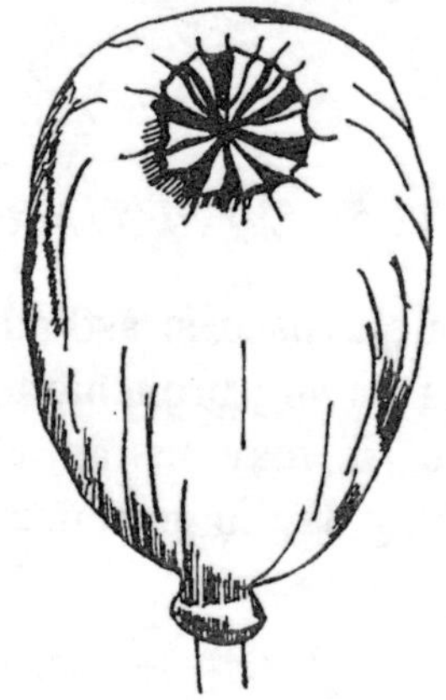

Fig. 7.26 : Capsule of *Papaver somniferum*

Chemical constituents : Opium contains about 25 alkaloids in which morphine, codeine, thebaine, noscapine, narceine and papaverine are important alkaloids. Generally these alkaloids are combined with meconic acid. Morphine, codeine and thebaine contain phenanthrene nucleus. These are strongly basic and highly toxic compounds whereas noscapine, narceine and papaverine are feebly basic in nature and less toxic compounds. Morphine contains both phenolic and alcoholic hydroxyl groups, on acetylatian converted into diacetyl morphine (Heroin). It also contain other constituents like citric acid, acetic acid, tartaric acid, protein, colouring matter, sugars, etc. Indian opium contains 9-12% of morphine, Turkish opium contains 10-16% of morphine and Yugoslavian opium contains 15-17% of morphine.

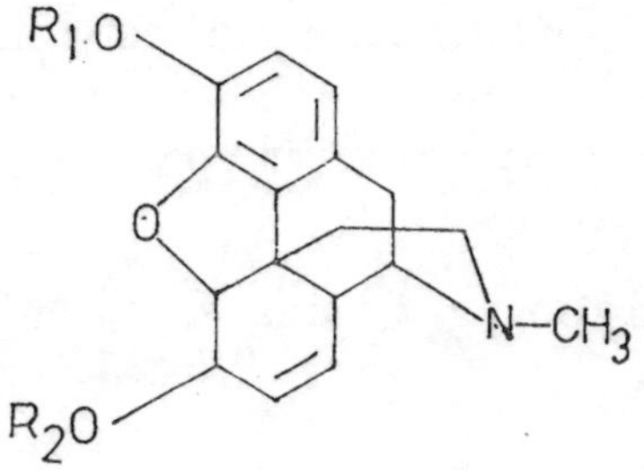

	R_1	R_2
Morphine	- H	- H
Codeine	$-CH_3$	- H

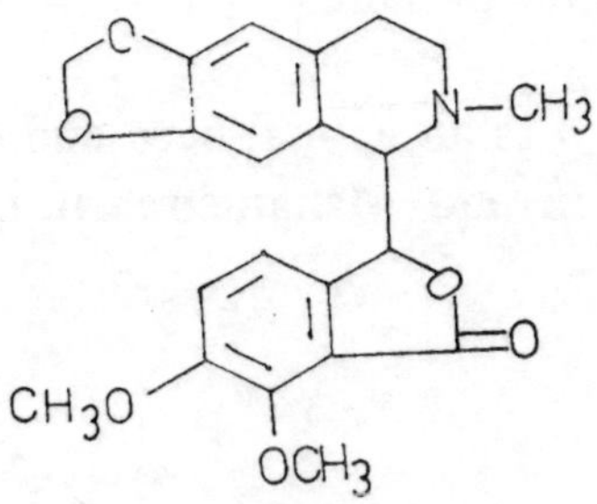

Noscapine

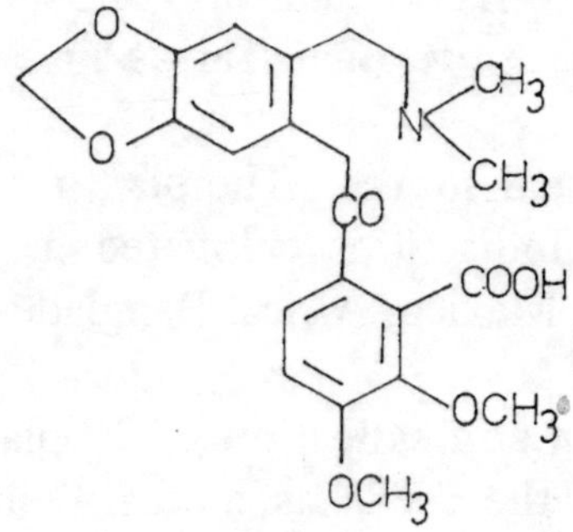

Narceine

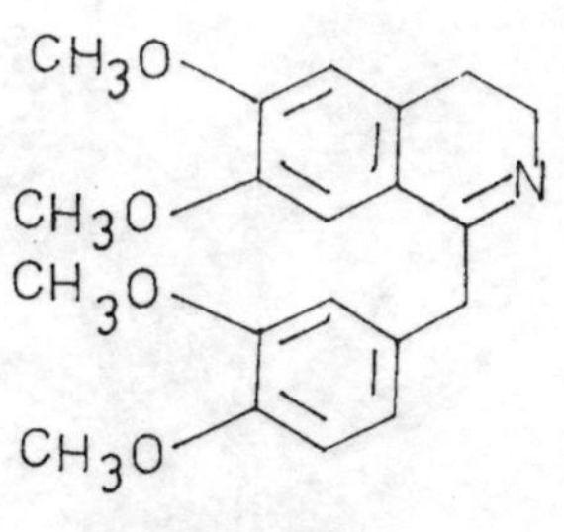

Papaverine

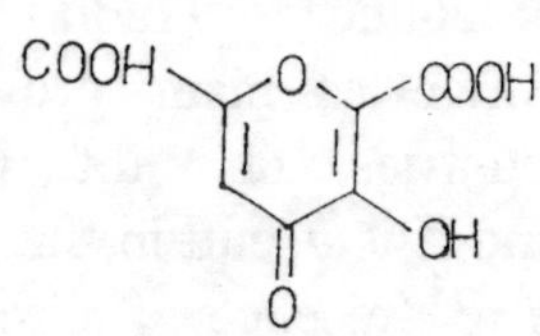

Meconic acid

Chemical tests

1. **Meconic acid test for opium** : Prepare a solution of opium in water, boil and filter. Add few drops of ferric chloride solution. Deep red coloured solution is obtained, colour even persists after adding few drops of dil. HCl.
2. **Test for morphine** : With concentrated sulphuric acid and formaldehyde, morphine gives dark violet colour.

Uses : Opium causes depression action on central nervous system, due to narcotic principle. It is also used as sedative, analgesic, hypnotic and anti-spasmodic drug. Codeine is less sedative than morphine and useful in cough preparations. Regular uses of codeine also produce constipation. Papaverine is useful in muscular spasms as smooth muscle relaxant action. Noscapine is a non-narcotic compound and useful as antitussive agent. Opium is also useful in diarrhoea, dysentery and diaphoretic disease. Opium, morphine and heroin cause drug addiction in which heroin (diacetyl morphine) is a more dangerous drug.

CANNABIS (INDIAN HEMP)

Vernacular names : English-Hemp; Hindi-Bhang, Charas, Ganja, Maxican-Marihuana; Tamil-Bangi; Telgu-Bangiaku, Ganzai.

Biological source : Cannabis consists dried flowering and fruiting tops of pistillate plants of *Cannabis sativa* Linn. This is a member of the *cannabinaceae* family.

Geographical source : The plant is indigenous to India. It is an annual herb and wildly grows. In India, it is cultivated in Bengal, M.P., Assam and Maharastra. It is also available in Mexico, Africa, Bangladesh and Pakistan.

Cultivation and collection : The plant is cultivated by sowing the seeds as a kharif crop. Seeds are sowing in June-July and harvested after six months, i.e., December-January. It is cultivated for various purposes like narcotic substances, stem fibre and drying oil (seed yield 30-35%). Plants growing in the tropical countries (India) produce narcotic substance where as plant growing in temperate climates countries do not produces narcotic substances and it is useful in the production of fibre and oil. Due to presence of narcotic substance it is cultivated under the government control. Resinous matter is formed, only in the unfertilized female plant of cannabis. Male plant is not collected beacuse it do not contain resin matter.

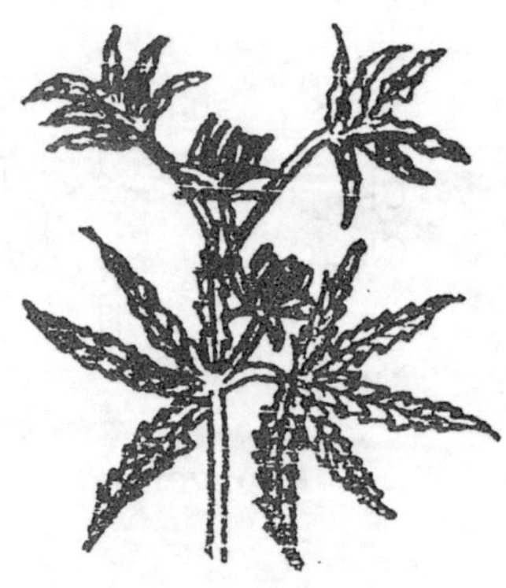

Fig. 7.27 : Cannabis herb

CANNABIS PRODUCTS

Bhang or Hashish : It consists of larger leaves and twigs of both male and female plants. It contains less amount of resin.

Ganja : It contains not more than 10 percent fruits, large foliage leaves and stems (3 mm in diameter).

Two types of Ganja are available :

(i) **Flat or Bombay ganja** : Flowering tops and fresh twigs are collected, arranged in flat heaps, and pressed. Resinous substance from flowering tops sticks together and form flat mass.

(ii) **Round or Bengal ganja** : In which every piece of flowering tops is rolled. In this way cylindrical mass is formed.

Charas : It contains crude resin; obtained by rubbing the flowering tops between the hands, beating them on clothes or carpets. A greenish brown soft mass adheres. These masses(resin) are then scrapped off. It is purified by pressing it through clothes.

Morphology : The flattened or cylindrical mass contains stem, branches, bracts, bracteoles,pistillate flowers and fruit stick together by resin. It is dull green to greenish brown in colour. It has strong characteristic odour and slightly bitter taste.

Description of plant : It is an annual,smelling, scarcely branched herb, usually 0.9 to 1.5 m in height. Female plant grows taller than male. Stem are straight, cylindrical with longitudinally furrowed. Bracts are numerous, alternate 1.5 to 2 cm long with narrow stipules. Bractioles are formed in pairs in the axil of bract. One yellow flower formed in the axil of each bracteole containing two brownish red hairy stigmas. Fruits are ovoid, glossy, green or yellowish-green in colour with a single seed.

Chemical constituents : Indian hemp contain 15-20% resin. It is a brown, amorphous semisolid, soluble in alcohol, ether and carbon disulphide. It contains more than sixty compounds. Cannabinol, tetrahydrocannabinol, cannabidiol,. cannabinol-carboxylic acid, cannabigerol and cannabichromene are priniciple active chemical compounds. The euphoric activity is present in the tetrahydro cannabinols (THC). It also contains volatile oil, trigonelline, choline, spermidine, flavonoid, alkaloid - cannabisativine, calcium oxalate, etc.

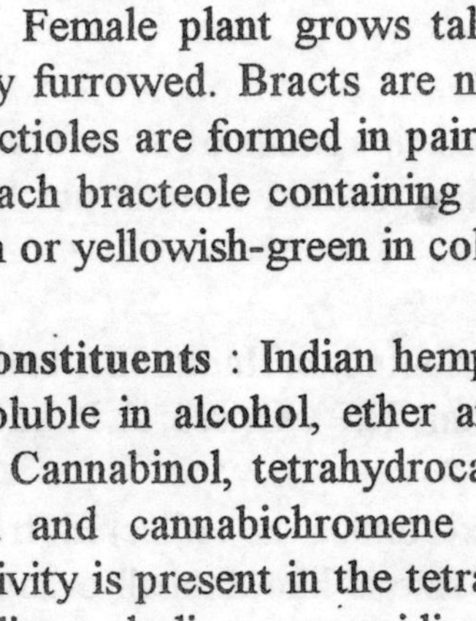

Tetrahydrocannabinol

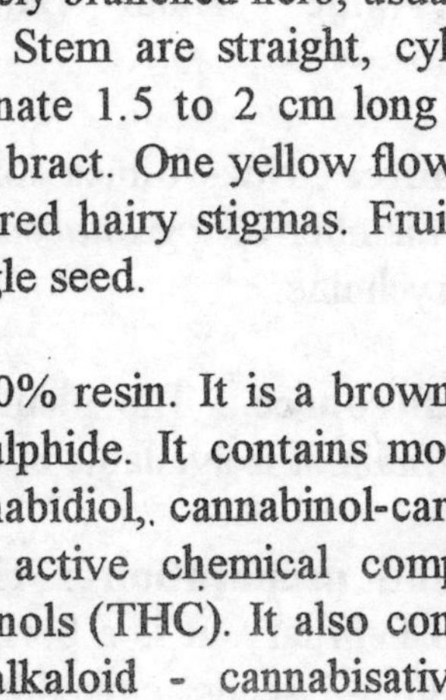

Cannabidiol

Chemical test : Extract the powder drugs with light petrolium ether, filter. In filtrate, add few ml solutions of hydrogen chloride in ethyl alcohol. A red colour is appeared at the junction of the two liquids. On shaking, upper layer becomes colourless and lower layer acquires orange-pink colour which disappears on addition of water.

Standards

Ash	:	$\leq$ 15%
Acid insoluble ash	:	$\leq$ 5%
Foreign organic matter	:	$\leq$ 2%

Uses : The drug is used as narcotic, anticonvulsant, anti-anxiety, antitussive, analgesic, stomachic and hypnotic. Cannabis first produces excitment and euphoria, later on one feel lithargy and sleep. Cannabis is a drug of abuse. It is also useful for cancer patient in relief nausea and vomiting produced by chemotherapy. Cannabis should be used within a year. Drug rapidly loose their activity. It become almost inert after two years.

NUX VOMICA

Vernacular Name : Hindi- Bailewa, kuchla; Sans.-Karaskara, Kapilu; Tam.-Etti; Tel.-Mushti.

Biological source : Nux-vomica consists of the dried ripe seeds of *Strychnos nux-vomica* Linn. It is a member of *loganiaceae* family. The drug should contain not less than 1.20 percent of strychnine.

Geographical source : The plant is widely distributed in India. Sri-lanka, Northern Australia. In India, it is available in the forest of Bihar, U.P., Orissa, A.P. and Mysore.

Collection and preparation : The fruit of nux-vomica is collected from forest in November to February. It is a berry, approximate size is like a small orange. Each fruit contains about 3-5 seeds, embedded in white pulp. Seeds are washed thoroughly with water, free from pulp and dried.

Morphology : The dried seeds of nux-vomica are very hard greenish-grey in colour, disc shaped 10-30 mm in diameter and 4-6 mm thick, flat, irregular bent and cancavo-convex type. The edge of a seed is acute and rounded. The testa of the seed is covered with numerous silky, closely appressed, radiating hairs. A distinct hilum is present in the centre of one of the flattened sides of seed and a small projection on the circumference represent the position of the micropyle. The micropyle is connected to the hilum by a radial ridge. A small embryo with two cordate cotyledons and a cylindrical radical directing towards micropyle is embedded in a grey horny endosperm of seed. There is a slit like cavity present in the centre of seed. The dry seeds are odourless but, when soaked in water for one or two days give unpleasant odour. The drug has a very bitter taste.

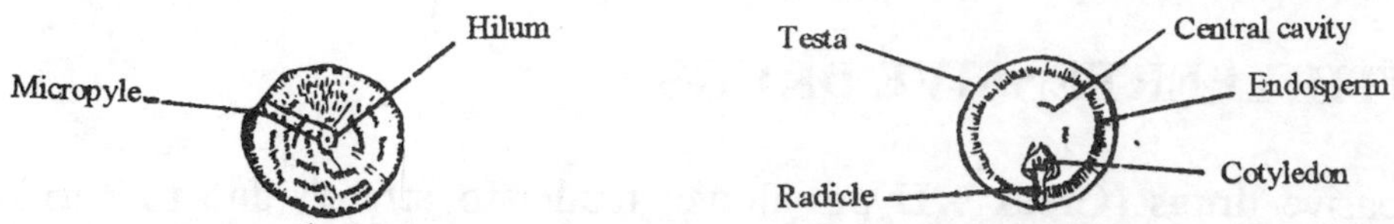

(a) External surface of seed (b) Seed section parallel to the flat faces

Fig. 7.28 : Nux - Vomica

Chemical constituents : Nux-vomica contain about 1.8 to 5.3 percent of indole alkaloid. The main alkaloids are strychnine (1.2%) and brucine(1.5%). Strychnine is most abundantly present in the inner portion of the endosperm and brucine in the outer layer. Strychnine is more physiological active than brucine. Nux-vomica also contain minor alkaloids like vomicine, novacine, ∝-colubrine, ß-colubrine, pseudostrychnine, isostrychnine, etc. It also cantain chlorogenic acid, loganin (glycoside) and about 3% of fixed oil.

Standards

Ash	:	≤ 3%
Sulphated ash	:	≤ 1%
Foreign organic matter	:	≤ 1%

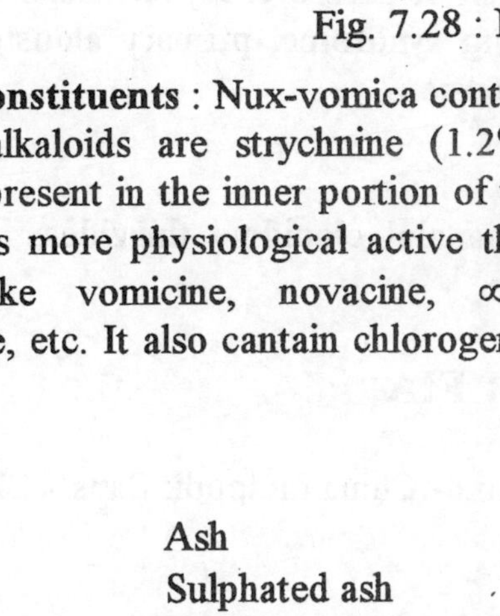

Strychnine ($R_1 = R_2 = H$)
Brucine ($R_1 = R_2 = OCH_3$)

Chemical tests

1. Cut a thick section of Nux-vomica seed, add few drops of a solution of ammonium vanadate and sulphuric acid, a violet colour is produced in the central part of endosperm indicating the presence of strychnine.
2. Cut a thick section of Nux-vomica seed, add few drops of nitric acid, crimson colour is observed near the circumsference indicating te presence of brucine.

Uses : The drug is used as bitter tonic and stimulant. Formerly drug was used as circulatory stimulant in case of surgical shock. It also improves apetite and digestion. The drug is also useful as aphrodiasic. Strychnine is a powerful CNS stimulant and produces convulsions. It is also utilized as vermine killer . Fatal dose of strychnine for human is 60 to 90 mg. Brucine is less toxic than strychnine and useful in alcohol denaturant.

7- F. ANTIHYPERTENSIVE DRUGS

Antihypertensive drugs (Greek : Hyper-above; tender-to stretch due to narrowing of peripheral blood vessel) are used to lower the abnormal high blood pressure. The abnormal blood pressure in young or middle aged person will be above 150 mm Hg as resting systolic pressure and 100 mm Hg as diastolic pressure. Hypertension is caused by some other diseases like renal disorder, cussing syndrome, primary aldosteronism and pheochromocytoma, is called secondary hypertension.
The drugs used as antihypertensive agents are

(I) **Synthetic** : Methyl dopa; guanethidine, propanalol, clonidine, thiazides.
(II) **Natural** : Reserpine (Rauwolfia); Veratrum.

RAUWOLFIA

Vernacular name : Bengali - Sarpagandha; Tamil- Chinanmdpodi; Sans.- Chhota-chand; Bihar - Pagla ka dawa; Hindi - Chandrika.

Biological Source : Rauwolfia consists of the dried roots and rhizomes of *Rauwolfia serpentina* Benth. e.g. Kurg. It is a member of *Apocynaceae* family.

Geographical source : It is widely distributed in West land and in shady forests in Punjab eastwards to Nepal, Sikkim and Assam in India; Bhutan, Pakistan, Java, Thailand, etc.

Cultivation, collection and preparation : The plant Rauwolfia grows not only in hot humid but also in shade conditions. Clay and loamy soil with large amount of humus and well drainage condition is ideal for growth. The plant is propagated by seeds, roots, cuttings, root stumps, etc. The seeds are sown in the month of May and seedlings are transplanted in August at a distance of 15-30 cm, chemical fertilizers like ammonium sulphate, urea, bone-meal are required for good growth. Soil pH should be 3.5 to 4.5. Large amount of sand should be avoided as it makes plant susceptible to diseases. For collection three to four years old plants are uprooted. The roots are washed and cut properly, washing helps in removing impurities. The cut roots are dried and packed.

Morphology : The roots and rhizomes closely resemble each other. The rhizome can be identified by the presence of small central pith. The drug occurs in cylindrical or slightly tapering, tortuous and rarely branched. The roots are 2-10 cm long and 0.5-2.2 cm in diametre. The external appearance of the root is greyish-yellow, light brown or brown. The old pieces contain longitudinal ridges while young pieces contain slight wrinkles and occasional circular scars of rootlets. The fracture of drug is short. The inner surface occupies 3/4 of diametre, is dense pale yellow wood at the transverse surface and yellowish-brown bark at narrow end. Fresh dried drug has slight odour, which decreases with age and has bitter taste.

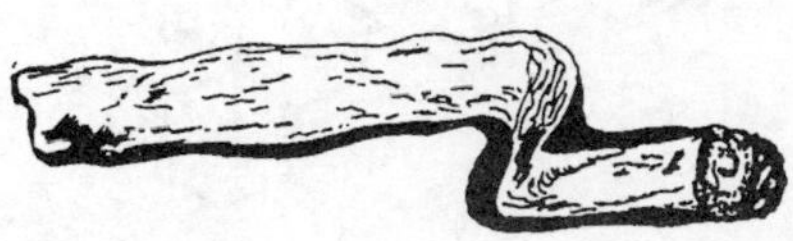

Fig. 7.29 : *Rauwolfia serpentina* root & rhizome.

Chemical constituents : The rauwolfia roots and rhizomes contain around 30-50 alkaloids which total some 0.7 to 2.4%, other organic matter like phytosterol, fatty acid, unsaturated alcohols and sugars are also present in rauwolfia. The most active tranquilizing and hypotensive alkaloids are reserpine and its trimethoxycinnamate

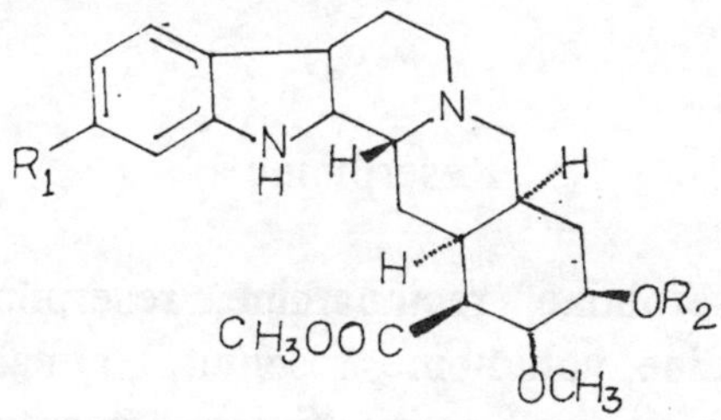

Compound	**R1**	**R2**
Rescimetol	- OCH_3	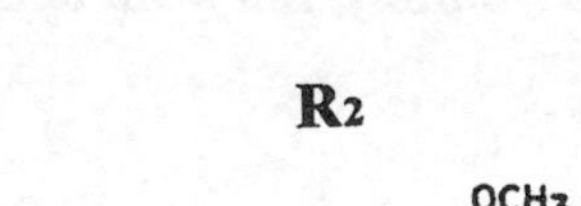
Rescinnamine	- OCH_3	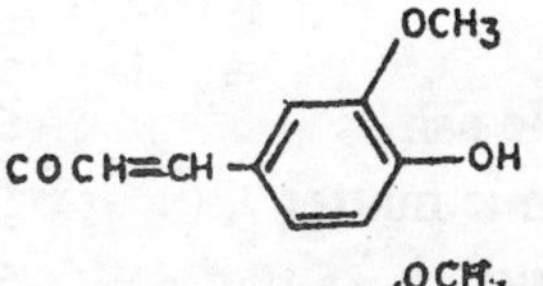
Reserpine	- OCH_3	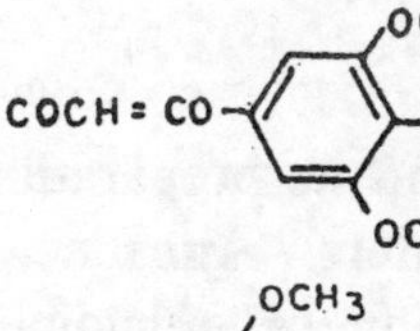

Deserpidine 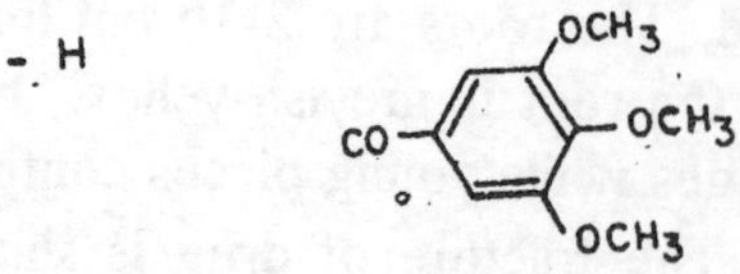

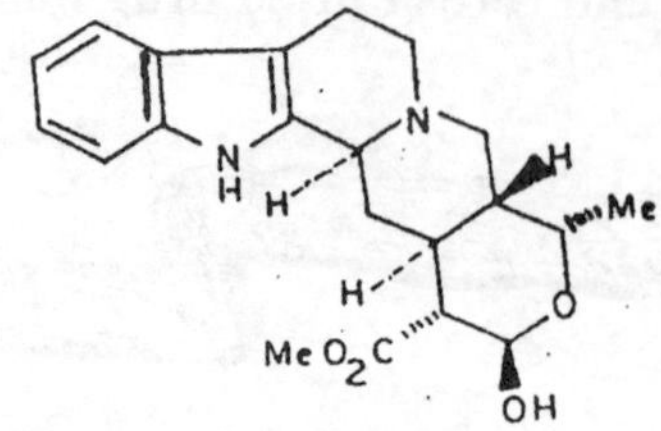

Ajmalicine

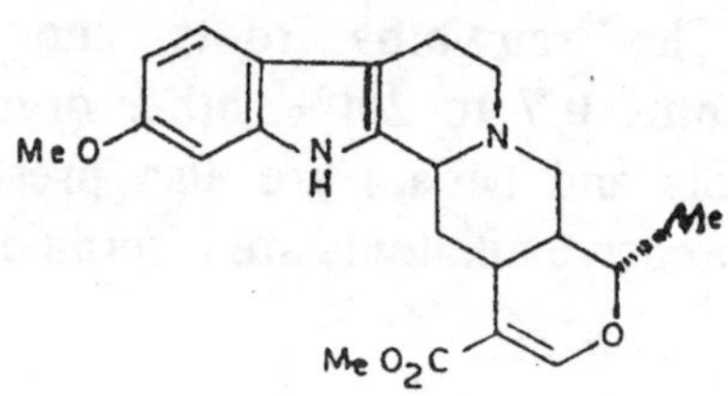

Reserpinine

analogue,rescinnamidine reserpinine, recinnamine, reserpiline. It also contains other indole alkaloids like ajmalicidine, yohimbine, rescimitol, ajmaline (rauwolfine), ajmalinine, ajmalicine, isoajmaline (isorauwolfine), rauwolfinine, serpentine and serpentinine.

Standards

Ash value	:	≤ 8%
Acid insoluble ash	:	≤ 2%
Foreign organic matter	:	≤ 2%
Loss on drying	:	≤ 12%

Uses : *Rauwolfia serpentina* and its preparations are used as hypotensive agent and in certain neuropsychiatric disorders. Ajmaline is used for the treatment of cardiac arrhythmias similar to the action of quinidine. Ajmalicine can also be isolated from *Catharanthus* species (vinca) and is used in circulatory diseases. The decoction of root is used to increase uterine contraction in difficult cases. The extract is used for intestinal disorders and as anthelmintic bitter tonic and fibrifuge.

7- G. ANTI TUSSIVES

Anti-tussive (Latins - tussis - cough.) drugs are the agents that suppress cough and make expectoration smooth. The irritation in pharynx or in respiratory tract stimulates coughing. It is a protective reflux that leads to expulsion of the bronchial mucous or secretion along with foreign matter. The main natural anti-tussive drugs are Vasaka, Tolu Balsam, Tulsi, Ephedra, Turpentine oil, etc. Expectorant is an agent that alters the rheological properties of sputum and enhances the removal of bronchial secretion.

VASAKA

Vernacular name : **Beng. - Bakas; Sans. - Bashika, Amalaka; Tamil -Adadodi; Guj.- Adsoga; Hindi & Urdu - Arusa; Marathi - Adulsa; Telugu- Addasarmu.**

Biological source : **Vasaka consists of dried and the fresh leaves of the plant *Adhatoda vasica* Nees. It is a member of *Acanthaceae*- family.**

Geographical source : **Vasaka is indigenous to India. It is found all over the country specially in sub Himalayan region and Konkon region of Maharastra. The plant is also available in Sri-Lanka, Malyasia and Myamar (Burma).**

Morphology : **The plant of Vasaka is dense shrub, 1.2-2.4 metre height. The leaves of the plant are 12.5-20 cm long and 3.8-6.3 cm. width, shape is elliptic and lanceolate; Apex is acuminate, minutely puberulous when young and becomes glabrous on maturity; Base is tappering and short petiole (1.3-2.5 cm). Colour of leaf is pale green when fresh; it turns pale brownish on drying. Venation is pinate. It has slight odour, acrid bitter in taste and gives cooling sensation.**

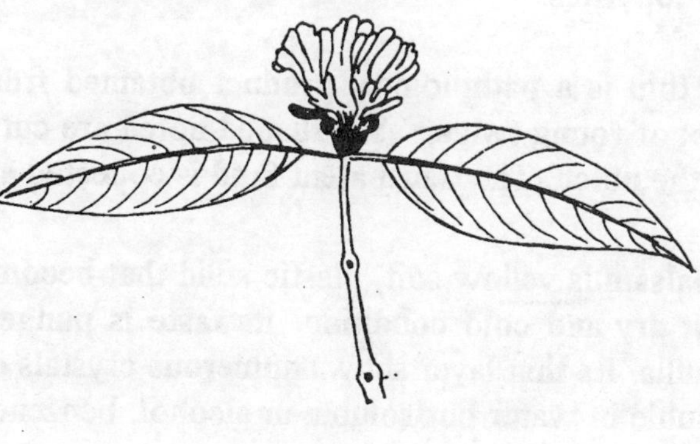

Fig. 7.30 : Vasaka twig.

Chemical Constituents : The drug contains quinazoline alkaloid and small amount of essential oil. The main alkaloids are Vasicine, (1 - Peganine) Vasicinone Vasicinol, 1-Vasicine, Betain and Vasakin. It also contains fats, resin, sugar, mucilage, adhatodic acid, ß- sitostesterol phytosterol and ascorbic acid.

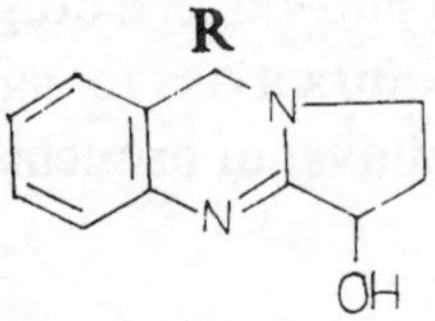

Compound	R
1- Vasicine	H
Vasicinone	=O

Uses : Vasaka is used as anti-tussive, expectorant, in chronic bronchitis, anti-spasmodic. Vasicine is reported to be bronchoconstrictor and selective uterine stimulant activity similar to methyl ergometrin and oxytocin. Its autooxidised form vasicinone is a bronchodilator. Traditionally leaves and roots of vasaka with ginger are used in all types of cough treatments. The dried leves are smoked in case of asthma and their juice is used in diarrhoea and dysentery.

TOLU BALSAM

Synonyms : Balsam of tolu, Resin Tolu, Balsamum tolutanum.

Biological source : Tolu balsam is obtained by incision of trunk of *Myroxylon balsamum* Linn; . It is considered as pathological product similar to balsum of Peru . It is a member of *Leguminosae* family.

Geographical source : The plant is indigenous to Colombia and cultivated in Venezuela and other South African countries.

Collection : Balsam of tolu is a pathological product obtained from the schizogenous duct present in the cortex of young twigs, " V " shaped notch are cut on bark and a small vessel is attached under the notch. The transparent fluid is collected and packed in tins.

Characters : The tolu balsam is yellow soft, plastic solid that becomes brown, hardened & brittle when placed in dry and cold condition. Its taste is pungent and the odour is aromatic, resembling vanilla. Its thin layer shows numerous crystals of cinnamic acid and is transparent. It is insoluble in water but soluble in alcohol, benzene, ether and partially soluble in carbon disulphide.

Standards :

Acid value	:	100 - 160
Reaction	:	Acidic to litmus (Alcoholic solution)
Ester value	:	40 - 95
Saponification value	:	170 - 230
Loss on drying	:	≥ 4%
Alcohol insoluble matter	:	≥ 5%

Chemical Constituents : Tolu Balsam contains about 80% resin. It contains 12-15% of free cinnamic acid, 8% free benzoic acid and 7-8% volatile oil. It has 35-50% of total balsamic acid. It also contains esters such as benzyl benzoate, benzyl cinnamate, vanilline, styrene, eugenol, ferulic acid, 1,2 di-phenyl ethane, mono and sesquiterpenes, hydrocarbon and alcohols.

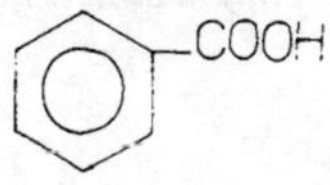

Benzoic acid

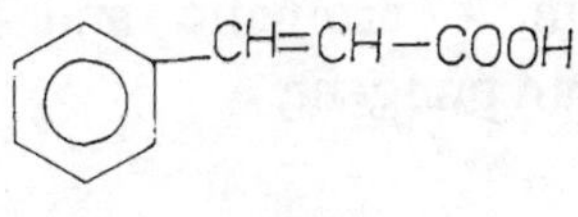

Cinnamic acid

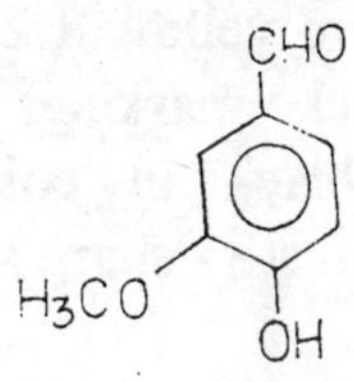

Vanilline

Chemical tests

1. To the alcoholic solution of tolu balsam, when a few drops of ferric chloride are added, green colour appears due to the presence of acidic group of benzoic and cinnamic acid.
2. Mix 1gm of balsam add 5 ml of pot. Permanagnate and boil, odour of bitter almond (due to formation of benzaldehyde) is produced.

Uses : It has antiseptic property. It is also used as an expectorant, flavouring agent in medicinal syrups, confectionery and chewing gum.

TULSI

Vernacular name : English - Holy Basil; Gujarati - Talaśi; Malayalam - Kunnakam; Tamil - Alangai; Sanskrit - Amriba, Brinda; Hindi - Tulsi.

Biological source :Tulsi is fresh and dried leaves of *Ocimun sanctum* Linn. This is a member of *Labiatae* family.

Geographical source : The plant of tulsi is strongly scented herb, shurb or under shrub, distribuited throughout India. It is also found in Malaya, Archilago, Australia, West Asia and Arabia.

Morphology : The plant is thickly branched and 30-60 cm in hight; stem and branches are usually purplish, sub-quadrangular and clothed with soft hair. The leaves are 2.5-5 cm long 1.6-3.2 cm broad; shape of leaf is elliptical oblong and acute or obtuse apex; Margin is entire or serrate and both the surfaces are pubescent with minute gland-dots. Flowers are purplish in colour; 15-17 cm long and in racemes in close whorls and bracts broadly ovate. Nutlets are yellow 1.25 mm long, ellipsoid, smooth with black marking. Seeds are subglobose and reddish black in colour, odour - aromatic and pleasant; taste - sharp aromatic and pungent.

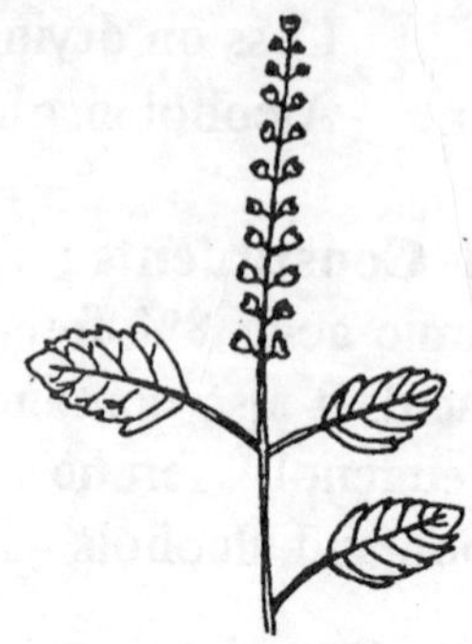

Fig. 7.31 : Tulsi (*Ocimum sanctum*) twig.

Chemical Constituents : The important chemical constituent of tulsi is volatile oil which is yellow coloured; leaves contain maximum contents of volatile oil (0.4 - 0.8%). The volatile oil contains eugenol (70%), methyl eugenol (20%) carvacrol (3%), caryphyllene (1.71%), cineole, linalool, etc. The seeds of tulsi contain fixed oil that has good drying properties. There are esters of palmatic, stearic, oleic, linoleic and linolenic acids.

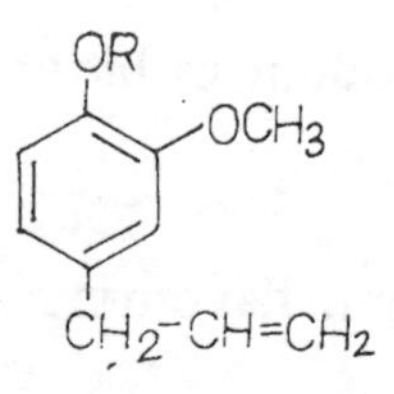

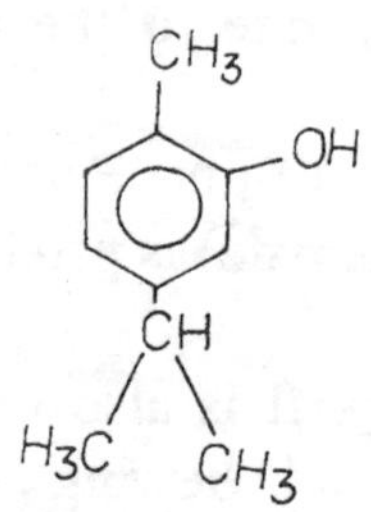

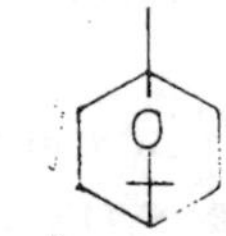

Eugenol R=H
Methyl eugenol R=CH_3

Carvacrol

Cineole

Uses : It is used as expectorant, antiseptic, antibacterial, insecticidal and in gastric disorder. The leaves of tulsi are also used as flavouring agent, aromatic, carminative and hepatic affections. The dried powdered leaves are used as snuff in ozaena. The decoctions of tulsi roots are given as diaphoretic in malaria fever. The juices of tulsi leaves are used in catarrh, bronchitis, applied on skin in ring worm and other cutaneous diseases.

7- H. ANTIRHEUMATICS

Rheumatism (Greek ; Rheuma flowing, and ismos - condition) is a disorder in which stiffness, soreness, aches and pain occurs in muscles joints, ligaments, tendons and bursae. The drugs used for the treatment of rheumatism are called antirheumatics. The different types of rheumatism are rheumatic fever, rheumatoid arthritis, spondilytis, osteoarthritis, etc.

The synthetic compounds used as antirheumatic have following therapeutic categories - antipyretics, analgesic, antiinflammatory, corticosteroid, antimalarials and ß- lactam antibiotics (Penicillin and its derivatives)
The plant products used in the treatment of rheumatism are -

Guggul : *Commiphora wightii* (Arnolt) Bhandari
Colchicum : *Colchicum luteum*
Jatamansi : *Nardostachys jatamansi*
Nirgundo : *Vitex nirgundo*
Fenugreak : *Trigonella foenum-graecum.*

GUGGUL [Indian Bdellium]

Synonyms : *Commiphora mukul* (Hook. ex stocks) Engl; *Balsamodendron wightii* Arnott.

Vernacular names : San.- Guggulu; Hindi & Beng.; Guggul; Tam, Maishakshi; Eng.; Indian Bdellium tree.

Biological source : Guggul is an oleo-gum-resin obtained by incision of the bark of the plant *Commiphora wightii* (Arnott) Bhandari. This plant is a member of *Burseraceae* family.

Geographical source: The tree is distributed in rocky and arid regions of South west (Mysore), North Western region (Rajasthan) of India, Bangladesh, Pakistan, Arabia and Sindh.

Characters : It is a small tree or shrub (2 to 3 metre height) with spinescent branches, silvery and paper like bark peelings, producing 0.5 to 1Kg of ole-gum-resin in the month of January to March. The oleo-gum-resin is a brown to pale yellow or dull green coloured substance possessing a balsamic odour and a characteristic bitter taste. It is partially soluble in alcohol and it forms emulsions when treated with water.

Standards

(a) Extractive values

Water soluble	: ≤	48%
Alcohol soluble	: ≤	39%
Petrolium Ether soluble	: ≤	13.3-16.6%

(b) Ash value

Total	: ≤	4.66%
Sulphated	: ≤	0.18%
Acid insoluble	: ≤	0.2%

(c) L.O.D (Loss on drying)	: ≤	8.46
(d) Acid value	:	35.7 to 37.2
(e) Ester value	:	46.8 to 48.5

Chemical constituents : The guggul contains essential oils (1.5%), gums (32%), resins (58%), mineral matter, amino acids , sugars, fatty acids, sterols and flavonoids.
The drug contains steroidal constituents like guggulusterols-I, II,III, IV, . & V and guggulusterone-I & II. Myrcene, dimyrcene, polymyrcene and caryophyllene are important constituents of essential oils. Alanine, arginine, aspartic acid, cystine, glutamic acid, histidine, leucine, lysine, proline, etc., are important amino acids and glucose, fructose are important sugars found in guggul.

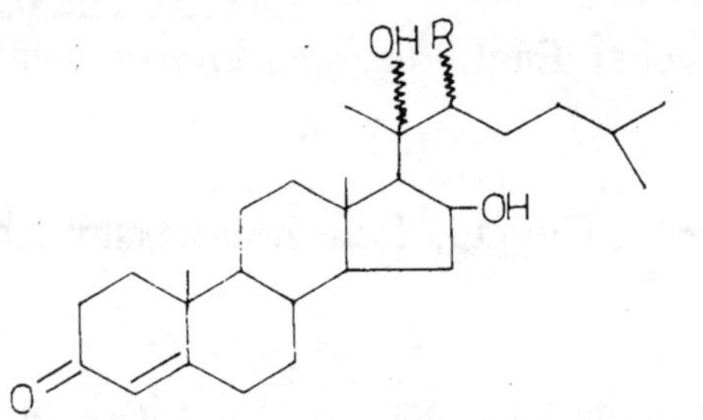

Compound	R
Guggulusterol I	-OH
Guggulustrol III	-H

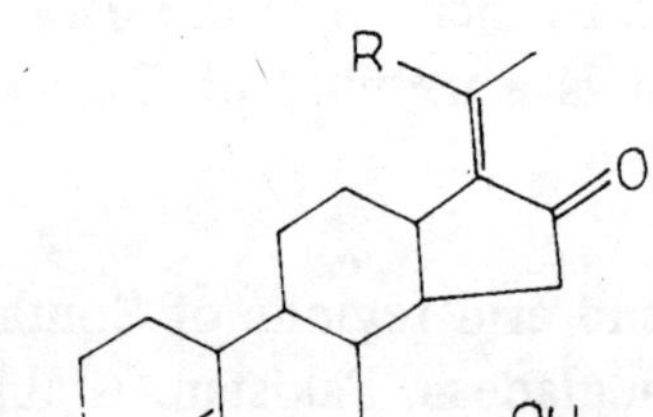

Compound	R
Guggulusterone I	-H
Guggulusterone II	$-CH_3$

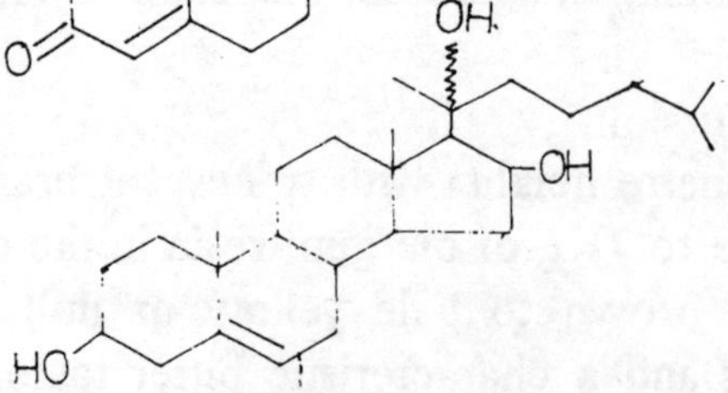

Guggulusterol II

Uses : It is used as antiinflammatory, antirheumatic, antiseptic, antispasmodic, aphrodisiac, appetizer, astringent, diuretic, carminative, expectorant and is specially recommended in urinary disorders. The fumes of burnt guggul are beneficial in chronic bronchitis, acute and chronic nasal catarrh, laryngitis and tuberculosis.

COLCHICUM

Vernacular name : Hindi-Hirantutiya; Sans. - Hiranyatutha; Punjab - Surinjan-i-talkh.

Biological source : Colchicum ripe seeds and corms are derived from *Colchicum autumnale* Linn. Indian colchicum is obtained from plant *Colchicum leutum* Baker. It is a member of *Liliaceae* family.

Geographical source : The Indian colchicum is found in North West Himalayas, Kashmir and chamba region of Himachal Pradesh. The plant is grown in England and many parts of Europe. It is a commercial crop in Yugoslavia, Poland, Czechoslovakia and Holland.

Morphology

Seeds : Colchicum seeds are ovoid or globular in shape, 2-3 mm in diameter. The seeds are reddish brown in colour and testa are minutely pitted. During drying, the seed darkens in colour and a covered with is sugary exudation. The seeds are hard. From a slight projection at the hilum, a well-marked strophiole extends for about 1/4th of the circumference . The small embryo is embedded in horny endosperm at the opposite end of hilum.

Corm : The fresh colchicum corm is conical in shape, 3-4 cm long 2-3 cm wide. One side of corm is flat and another is convex. It is yellow to brown in colour and slightly wrinkled. The dried colchicum corm occurs as conical, elongated pieces and as transverse and longitudinal slices. The interior part of the slices is starchy and white in colour. The slices are 2-5 mm thicken and sub-reniform, in shape. It breaks with short and mealy fracture. It possesses a slight odour and slightly bitter and acrid taste.

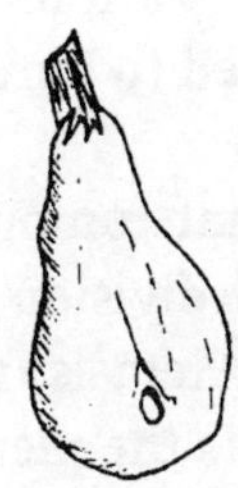

Fig. 7.32 : Colchicum corm

Chemical constituents : Colchicum contains tropolone type of alkaloids colchicine'(0.3-0.8%),colchciein, colchicoresin and demecolcine. Colchicine is a weak base, readily dissolves in water, alcohol or chloroform.

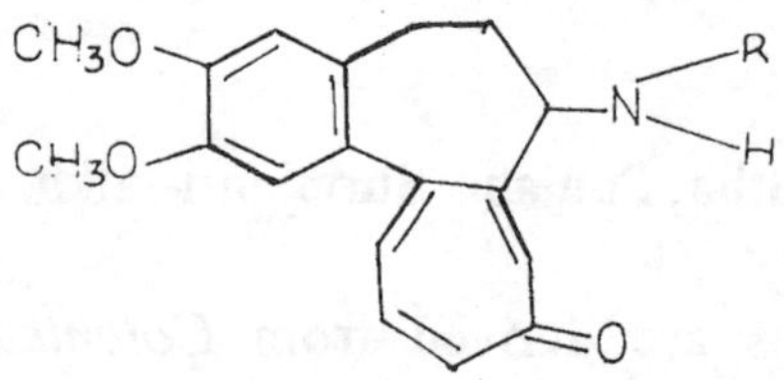

Compound	R
Colchicine	$-COCH_3$
Demecolcine	$-CH_3$

Chemical test :Colchicum corm on treatment with 70% sulphuric acid or hydrochloric acid becomes yellow due to the presence of alkaloid colchicine.

Uses : Colchicum preparations are used to relieve pain, and inflammation in gout. It is also used in biological experiment to produce polyploidy. It is also reported to have antitumor activity.

7- I. ANTITUMOUR DRUG

The drugs used for the treatment and cures of cancerous tissues (tumors) are known as Antitumour drugs. Cancer is an abnormal growth of new tissues in any part of the body. It is carcinogenic. This disease is incurable in the secondary stage, various types of cancer are reported like Hodgkin's disease, leukemia, breast cancer, lung cancer, blood cancer, etc. Various radioactive substances, metal compounds and chemotherapeutic drugs are used to cure cancer.

Any malignant tumour including carcinoma and sarcoma arises from the abnormal and uncontrolled division of cell that invade and destroy the surrounding tissues. Spread of cancer cell (Metasis) may occur via the blood stream or lymphatic channel or across body cavity such as the pleural and peritonial spaces, thus setting up secondary tumour at sites distant from original tumour, this stage is called secondary stage and is incurable. Anticancer therapy depends on the type of tumour, site and extent of spread of malignant cells.

The following plants are reported as anti tumour drugs

1. Colchicum : *Colchicum autumnale*
2. Podophyllum : *Podophyllum hexandrum*
3. Taxol : *Taxus baccata* Linn
4. Vinca : *Vinca rosea*

VINCA

Synonyms: *Vinca rosea* L; *Lochnera rosea* (L) Reichb.

Vernacular name : Hindi- Sadabahar ; Eng.- Periwrinkle; Sans.- Sadampuspa; Tam.- Sudukadu, mallikai; Beng.- Nayantara.

Biological source : It is a dried whole plant of *Catharanthus roseus* (L) G. Don. It is a member of *Apocynaceae* (*Cantharaceae*) family.

Geographical source : It is indigenous to Madagascar. This plant is cultivated as an ornamental plant and found in tropical regions like Africa, Australia, Eastern Europe, South Florida, India, Taiwan and Thailand.

Morphology : Vinca is an erect ever blooming pubescent herb or sub-shrub. The plant is woody at base and 0.4-0.8 metre in height. The leaves are oblong with petiolate acute base and are oppositely arranged, have rounded or mucronate apex with entire margin. The flowers are generally white with red eyes, violet and rose. It has bitter taste and slight odour.

Chemical constituents : Catharanthus contains terpenes and more than 100 different alkaloids. The alkaloids are of indole; dihydroindole and dimeric (indole and dihydroindole moieties) type. The indole or dihydroindole derivatives are ajmalicine, tetra hydro alstonine, serpentine and lochnerine. The dimeric alkaloids are active against malignant tumour namely vincristine and vinblastine. The vincristine is available in 0.0002% and vinblastine is 0.003% in crude drug. The vinblastine is an N-methyl

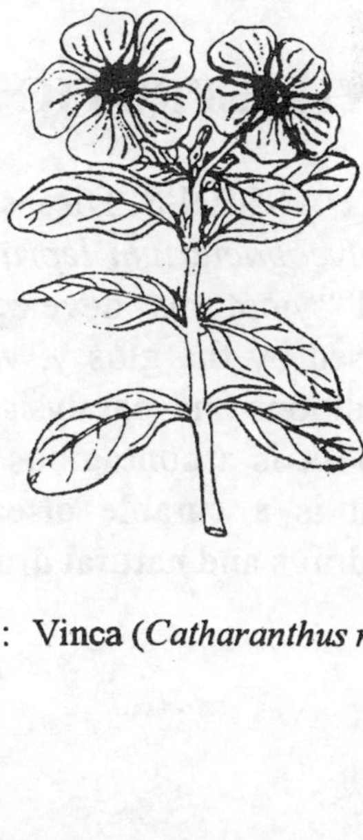

Fig. 7.33 : Vinca (*Catharanthus roseus)* herb.

derivative. The vinblastine is converted into derivative while vincristine is N-formyl vincristine.

COMPOUND	R_1	R_2	R_3
Vinblastin (vincaleukoblastine)	$-CH_3$	$-OCH_3$	$-COCH_3$
Vincristine (leurocristine)	$-CHO$	$-OCH_3$	$-COCH_3$
Vindesine	$-CH_3$	$-NH_2$	$-H$

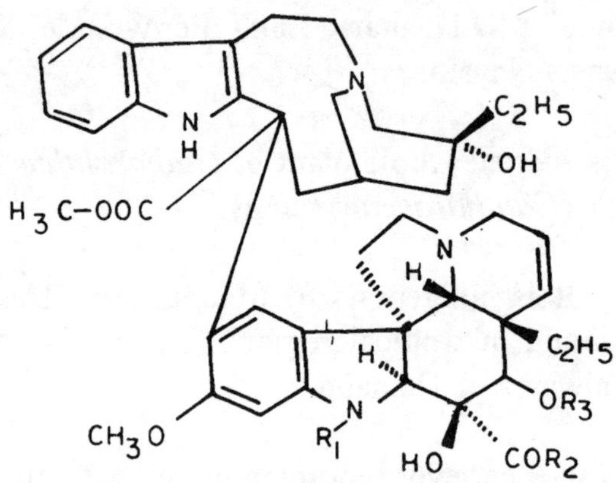

Uses : Vinca is used in cancer and hypertension. The Vincristine is used in leukemia while vinblastin is used in Hodgkin's disease and chlorionepithelioma.

7 - J. ANTILEPROTIC AGENT

Leprosy (HANSEN'S Disease) is a chronic disease caused by an acid fast bacillus bacteria-*Mycobacterium leprae*. The incubation period of these bacteria is around 1-30 years and symptoms develop gradually and mainly involves skin & nerves. It is characterised by the glossy, widely distributed lumps on the skin; numbness of skin in sever conditions and paralysis leading to disfigurement and deformity. It is confined to tropics and it is a contagious disease. Antileprotic drugs are used for the treatment of leprosy. It is a curable disease but requires a longer duration of therapy. Various synthetic drugs and natural drugs are used in the treatment of leprosy.

Synthetic drugs

(I) Sulphone	:	Dapsone
(II)Non sulphone	:	Streptomycin, Rifampicin, Thiambutosine, Chofozimine
Natural drugs	:	Brahmi, Chaulmoogra oil.

CHAULMOOGRA OIL

Synonyms : Gynocardia oil, Hydnocarpus oil

Vernacular Name : Hindi & Beng.-Chaulmoogra; Tamil-Maravattai, Mal.- Niradi.

Biological source : Chaulmoogra oil is a fixed oil obtained from the cold expression from fresh ripe seeds of plant *Hydnocarpus laurifolia* (Dennst.) sleumer (Syn. - *H. wightiana* Blume; *Munnicksia leurifolia* Dennst.) and *Hydnocarpus kurzii* (king) Warb. [Syn. - *H.heterophyllus* Kurz; *Taraktogenos kurzii* king). It is a member of *Flacourtiaceae* family.

Geographical source : The plant *H. laurufolia* is widely distributed in tropical forests of Western Ghats from Konkan Southwards and plant *H. kurzii* is widely distributed in North east forest of Assam and Tripura in India. The plant is also available in Thailand & Burma.

Characters : Chaulmoogra oil is yellow or brownish-yellow liquid which turns into soft solid mass at temperature below 25°C. It possesses characteristic odour, acrid taste and is soluble in benzene, chloroform, ether and carbon disulphide while sparingly soluble in alcohol.

Standards

Specific gravity	:	0.93 to 0.96 gm/ml at 25°C
Specific rotation	:	+48° to + 60°C
Refractive index	:	1.427 to 1.476
Acid value	:	≤ 13
Iodine value	:	93-104
Saponification value	:	195 - 213

Chemical constituents : Chaulmoogra oil contains glycosides of cyclopentenylfatty acids like chaulmoogric acid (about 27%), hydnocarpic acid (about 48%), gorlic acid (15%), oleic acid and palmitic acid along with a apigenin, luteolin, chrysocresol, hydrnocarpin, isohydnocarpin and methoxyhydnocarpin (flavonon lignans). The cyclopentanyl derivatives of acids are strongly bactericidal towards the micrococcus of leprosy and are biosynthesized in the last 3-4 months of the maturation of fruits.

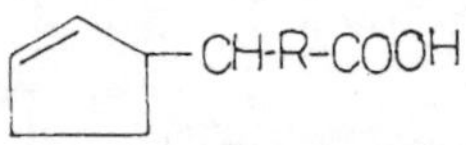

R	Compound
$(CH_2)_{10}$	Hydnocarpic acid
$(CH_2)_{12}$	Chaulmoogric acid
$C_{12}H_{22}$	Gorlic acid

Uses : The chaulmoogra oil is used in the treatment of leprosy, tuberculosis and rheumatism. It is applied externally on affected areas. Its unsaturated acids are effective bactericidal against *Mycobacterium leprae* and *M. tuberculosis*.

7 - K. ANTIDIABETIC DRUGS

The substances used in the treatment of *Diabetes mellitus* are called antidiabetic drugs. The diabetes is a disease in which glucose utilization in body is reduced. It is either by reduction of insulin secretion by β cells of pancreas or by the death of β cells of pancreas (insulin secreting cells). Insulin is a protein hormone plays a vital role in the metabolism of glucose or in the generation of energy from glucose. It helps in phosphorylation of glucose to glucose 6 phosphate.

Natural antidiabetics drugs are Gymnema *(Gymnema sylvestre)*, Pterocarpus *(Petrocarpus marsupium)*, Jamun (*Eugenia jambolana*), Bitter gourd (*Momordica charantia*),, etc.

PTEROCARPUS

Vernacular names : Sans. - Pitasara; Hindi- Bijasar; Bengli- Pitashal; Tamil- Vengai; Eng. - Indian kino tree.

Biological source : It consists of the juice of the plant *Pterocarpus marsupium* Roxb and is obtained by making incision on stem bark. Plant is a member of *Papilionoideae (leguminosae)* family.

Geographical source : The plant is commonly distributed in the hilly region throughout Southern India, Gujarat, Madhya Pradesh, Bihar, Orissa and U.P.

Characters : The plant is a moderate to large deciduous tree about 30 metre in height, 2.5 metre in width with a straight clean bole (trunk). Bark is rough, grey in colour, scaly and longitudinally fissured. Older tree of *P. marsupium* exudates gum (kino) when an incision is made in the bark upto the cambium. The gum occurs in small (3.5 mm), angular, glistering, brittle fragments, appearing almost black in colour . The edge looks transparent and ruby-red in colour. Taste is astringent and odourless.

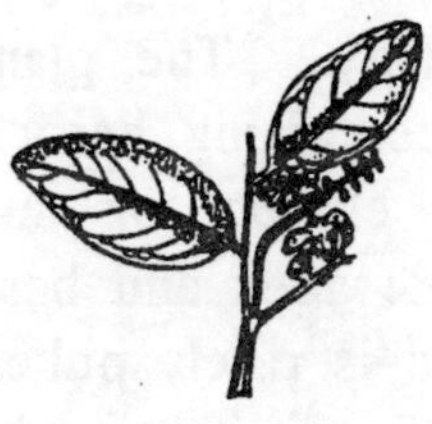

Fig. 7.34 : *Pterocarpus marsupium* herb.

Chemical constituents : Kino contains non-glycosidal tannin, Kinotannic acid, kino red ($C_{28}H_{22}O_{11}$), kinoin ($C_{28}H_{24}O_{12}$), kino red catechol, gallic acid, levoepicatechin,, etc. The heart wood contains tannins, marsupole, marsupinol, marsupin; phenolic compounds, steroids, reducing sugar, pectin, protocatechuic acid, resins, liquiritigenin, isoliqiuiritigenin,, etc.

Chemical tests

(1) PPt. is obtained by addition of mineral acid.
(2) With ferrous sulphate, it gives green colour.
(3) With potassium hydroxide, it gives violet colour.

Uses : The aqueous cold extract of the wood is used in diabetes. It is a powerful astringent and also used in diarrhoea, dysentery and pyorrhea of tooth ache. It is used in tanning,printing and dyeing.

GYMNEMA SYLVESTRE

Synonym : *Asclepias geminata* Roxb.

Vernacular names : Sans - Meshasringi; Hindi- Gur-mar; Beng. - Mera-sringi; Tam. - Cherukurinja.

Biological source : The drug consists of leaves of plant *Gymnema sylvestre* R.Br. This is a member of *Asclepiadaceae* family.

Geographical source : It is commonly distributed in the hills of Bihar, M.P, Orrisa and Deccan peninsula.

Morphology : The plant is a large stout woody climber containing hairy branchlets. The leaves are opposite elliptic or ovate containing acute or accuminate apex and base is rounded or cordate in shape and is rarely pubescent on upper surface but lower surface is more pubescent. It has a pleasant and aromatic odour; and is tasteless. It is 5-7 cm in length. The taste glands are paralysed for some time when leaf is chewed against sweet and bitter taste for few hours.

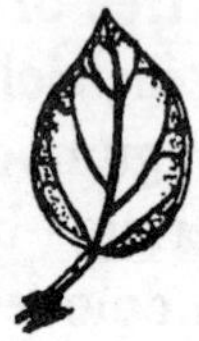

Fig 7.35 : *Gymnema sylvestre* leaf.

Chemical constituents : Leaves contain pararabin, albumin, organic acids, hentriacontane, pentatriacontane, phytin, α & ß chlorophylls, resin, mucilage, gymnemic acid, inositol. It also contains anthraquinone derivative and alkaloids, valine, adenine, stigmasterol, etc.

Uses : It is useful in hypoglycemia, cough and fever and is used as stomachic, stimulant, antiperiodic. The hypoglycemic action is due to stimulation of insulin secretion. It is mixed with castor oil and applied on swollen glands and enlarged spleen.

Allied drug : *Gymnema hirsutum* is found in Bihar and Konkan (Western Ghat), and used as substitute for Gymnema.

7 - L. DIURETICS

Diuretics are the drugs that increase the volume of urine by promoting the excretion of salts and water. The diuretics are clinically used in the treatment of glaucoma, regulation of osmotic pressure, prophylaxis of acute renal failure and management of different types of oedema. Various plants are used as diuretic, like Gokhru, Punarnava, Tea, Coffee, etc. The mechanism of diuretic action is either of the following types.

(i) Few agents increase the solute excretion in the glomerular filtrate and tubuluar fluid. They are called osmotic diuretic. These are filtered at glomerulus and are very less reabsorbed through renal tubule. There are few agents that inhibit sodium reabsorption from glomerular filtrate and increase the amount of solute and water excreted.

(ii) Another class of drug increases the renal blood flow and glomerular filtration rate leading to diuresis. It is the secondary effect by such drugs. The examples of this group are xanthine derivatives, cardiac glycosides, plasma expanders, etc.

The diuretics are classified in following manner.

1. **Acidifying diuretics** : These diuretic increase formation of urine by producing acidosis, i.e., kidney excretes excess of acid with extra water.
2. **Alkaline diuretics** : They increase urine formation by potassium salt because they are not retained by kidney.
3. **Cardiac diuretics** : These diuretics are cardiotonic drugs which increase blood circulation and hence they increase blood filtration through kidney and produce diuresis.
4. **Mercury diuretics** : These are mercury compounds which causes irritation to kidney and tubules and inhibite reabsorption. They are clinically not used because they damage the kidney.
5. **Osmotic diuretics** : These agents act by osmosis. Due to osmotic effect they diminish tubular reabsorption of water and enhance urine formation.
6. **Purine diuretics** : These agents are alkaloids containing purine nucleus. They act as central nervous system stimulant and diuretic.
7. **Saline diuretics** : These agents have low renal threshold and cause diuretic action e.g. Neutral salts.

GOKHRU

Vernacular names : Sans. & Beng. - Gokshura; Hindi - Chhotagokhru; Tamil - Nerinji; Eng. - Puncture - Vine.

Synonyms : *Tribulus terrestris* acute. non L.

Biological source : The drug consist of dried fully ripe fruits of *Tribulus lanuginosus* L. It is a member of *Zygophyllaceae* family.

Geographical source : The plant is found in waste places and dry habitats in the warmer region of India including Gujarat and West Rajasthan.

Morphology : The plant is a small prostrate annual herb bearing silky hair. The plant is flowering in rainy season and fruits are collected in October and November.The fruits are yellowish, globose & hairy. It is about 1-2 cm in diameter containing fine woody spiny cocci. Each coccus bearing two large sharp and pointed spines, directed towards the apex.. Two smaller spines are directed downwards.

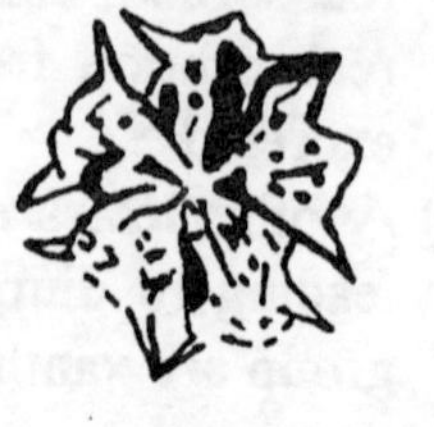

Fig. 7.36 : Chota Gokhru (*Tribulus lanuginosus)* fruit.

Chemical constituents : The drug contains saponin, which on hydrolysis yield diosgenin, ruscogenin, gitogenin, chlorogenin, hecogenin, dioscin, acoginin, gracillin, neogitogenin, quercitin,, etc. It also contain alkaloid as harman and harmine; flavonoids e.g. Kampferol and its glycoside e.g. tribuloside, traces of resins, fixed oils, essential oils, enzymes, etc.

Uses : The drug is used as diuretic, aphrodisiac, demulcent, stomachic and tonic. It is an important constituent of Ayurvedic preparation like *Dashmoolarishtha* and *Chayavanparash*. It is also used in the gonorrhea, gout, kidney diseases, painful micturition and in affections of urinary calculus.

BARA GOKHRU

Vernacular name : Hindi- and Beng. - Bara Gokhru; Guj. -Motto Gokhru; Tel.- Enugu-palleru; Tam.- Anai-nerunji.

Biological source : The drug consists of dried fruits of *Pedalium murex*. This is a member of *Pedaliaceae* family.

Geographical source : The plant is found near sea coast of India. It is also available in Rajasthan, Punjab, Delhi and Gujarat.

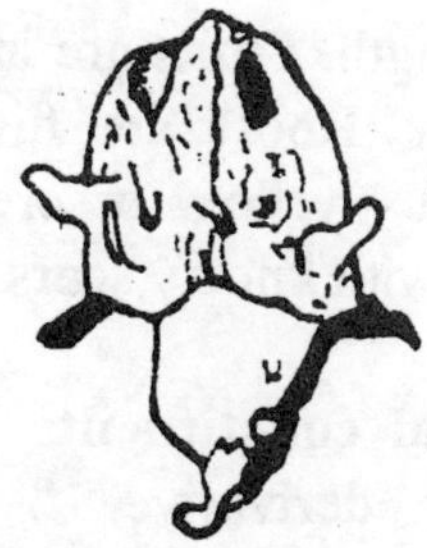

Morphology : The plant is a succulent annual herb containing pyramidal ovoid fruits. The fruits are four angled and tapering at base and apex, bearing four short stouts and horizontal spines. It is odourless and slightly mucilaginous.

Fig. 7.37 : Bara Gokhru (*Pedalium murex*) fruit.

Chemical constituents : Fruit contain fatty oil of tetra to hepta-triacontanes, hexa-triacontanoic, hentriacontanoic acids and sitosterol. The other chemical constituents are alkaloids, traces of resins, mucilages, and vanillin.

Uses : The fruits are used as diuretic, demulcent, antiseptic, tonic, aphrodisiac and in gonorrhoea, , spermatorrhoea, impotency and kidney stones.

PUNARNAVA

Synonym : *Boerhaavia repens* L.

Vernacular name : Sans. -Rakta punarnava; Hindi -Biskhafra; Beng.- Punarnava; Tam. - Mukaratte- kirei; Eng. -Spreading Hog-weed.

Biological source : The drug consists of herb of *Boerhaavia diffusa* Linn. It is a member of *Nyctaginaceae* family.

Geographical source : The plant is a weed and found throughout India especially in rainy season.

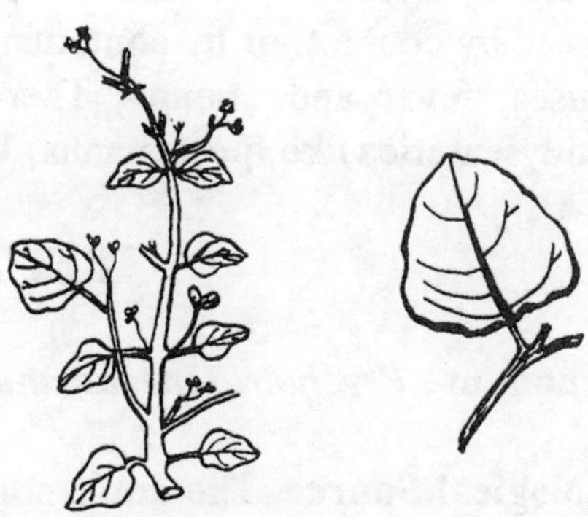

Morphology : The plant is a perennial cripping herb. Stem is greenish - purple, stiff cylindrical thick at node and is minutely pubescent. Large leaves are 2.5-3 cm long and small are 1 to 2 cm long. It is ovate, oblong or sub-orbicular in shape. Apex is slightly pointed and base is rounded or subcordated with entire margin. The upper surfaces of leaves are green and the lower surface is whitish. Flowers are pink in colour, sessile, small umbels and about 1 to 2.5

Fig. 7.38 : (a) Herb of Punarnava (b) Leaf of Punarnava.

cm in length. Fruits are indehiscent, one seeded nut about 0.5 cm long. Seeds are brown in colour. Roots are fusiform, stout, woody, tapering and tuberous. They are light brownish - yellow or cream in colour. The root contain very soft skin, old roots are marked with knotty scars.

Chemical constituents : Punarnava contains 0.04% alkaloid known as punarnavine, xanthene derivative, ß - sitosterol, ursolic acid, myricyl alcohol, myristic acid. punarnavoside, The plant also contains inorganic salts like potassium nitrate, pot. sulphate, etc.

Uses : Punarnava is used as diuretic, expectorant and stomachic. It is also prescribed in the treatment of jaundice, nephritic symptoms, oedema, anemia and heart diseases.

7 - M ANTIDYSENTERICS

Dysentery is an infection of the gastro intestinal tract which causes severe diarrhoea with blood and mucosa. (dys-bad or difficult; enteron- intestine). The dysentery is caused by the endotoxins secreted by certain protozoa like Amoeba, ciliate protozoas, schistosoma, shigella, etc. The treatment of dysentery depends upon the causing protozoan like Amoebic dysentery. Bacillary dysentery (shigella), etc.

Amoebic dysentery : This is caused by *Entamoeba histolytica* type of protozoa. It may cause ulceration in the intestine or abscesses in the liver, lungs, brain, etc. Symptom of this infection includes diarrhoea, indigestion, loss of weight and anemia. It is mainly present in tropical and subtropical regions.

Bacillary dysentery : This is caused by bacteria of genus *Shigella*. The infection may be spread by contact, or by contaminated food and water. The symptom includes diarrhoea, nausea, fever and cramps. There are certain plants, used in herbal formulations as antidysenterics like Ipecacuanha, Kurchi,, etc.

IPECACUANHA (IPECAC)

Synonym : *Psychotria ipecacuanha* Linn.

Biological Source :The drugs consist of dried roots or roots and rhizomes of *Cephaelis ipecacuanha* Brot. (Rio or Brazilian ipecac) or *Cephaelis acuminata* Karsten (Cartagena or Nicaragua or Panama Ipecac). The plant is a member of *Rubiaceae* family.

Geographical source : Ipecac (Rio Variety) is indigenous to Brazil and plant is widely cultivated in Malaya, Burma, Brazil and West Bengal in India. The Cartagena variety is indigenous to Colombia and cultivated in Panama & Nicaragua.

Cultivation & collection : The plant can be raised both from seeds and cuttings. Humid weather enhances the growth of Ipecac. Roots and rhizomes are collected from 2-3 years old plants in dry weather by removal of soil. The adhering soil on roots and rhizomes is removed and dried in the sun light for 2-3 days.

Morphology

Rio Ipecac

(a) **Roots** : The roots are dark brick red to brown in colour. It is about 5-15 cm in length and 6 mm in diameter. It is found as tortuous pieces. The roots are closely annulated externally (about 8 annulation per cm) ridges are rounded and completely encircle the roots. The fracture of root is short showing a thick greyish bark and a small dense wood but pith is absent.

(b) **Rhizomes** : The rhizomes are brick red to dark brown in colour, about 2mm in diameter. It is cylindrical non annulated in shape and attached with roots. It is finely wrinkled longitudinally and shows the presence of pith. It possesses irritating odour and bitter taste.

Cartagena Ipecac : It is greyish brown in colour about 4-6.5mm in diameter. They contain lesser annulations and are less projecting. It is cylindrical in shape. Odour and taste are similar to Rio Ipecac.

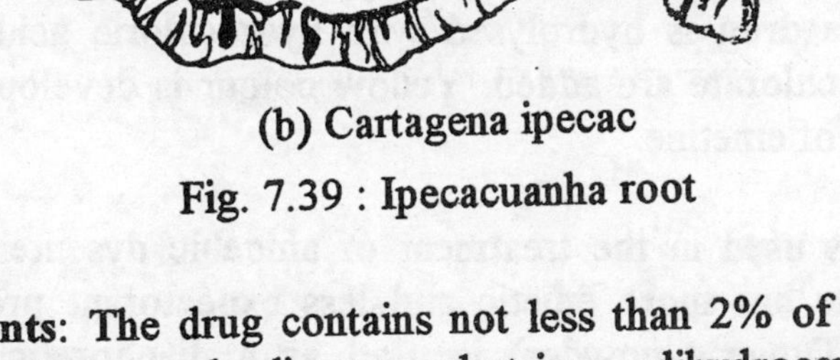

(a) Rio ipecac

(b) Cartagena ipecac

Fig. 7.39 : Ipecacuanha root

Chemical constituents: The drug contains not less than 2% of isoquinoline group of alkaloid, like emetine, cephaelin, psychotrine, dihydrocephaeline, emetamine, protoemetin, psychotrine methyl ether. The root also contains a crystalline glucosidal tannin i.e., ipecacuanhin or ipecacuanhic acid. It also contains ipecoside, ipecamine, calcium oxalate. A 3 to 4 year old plant contains maximum alkaloid.

Rio ipecacuanha contain about 2.5% alkaloids in which 50-70% is emetine whereas Cartegena contains about 2.8% of alkaloid in which 30-50% emetine.

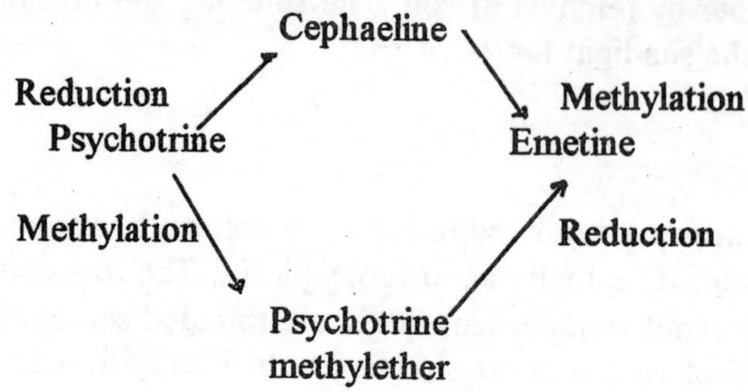

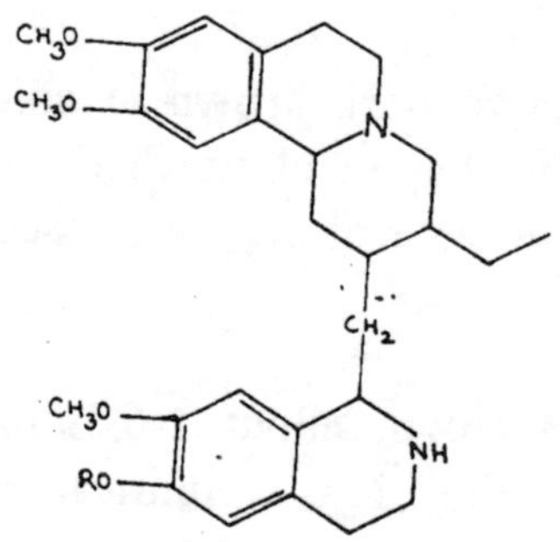

Compound	R
Cephaeline	H
Emetine	CH_3

Standards

Ash value	:	$\leq$ 5%
Acid insoluble ash	:	$\leq$ 2%
Ether soluble extract	:	$\geq$ 2%
Foreign organic matter	:	$\leq$ 2%

Chemical Test : The drug is hydrolysed with hydrochloric acid and filtered, a few crystals of potassium chlorate are added. Yellow colour is developed which changes to red showing presence of emetine.

Uses : Ipecacuanha is used in the treatment of amoebic dysentery, as an emetic and expectorant. Cephäline has more emetic and less expectorant property than emetine. Ipecac with opium (Dover's powder) is used as a diaphoretic, It has also shown antitumor property but it has marginal usefulness.

7- N. ANTISEPTICS AND DISINFECTANTS

Antiseptics are the agents that sterilize the living surface, i.e., kills all the bacteria over living organism. These are generally applied on broken skin, wounds and burns to prevent the sepsis (growth of bacteria). It may also be applied to mucous membranes to prevent conjunctiva or to treat superficial infections. The volatile oils, resins,, etc. are used as antiseptic. These agents should be non-toxic, non-irritant and does not cause allergic reactions.

The term disinfectant is used for those chemicals that kill bacteria and spores present over nonliving surface. These agents produce harmful effect over skin and are toxic on living surface. These agents are used to sterilize nonliving surface, for decontaminating drains and fecal matter.

BENZOIN

Vernacular name : Hindi, Beng., Guj. and Mar.- Loban; Tam. & Kan.- Sambirani.

Biological Source : The drug consists of balsamic resin obtained from incision on stem of *Styrax benzoin* Dryand (Sumatra benzoin) and *Styrax tonkinensis* Craib (Siam benzoin). This is a member of *Styracaceae* family.

Geographical source: Sumatra Benzoin trees are native of Borneo and Java, cultivated throughout Sumatra. Trees of Siam benzoin are grown in Thailand, Tonkin Vietnam and N. Annam.

Collection and preparation : Benzoin is a pathological resin obtained from seven years old wild or cultivated tree. The triangular incisions are made in a vertical row about 40 cm apart on the trunk of tree. The bark between the wounds is scraped smooth. The first exudate is yellow in colour and very sticky and is rejected for medicinal purpose. The subsequent flow is white & viscous. The outer part is finest in quality and forms the almond of benzoin. The fresh triangular cuts are made just above the previous incisions at three month intervals. The darker exudation are inferior and are mixed in definite proportion.

Characters : Sumatra benzoin occur as opaque, whitish, reddish block or tears, brittle mass and the surface is dull uneven. It softens on warming and gritty on chewing. Fumes of benzoic acid and cinnamic acid are produced by heating the mass. It has a characteristic odour, sweetish and slightly acrid taste.

Siam benzoin occurs as yellowish-brown to rusty-brown coloured mass, made of tears. Tears are flattened and sometimes concavo convex; externally yellowish or reddish-brown but internally milky white in colour. They are opaque and brittle. It has vanilla like agreeable odour, containing sweetish, acrid taste. On heating, Saim benzoin becomes soft like plastic.

Chemical constituents : Sumatra benzoin contains free balsamic acid and their esters. The Balsamic acids are benzoic and cinnamic acids. It also contains triterpenoid acids like Sumaresinolic acid, Siaresinolic acid,vanillin, styrol, free benzoic acid, etc.

The Siam benzoin contains mainly conferylbenzoate and cinnamyl benzoate and sufficient amount of cinnamic acid to give the odour of bitter almond due to presence of benzaldehyde, when heated with potassium permanganate ($KMnO_4$.)

Standards

		Siam benzoin	Sumatra benzoin
Acid insoluble ash	: ≤	0.5%	1.0%
Benzoic acid	: ≥	12%	6%
Foreign organic matter	: ≤	1.0%	-

Chemical tests

1. In the powdered drug, add solution of potassium permanganate and heat, Saim benzoin does not give bitter almond odour while Sumatra benzoin gives odour of bitter almond.
2. Heat the benzoin in dry test-tube, white fumes condense on the cool surface as crystalline sublimate.
3. In the alcoholic solution of benzoin, add alcoholic solution of ferric chloride, Siam benzoin gives green colour.
4. In the ethereal extract of benzoin, add few drops of sulphuric acid, sumatra benzoin gives deep reddish brown colour while Saim benzoin gives deep purplish red colour.

Uses : Benzoin is used internally as diuretic, carminative and expectorant and externally as antiseptic and protective. It also prevents the rancidity of fats in the preparation of benzoated lard. It is also included in the cosmetics to mask the taste and as perfumes in incense sticks, soaps,, etc.

MYRRH

Synonyms : *Commiphora schimep, Commiphora abyssinica.*

Biological source: Myrrh is an oleo-gum-resin obtained from stem of *Commiphora molmol* Eng. and other species of *Commiphora.* This is member of *Burseraceae* family.

Geographical source: It is found in Sommaliland, Arabian pennisula.

Collection : Myrrh is a small tree or shrub about 10 metre in height. The oleo-gum-resin is formed in schizolysigenous cannal of pholem in the stem bark of Myrrh. When incisions are made in the bark, the plant exudates oleo-gum-resin, which is a yellowish-white viscous fluid. After some time the gum resin solidifies and produces reddish-brown mass. This coagulated mass is collected by the tribals in a goat skin and sent to the market.

Characters : It is available as an irregular mass or tears. Externally it is reddish-brown in colour and internally brown in colour. The surface of oleo-gum-resin is covered with fine dust (powdery). It is about 2.5 cm in diametre. It contains an aromatic odour and bitter and acrid taste.

Chemical constituents : Myrrh contains oleo-gum-resins in which (7-17%) volatile oil; (57-61%) gum, about (26-40%) resin and (3-4%) impurities are present. Volatile oils mainly contain terpenes, sesquiterpene cuminaldehyde ester and eugenol. Resin contains α, ß & γ commiphoric acid, α & ß herabomyrrholic acid and gum contains about 18% of protein and 64% carbohydrate which includes arabinose, lactose, glucoronic acid and associated with oxidase enzyme.

Standards

Ash value	:	$\leq 9\%$
Volatile oil	:	$\geq 7\%$
Foreign organic matter	:	$\leq 4\%$

Chemical test : The etherial extract of myrrh is exposed to bromine vapours, red colour develops which turns violet in contact with nitric acid.

Uses : It is used as antiseptic, astringent, anti-inflammatory, antispasmodic, diuretic, anti-rheumatic, dermatology, etc. Fume of burnt Myrrh is beneficial in chronic bronchitis, laryngitis and tuberculosis. Myrrh is also used as carminative and in incense sticks as perfume. It is used in tooth powder and as mouth wash.

NEEM

Synonyms : *Melia azadirachta, Melia indica* Bran.

Vernacular name : San.; Nimba; Hind & Beng.- Nim; Tamil- Vepa; Eng.-Margosa tree.

Biological source : It consists of leaves and seed oil of *Azadirachta indica* J. It is a member of *Meliaceae* family.

Geographical source : It is indigenous to India and widely grows in various tropical and subtropical parts of the world.

Characters : Neem is a large tree upto 20 metre height containing a straight trunk and long spreading branches. The leaves are pinnate, crowded at the ends of branches. Leaves are alternate, opposite, lanceolate, very shortly stalked about 1-1.5 cm long. Leaf is attinuated at the apex and unequal at the base, margin blunlty serrate. Leaves are smooth and dark green in colour containing bitter taste and typical odour.

Fruit is a drupe, 1.2 to 1.8 cm long bluntly pointed. It is greenish-yellow when fresh & unripe but becomes yellow to brown when mature and ripe. It has scanty pulp and hard bony endocarp. The seeds are deep greenish, yellow-brown in colour about 1 cm in length and 0.5 cm wide.

Chemical constituents : The neem leaves contain azadirachtin, meliacin, quercitin, nembosterol, ß setosterol, ascorbic acid, Carotenoids, amino acid, etc. The seeds of Neem contains azadirachtin, azadirachtol. The Kernels yields about 40 to 49% oil of Margosa. Neem barks contain nimbin, nimbinine, nimbidine, nimbosterol, nimbidol and margosin (bitter principle). Neem oil(oil of Margosa) contains mainly glycerides and 2% bitter principle.

Uses : Neem oil is used as antiseptic, stimulant, antirheumatic and in skin diseases. The paste of Neem leaves is used as externally in small pox. It is commercially used as insecticidal agent. Margosa is used as antifertility, antifungal and antimicrobial against gram-positive and gram-negative type of bacteria. It is used as tooth brush for its antipyrorrhoeal property. It may be useful for the treatment of AIDS.

CURCUMA

Synonym : *Curcuma domestica* Valeton.

Vernacular name : Hindi, Beng.; Mar. and Gujrati-Haldi; Tam.-Manjal; Tel.-Pasupu.

Biological source : Turmeric consists of fresh, dried rhizomes of *Curcuma longa* Linn. This is a member of *Zingiberaceae* family.

Geographical source : The plant is cultivated throughout the tropical countries e.g. West Indies, Malasia, China, India, etc. In India, it is largely cultivated in Maharastra, Punjab, Tamilnadu, U.P & West Bengel.

Morphology : It is found in the form of bulb or round or fingers containing primary and secondary rhizomes. The primary rhizomes are ovate or pear shaped or cylindrical often short branched known as bulb or round turmeric. The secondary rhizomes are more cylindrical, lateral branched tapering on both ends. It is about 4-7 cm long, 1-1.5 cm wide known as fingers. Fingers contain more yellowish colouring matter than bulb. The external surface of turmeric is yellowish to yellowish-brown and longitudinally wrinkled and marked with transverse rings (leaf scars). Internal surface is yellowish-orange or orange. The fracture is horny and cuts surface showing waxy and resinous appearance. The drug contains aromatic odour and bitter taste.

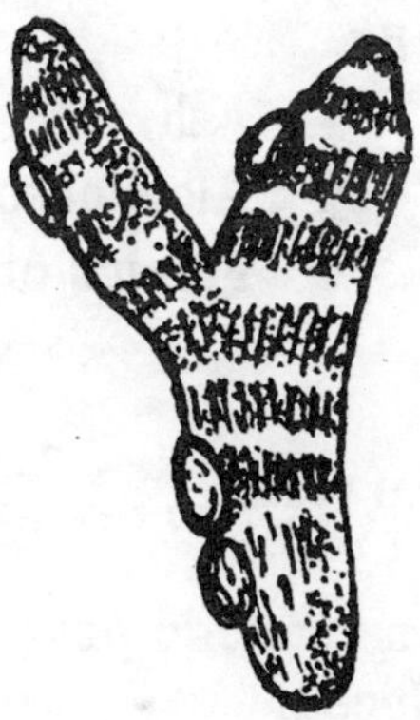

Fig. 7.40 : Turmeric (*Curcuma longa*)

Chemical constituents : Turmeric contains about 5% curcumanoids (diaryl heptanoid) as a colouring matter. The curcumanoid contains curcumine-I (diferuloylmethane), curcumine-II (caffeoylferuloylmethane) and curcumine-III (dicaffeoylmethane). Turmeric contains about 5% volatile oil. Their volatile oil contains sesquiterpenes, alcohol and ketone and monoterpene e.g. zingiberone, turmerone, arturmerone, alcohol-p-tolylmethyl, carbenol, cineole, broneol, etc. It also contains arabinose, fructose, glucose and starch grains.

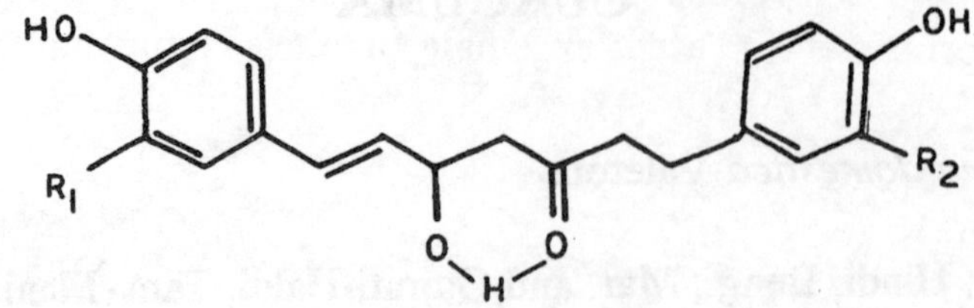

R_1	R_2	Compound
$-OCH_3$	$-OCH_3$	Curcumin I
- H	-H	Bis (4-hydroxycinnamoyl) methane (Curcumin III)
- H	$-OCH_3$	Feruloyl- (4-hydroxycinnamoyl)methane (Curcumin II)

Standards

Ash	: $\leq 9\%$
Alcohol soluble matter	: $\geq 8\%$
Foreign organic matter	: $\leq 2\%$

Chemical tests

1. When turmeric powder is treated with sulphuric acid a deep crimson-red colour is produced.
2. When turmeric powder is treated with boric acid solution, a reddish-brown colour is produced. On addition of alkali, the colour changes to greenish-blue.

Uses: It is used as stomachic. carminative, aromatic, antiperiodic, blood purifier and stimulant. It is also used in menstrual pain, liver diseases and to produce choleritic and chologogue action. Turmeric is used in curry powders, sauces and paper impregnated with its tincture is used for the borate and boric acid detection.

7 - O. ANTIMALARIAL

The disease malaria is characterised by intermittent fever, spleen enlargement and anaemia. The disease attack starts with headache, nausea, vomitting followed by shivering with fever and profuse sweating. It is caused by protozoa of the genus *Plasmodium.* This protozoa is present in female anapheles mosquito (primary host) and is transferred to man (secondary host) via. mosquito bite. There are four species of Plasmodium which can cause malaria in man. They are *P. malariae, P.vivax P. ovale* and *P. falciparum.* The life cycle of these species is completed in female anapheles mosquitoes and humans. Plasmodium does not produce any harmful effect on primary host. The most important and commonest infections are caused by *P.falciparum* and *P. vivax.* Cinchona bark is very effective against malaria fever.

CINCHONA

Biological source : Cinchona consists of dried bark of stems and roots of various species and hybrids of Cinchona such as *C. succirubra. C calisaya, C. ledgeriana, C. officinalis C. micrantha.* It is a member of *Rubiaceae* family.

Geographical source : It is indigenous to Columbia, Equador, Peru and Bolivia. It is also cultivated in Indonesia, Java and India. In India, it is cultivated in valley of Sikkim, Nilgiris, Satpura range in Madhya Pradesh and in hills of Anamalai.

Cultivation : The plant grows well at high altitude, acid soil and good rainfall. Cinchona is generally cultivated by seed or by budding and layering. For the germination of seed, it is supplemented with sand. It takes about 3-5 weeks for germination in the nursery. Seedlings are protected from sunlight and bacterial infection. The young seedlings are transplanted in the forest after 14-15 months. Maximum alkaloids are present in the 10-12 year old plants. The hybrid of *C. calisaya* and *C. ledgeriana* produces maximum amount of alkaloid. The lower branch of stem die and the main trunk grows tall. The bark collected from young plants contains three fold alkaloids than the older plants. The bark is collected from trunk and root by choping.

Character : The stem bark is available in the form of coils upto 30 cm length and 2-6 mm thickness. The outer surface bears greyish patches of moss or lichens, contains longitudinal and transverse cracks, fissures, ridges and protuberences. The inner surface is striated and yellowish brown to deep reddish brown in colour. The fracture is short but fibrous in the inner part. The drugs contain slight odour and bitter to astringent taste. Generally root bark occurs as channeled pieces. It is about 2-7 cm long, outer surface is scaly and inner is striated, both surfaces possess similar colour.

Chemical constituents : Cinchona bark contains quinoline group of alkaloids. The most important alkaloids are quinine, quinidine, cinchonine, cinchonidine. It also contains quinicine cinchonicine, hydroquinine and hydrocinchonidine. These alkaloids are associated with quinic acid and cinchotannic acid, present in the parenchymatous tissue of the bark. Cinchona red is formed by the decomposition of cinchotannic acid and it is present in the bark. It also contains quinovin (glycoside) which on hydrolysis produces quinovic acid and quinovose.

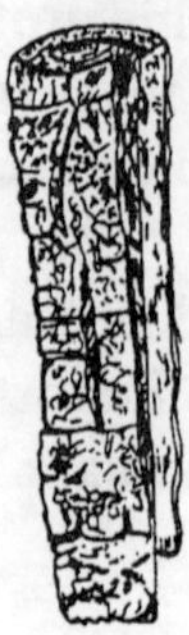

Fig. 7.41 : Cinchona bark.

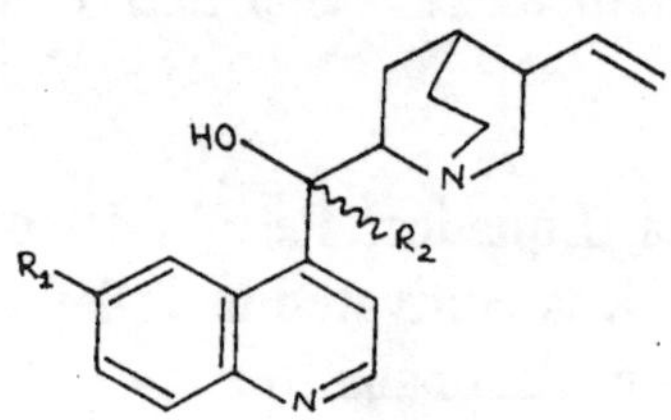

Compound	R1	R2
Quinine	OCH_3	α -H
Quinidine	OCH_3	ß - H
Cinchonidine	H	α - H
Cinchonine	H	ß - H

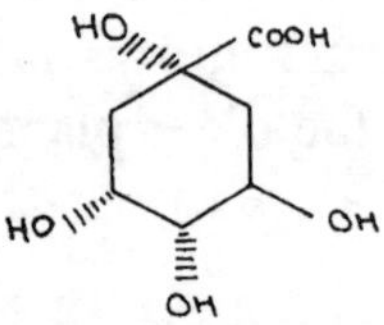

Quinic acid

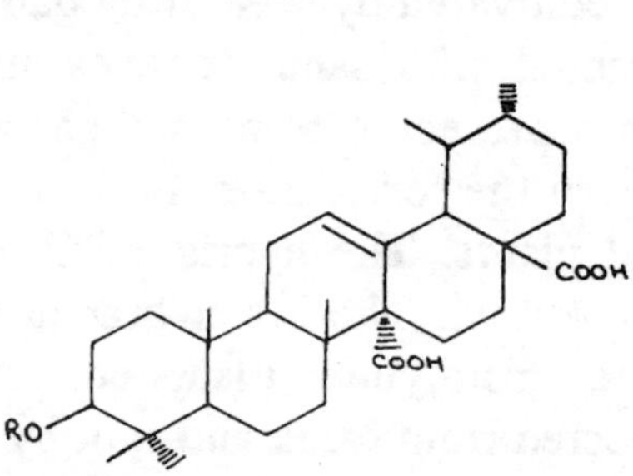

Quinovic acid (R=H)
Quinovin (R= quinovose)

Standards

Ash value	: ≤ 10%
Acid insoluble ash	: ≤ 2%
Foreign organic matter	: ≤ 2%
Water soluble extract	: ≥ 10%

Chemical tests

1. The drug is moistened with sulphuric acid, blue fluorescence is observed in U.V. light.
2. The drug is moistened with glacial acetic acid and heated in a test tube, reddish fumes are formed and condensed on the side of test tube.

Uses : The cinchonna bark is used as antimalarial, antipyretic and analgesic, quinidine is used for the treatment of atrial fibrillation, cardiac arrhythmias and as a bitter tonic and stomachic. Cinchonidine is used in rheumatism and neuralgia.

7 - P. OXYTOCIS

Oxytocics are the drugs which stimulate the motility of the uterus. The uterus is composed of smooth muscles. It shows rhythmic and spontaneous contraction activity exhibited .even in the pre-puberty age but more pronounced on maturity. Uterine contractions and foetal heart rate should be monitored during use of oxytocin. The physiological function of oxytocin is to help in labour and release of milk during suckling by the baby. The contraction due to oxytocin is periodical but highest contraction is in the second stage of labour and causes fundal contraction and dilation of cervix. The plant ergot contains ergotamine which possesses oxytocic activity.

ERGOT (ERGOT OF RYE)

Biological source : It is a dried sclerotium of a fungus *Claviceps purpurea* Tulasna arising in the ovary of the rye plant *Secale cereale* (family - *Graminae*). Ergot is a member of family *Clavicipitaceae*.

Geographical source : It is found in Yugoslavia, Spain, Germany, Switzerland, Czechoslovakia, Russia and India. In India, it is cultivated in Kodaikanal.

Cultivation and collection of Ergot : Ergot is a fungal growth and is found in infestation of the crop of cereal rye. Ergot is cultivated in sandy soil. The rye plant ,becomes infected in the spring season or in early summer. The ascospores are developed on different colonies in the presence of a nutrient medium in petridishes. For the development of large number of spores, the colonies are cut and transferred to liquid medium in a large flask. The spores are then diluted in water and sprayed on rye crop at flowering stage. A large number of sclerotia are produced on each spike of rye which are collected either by hand or by threshing the crop. Special machinaries are used for the separation of sclerotia. These are also separated by using 20 to 30% solution of sodium chloride where erogt floats and rye sinks. After separation and collection, the sclerotia are dried thoroughly and stored in suitable containers. The moisture content should not exceed 8.0%. The drug is sprinkled with carbon tetrachloride to prevent the attack of mites, insects, moulds and bacteria The drug is defatted to preserve its activity for longer duration.

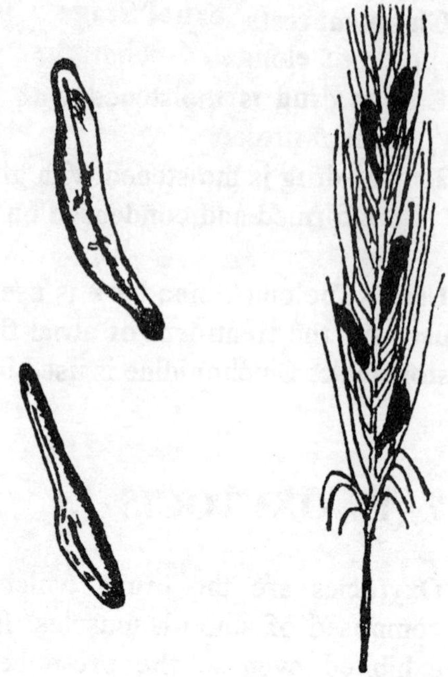

Fig. 7.42 : (a) Ergots (b) Rye ear with ergots.

Life cycle of Ergot : Ergot is a fungal growth. It a parasite in nature and requires one host to complete its life cycle. The life cycle of ergot is described in three stages.

(i) Honeydew or asexual stage.
(ii) Ascigerous or sexual stage.
(iii) Ascospore stage.

Honey dew or asexual stage : The rye plant gets infected in the spring or early summer at the flowering stage which lasts about one week, by the ascospore of the fungus. The spores are carried out either by insects or by the wind to the flowers at the base of the young ovary. The germination of the spore takes place in damp weather. After germination they form filamentous hyphae, which enter into the wall of the ovary due to enzymatic action and form sphacelia. They are soft and white mass over the surface of the ovary. In this stage the sphacelia produces viscous yellowish saccharine secretion known as " honey dew" which is a reducing sugar (as it reduces Fehiling's solution). Some of the hyphae contains chains of small oval conidiospores. The honey dew is sweet in taste and attracts ants, weevils and other insects which carry the conidia to other plants and this helps in the spreading of disease. So this stage is called either honey dew stage or sphacelia stage.

Ascigerous or Sexual Stage : In this stage the hyphae penetrate deeply into the ovary and form elongated sclerotium. It is the resting stage of the fungus. The sclerotium develops and attains the maximum size and falls on the ground in summer season. The sclerotium projects on the rye having sphacelia at its apex. They are collected either by hand or by using machine.

Ascospore stage : If ergot is not collected then it falls to the ground in autumn. In the following spring season after getting suitable condition they produce stalk like projections which are known as stromata. The stromata have globular heads. The head of stromata contains a number of flask shaped cavities that are known as perithecia. Each perithecia possesses many sacs (asci) which contains eight threads like ascospores. These ascospores are spread by the help of insects or wind or ants to the flowers of the rye crop in spring season. This is the way by which life cycle of ergot is completed.

Chemical constituents : Ergot contains indole group of alkaloids. The water soluble indole alkaloid is ergometrine (ergonovine) and water insoluble are ergotamine and ergotoxin.

(A) Water soluble

Ergometrine group	**Ergometrine.** **Ergometrinine**

(B) Water insoluble

(I) Ergotamine group	**Ergotamine** **Ergotaminine** **Ergosine** **Ergosinine**
(II) Ergotoxin group	**(l) Ergocristine** **(d) Ergocristinine** **(l) Ergocryptine.** **(d) Ergocryptinine.** **(l) Ergocornine** **(d) Ergocorninine**

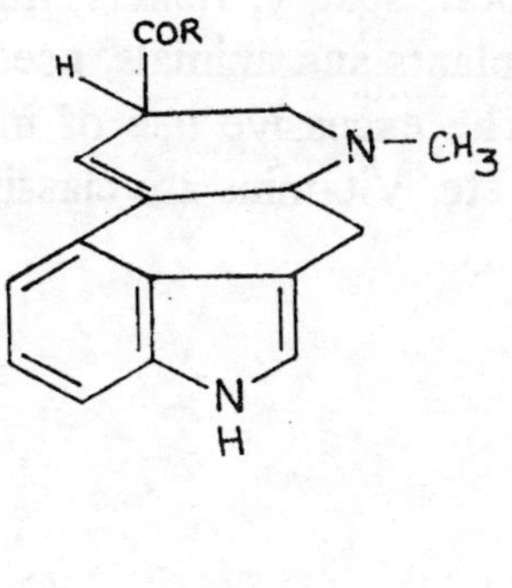

Lysergic acid, R =OH
Ergine, R= NH_2
Ergometrine, R= $NH(CH_3)$- CH_2OH
Methylergometrine, R= $NHCH(CH_2CH_3)CH_2OH$

Ergotamine, R' = 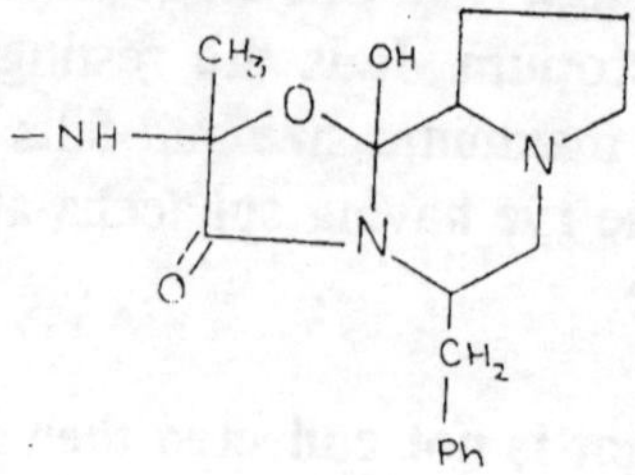

Chemical tests

1. The drug shows red fluorescence in U.V. light .
2. Powdered ergot is extracted with a mixture of chloroform and sodium carbonate, to the chloroform layer added a mixture of p-dimethyl aminobenzaldehyde (0.1 gm), H_2SO_4 (35% v/v) and 5% ferric chloride (1.5% ml). A deep blue colour is produced.

Uses : Traditionally ergot preparation is used in labour to assist delivery and to reduce postpartum haemorrhage. Ergometrin produce oxytoscis effect. Ergotamin and di-hydro ergotamin salts (semi synthetic) are used in the treatment of migrane. Lysergic acid diethylamide (LSD-25), is a semi synthetic derivative of lysergic acid and is potent psychotomimetic.

7 - Q. VITAMINS

Vitamins are organic nitrogenous or non nitrogenous compounds, not synthesized within the body, hence they are essential in small amount for the maintenance of life and normal growth in human beings and animals. They are not the source of energy or building blocks of the body but are very essential for regulation of metabolic processes. The deficiency of vitamins causes a number of diseases like beri-beri, scurvy, rickets, night-blindness; etc. Vitamines are isolated from both sources, i.e.; plants and animals, used as therapeutic agent in prophylaxis and treatment of diseases. The excessive use of many vitamins causes toxic and adverse effect such as vitamin A, D, etc. Vitamins are classified into two groups

(a) **Fat soluble** : Vitamins A, D, E & K.

(b) **Water soluble** : Vitamin B complex, Vitamin C.

Sources of Vitamins

Animals : Shark liver oil, Egg yolk, Cod liver oil, Halibut liver oil, Milk and Milk products.

Plants : Amla, Potato, Carrots, Rice, Cereals, Legume, Citrus fruits. Spinach, Onion, Chilli, Cabbage, etc.

SHARK LIVER OIL

Synonym : Oleum selachoide

Biological source : Shark liver oil is obtained from the fresh and healthy livers of shark fish of various species mainly *Hypoprion brevirostris*.

Geographical source : Shark is found on sea coast of many European countries and India. In India, it is found in Madras, Malabar and Maharastra. Commercially the shark oil is obtained from shark fish in Maharastra, TamilNadu and Kerala.

Preparation : Shark liver oil is prepared from fresh and healthy or carefully preserved livers without gall bladders of shark fish. The livers are cleaned thoroughly, fatty substances are removed and then minced. The minced mass is heated in water at 80°C. The oil exudes, floats on top which is filtered, washed and water is removed by using dehydrating agents. The dehydrated oil is chilled to separate stearin. The suspended particles present in oil is separated by centrifugation. Now the pure oil is manipulated to adjust the desired strength of vitamin A and D. Since the oil is very sensitive to light. It is stored in full filled, air tight dark containers which should be filled with oil right up to the top. These containers should be kept in a cool and dark place.

Characters : Shark liver oil is pale yellow to brownish yellow in colour. It is viscous liquid containing characteristic fishy odour and bland taste. It is soluble in ether, chloroform and light petroleum, insoluble in water and slightly soluble in alcohol.

Chemical constituents : Shark liver oil is rich in vitamin A which varies from 15000 to 30,000 IU per gram. It also contains glycerides of both saturated and unsaturated acids.

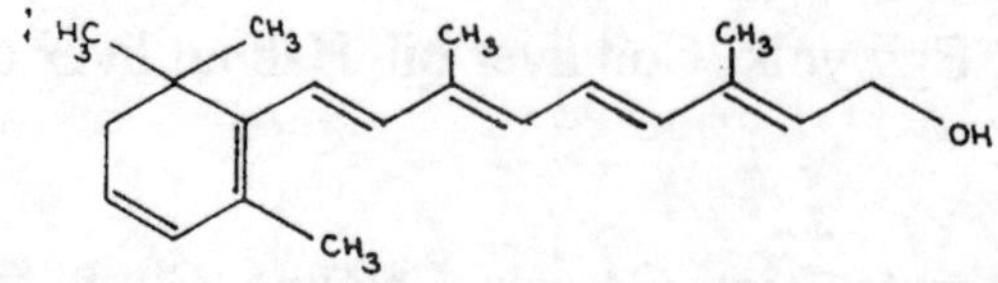

Vitamine A

Standards

Specific gravity	:	0.912 to 0.916
Refractive index	:	1.45-1.47 at 40°C.
Saponification value	:	≤ 200
Acid value	:	≤ 2
Iodine value	:	≥ 90

Chemical tests

1. Dissolve 1 gram of shark liver oil in 1 ml of chloroform and add 2-3 drops of sulphuric acid. It produces pale violet colour, changing to purple and finally to brown due to the presence of Vitamin A.
2. Dissolve 1 ml of shark liver oil in 10 ml of chloroform and treat with few drops of saturated solution of antimony trichloride in chloroform and shake well. A blue colour is formed due to the presence of vitamin A.

Uses : It is used in the deficiency of vitamin A and is also known as antixeropthalmic factor because it cures night blindness. It is used in prevention of hyperkeratosis of skin, promotes growth and development and increases resistance of body to infection. When shark liver oil is mixed with vitamin D, it acts as a substitute of cod liver oil and acts as tonic. It is also used in tuberculosis, burns and sunburn ointments.

AMLA (Indian gooseberry)

Synonyms : *Phyllanthus emblica* Linn. *Cicca emblica* Kurz.

Vernacular name : Sans. & Beng.- Amalakee; Hindi-Amla, Aonla, Guj.- Amali; Tam-Nelli; English-Indian Gooseberry.

Biological source : Amla consists of fresh & dried fruits of *Emblica officinalis* G. This is a member of *Euphorbiaceae* family.

Geographical source : Widely distributed throughout tropical and subtropical countries like Ceylon, China, Malaya and India. In India, wild or cultivated plants are available throughout the country.

Morphology : Amla is a large decidous tree with spreading branches. It contains greenish-grey or red bark, leaves are pinnate distichously close-set. The fruit is fleshy, globous, green, when unripe but turns yellow or pink on maturity. Fruits are tricarpellary drupe having edible mesocarp and stony endocarp. The outer surface of the fruit is smooth and shining with six lobes. The seeds are trigonous. Amla is sour and astringent in taste.

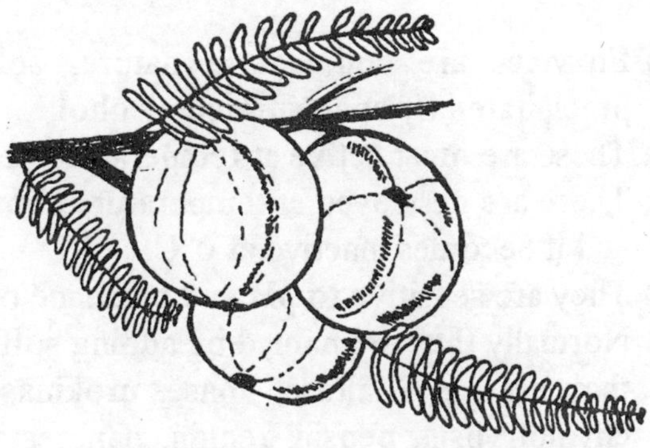

Fig. 7.43 : Amla fruits.

Chemical constituents : The Amla is the richest natural source of vitamin C containing 650-900 mg/100 gm. It contains polyphenolic tannins like ellagic acid, corialgil 1,3,6 trigalloyl glucose, etc. like phyllantidine and phyllantine are also present in Amla. It also contains emblicol, phyllembic acid, fixed oils, carbohydrates, pectin, minerals like calcium, iron and phosphorous.

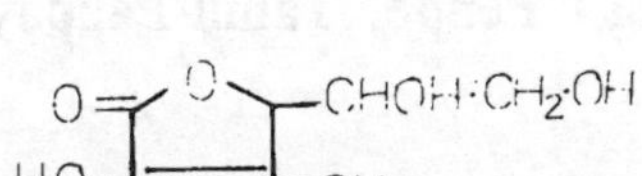

Ascorbic acid (Vitamin C)

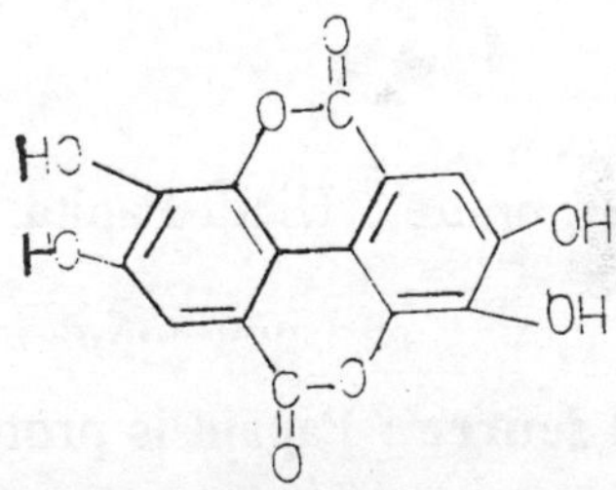

Ellagic acid

Uses : Amla fruits are astringent, antiviral, antibacterial, cardiotonic, antipyretic and anticancerous. It is used in treatment of scurvy, asthma, urinary troubles, bronchitis, toothache, gonorrhoea, tuberculosis and liver diseases. In combination with iron it is used to treat anaemia, jaundice and dyspepsia. Amla is an important ingredient of Ayurvedic formulation like **triphala** and **chyavanprash**. It is used in preparation of hair oil and shampoo. The leaf is used in opthalmia and incipient blindness.

7 - R. ENZYMES

Enzymes are organic catalyst, proteinous in nature, non living (lifeless), high molecular weight substances produced by living organism. It serves as catalyst in many complex chemicals' reactions that make up life processes. The enzymes contain several common properties.

(a) Enzymes are colloidal in nature, soluble in water and dilute alcohol but are precipitated by concentrated alcohol.
(b) These are most active at temperature between 35 to 40°C.
(c) These are destroyed at temperature.above 65°C especially in the presence of moisture and it becomes inactive at 0°C.
(d) They are sensitive to pH and presence of other substances in medium.
(e) Normally they are named by adding suffix -ase or-in to specific substrates upon which they act e.g. Maltase, lipase, urokinase, pectase, invertase, phospholipase, papain, chymotrypsin, pepsin, rennin, pancreatin, etc. Enzymes occur in combination with inorganic or organic substances. The non protein organic compounds are known as *co-enzymes*. Several vitamins such as thiamin, riboflavin, nicotinic acid, etc. are known as coenzymes. If they are inorganic ions they are known as activators. Renin, pancreatin, pepsin, trypsin, etc. are the examples of animal enzymes whereas papain, emulsin, myrosin, zymase, maltase, etc. are examples of plant enzymes. Enzymes are classified into following categories. Transverses, Hydrolyses, Lyases, Isomerases, Synthetases (ligases) and Oxidoreductases.

PAPAYA

Vernacular name : Hindi-Papita; Sans.- Parisha; Beng.- Penpe; Tamil-Pappayi; Eng.- Papaya tree.

Biological source : Papain is proteolytic enzymes obtained from the dried and purified latex of the unripe fruit (papaya) of *Carica Papaya* Linn. It is a member of *caricaceae* family.

Geographical source : Papaya is indigenous to America and cultivated in Sri-Lanka, Tanjania, Florida, Hawai and India. In India, it is cultivated throughout the country.

Collection and Preparation : It is an erect tree 6-7 metre in height with spongy trunk and milky sap bearing cylindrical or spherical fruits near the top of the trunk. It is about

30 cm. in length and 5 kg in weight. The unripe fruits are injured deeply on all the sides at weekly interval. Latex flows out freely from the fruit within few seconds, is collected and dried in sunlight or by artificial heat. The process is repeated until secretion of latex ceases. The crude papain is purified by dissolving in water and it is precipitated with alcohol. This is also called as "vegetable Papain".

Description : Papain occurs as light brown or white coloured amorphous powder. It is soluble in water and insoluble in alcohol, chloroform and ether. The papain may digest about 35 times, its weight of lean meat. The best quality of papain digests 300 times of their weight of coagulated egg albumin. The enzyme shows maximum proteolytic activity at pH 5 and temperature between 60 to 90°C.

Chemical constituents : Papain contains several enzymes like papain and chymopapain which hydrolyses polypeptides, amides and esters. These proteolytic enzymes convert proteins into Dipeptide, Polypeptides, etc.

Use : It is used to tenderize meat, protein digestant, clearance of protein from the surface of soft contact lenses and in clearance of beverages.

DIASTASE

Synonym : Amylase.

Biological source : Diastase is an amylolytic enzyme found in saliva or pancreatic juice of animals, so it is also known as animal diastase. Malt diastase is found in germinated barley grains, *Hordeum vulgare* (family: *Gramineae*) and converts starch into maltose. The cultivation of barley is done throughout the world. The dry malt contains dextrins (2 to 15%), proteins (8%) sugar (50 to 70%), diastase and peptase enzymes. The extraction of malt is carried out by extracting partially greminating grains of *H. vulgare*. It contains glucose, maltose and amylolytic enzyme. In animals diastase is found as ptyalin or salivary diastase and amylopsin or pancreatic diastage. Diastase is a yellowish white amorphous powder. It catalyses the hydrolysis of α-1, 4- glucosidic linkages of polysaccharides such as starch and glycogen. It converts 50 times of its weight of potato starch into sugars (dextrin and maltose).

Uses : Diastase is used as digestant and in manufacture of starch, converts starch into sugar. It is also used in the production of predigested starchy food and brewing industries.

YEAST

Synonyms : Dried yeast, Cerevisiae fermentum.

Biological source : Yeast consists of unicellular fungal microorganisms obtained from *Saccharomyces cerevisiae*. It is a member of *saccharomycetaceae* family, a subdivision of Ascomycetes.

Fruit juice, bread and several fermented or fermenting media are the natural habitat of yeast. On large scale, it is produced by molasses, molasses wort, grain wort and citrus fruits, etc.

Collection and preparation : Yeast is commercially produced by using malt or a mixture of malted or unmalted grains. These are soaked in water keeping the temperature in between 60 to 65°C. This medium is known as Distiller's wort or Brewer's wort. This medium contains inorganic salts and appropriate proportions of nitrogenous matter. Now the yeast is transferred to this medium and the temperature is maintained between 20 to 25°C for rapid multiplication. The yeast is separated from medium, washed thoroughly in water and passed through filter press. This type of yeast is known as baker's yeast or compressed yeast. It contains about 70 to 75% of moisture. When the yeast cells are dried by heating at a temperature below 30°C till the moisture content is about 9%. This type of yeast is known as dried yeast.

Characters : Dried yeast is pale buff to light yellowish in colour. It is found in form of powder, granules or flakes. It has characteristic odour. It is inactive in fermentation process due to presence of dead cells. It is unicellular microorganism having elliptical ovate or subspherical in shape.

Chemical constituents : Yeast contains vitamin B complex group such as nicotinic acid, riboflavin, aneurine, folic acid, thiamine, pyridoxine and B_{12}. Yeast is rich in enzymes like zymase, maltase, invertase, endotryptase, diastase, etc. It contains about 65 to 85% of moisture, 46% proteins, 36% carbohydrates (mainly glycogen), fat and other constituents.

Uses : Yeast is used in manufacture of beer, preparation of alcohol, in bread making, etc. It is also used in the treatment of vitamin B deficiency and furunculosis. It is a rich source of biologically complete protein and is used in manufacture of nucleic acid.

7 - S. PERFUMES AND FLAVOURS

PERFUMES : Perfumes are used for creating particular pleasant odour. It may be natural, synthetic or a combination of natural and synthetic materials. Volatile oils obtained from plants are also used as perfumes. These are also known as essential oils. Certain oils used in perfumery are prepared by steam distillation, enfleurage method or solvent extraction. Certain perfumes are also obtained from different animals such as musk. Musk is an important ingredient of various high class perfumes and acts as a fixative. The chief odourous consistent of musk is muskone. Perfumes are widely used in various preparations such as toilet preparations, lipsticks, body lotions, powders, etc. to create a pleasant odour. Perfumes are also used as industry odorants. Sometime perfumes are used for masking the odour and to provide particular odour in various preparations like polishes, insecticides, etc.

Some perfumes are derived from natural sources, these are given below.

1. Citronella : Leaves of *Cymbopogon Spp.*
2. Jasmine : Flowers of *Lavandula officinalis*
3. Rose : Flowers of *Rosa gallica*
4. Sandal wood : Heart wood of *Santalum album*
5. Styrax : Balsamic resin of *Styrax benzoin*
6. Vetiver : Roots of *Vetiveria zizaniodes*
7. Civet : Odorous secretion obtained from the perineal follicles of African or Indian Civet cats *Viverra spp.*
8. Musk : Dried secretion from preputial follicles of musk deer *Muschus moschiferus.*

FLAVOURING AGENTS

Flavouring agents are used to mask the unpleasant taste and odour of drugs and make medicines more acceptable to patients. The word flavour refers to a combined sensation of taste, smell, touch and sight. Children are very sensitive to taste because they have more taste buds than adults. Women are more sensitive to odour than men. Flavour is usually choosen according to the taste to be disguised or masked. Flavouring agents have an important role in the development of a pharmaceutical formulation. An ideal flavouring agent must be soluble, non toxic, stable and compatible with the drugs and adjuvants. At the time of selection of flavours, the taste and colour should match and relate to drugs. A large number of flavours are derived from natural sources like Rose, Mint, Lemon, Orange, etc.

Natural Flavours

Cherry, Rose, Strawberry	: Red Colour
Lemon, Orange	: Yellow to orange colour
Vanilla, Mint	: White colour
Lemon, Orange	: Sour taste (Acid)
Cinnamon, Cherry, Mint	: Bitter taste.

PEPPERMINT OIL

Synonym : Oleum *Mentha Piperata*

Biological source : Peppermint oil is obtained by steam distillation of fresh flowering tops of the plant *Mentha piperata* Linn. or other species of *Mentha*. The plant is a member of *Labiatae* family.

Geographical source : The plant Mentha is cultivated in Japan, England, Bulgaria, U.S.A, USSR, India, etc. In India, it is cultivated in Bihar, Uttar Pradesh, Jammu.

Cultivation & Preparation : The Plant Mentha is perennial herb. It is cultivated in fertile and well irrigated lands. Good sunlight enhances mentha production. Several varieties of mentha are cultivated in this country. The plants of mentha are cultivated by vegetative propagation method by using cuttings and suckers. The leaves and flowering tops are cut down and dried in sun-light for a day and the oil is extracted by steam distillation. The average yield of oil is 0.5 to 1.0% v/w.

Characters : Mentha oil is colourless to yellowish in colour. It has pleasant characteristic odour; containing pungent taste followed by cooling sensation.

Chemical constituents : Peppermint oil mainly contains menthol (about 70%). It also contains menthone, menthyl acetate and other terpene derivatives like cineole, pinene, isopulegone, camphene, limonene, Zasmone, menthofurone, menthyl isovalerate, etc.

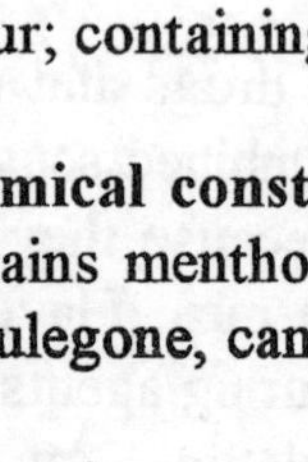

Menthol

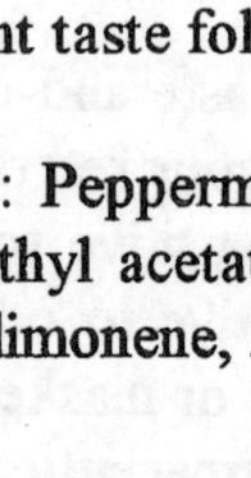

Menthone

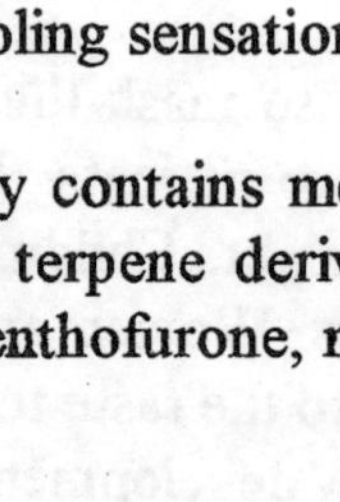

Menthyl acetate

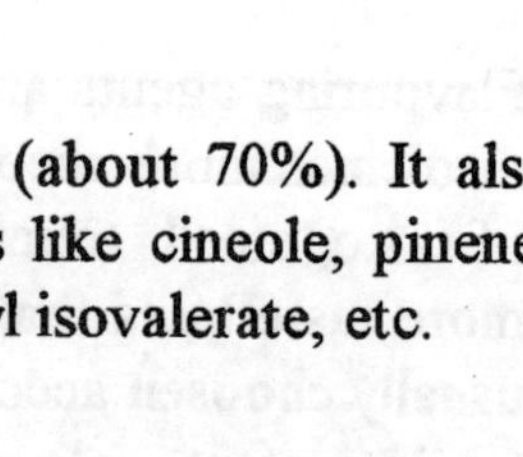

Jasmone

Standards

Optical rotation : - 18° to - 33°C
Refractive index : 1.4590 to 1.4650
Specific gravity : 0.896 - 0.908

Uses : Peppermint oil is used as carminative, aromatic, stimulant and flavouring agent. It is widely used as an antiseptic in various preparations and in mouth freshness. It is also used as antipruritic and counter irritant over skin and mucous membrane.

LEMON OIL

Synonym : Oleum Limonis.

Biological source : Lemon oil is obtained from the peels of *Citrus limon* (L.) Burm .f. It is a member of *Rutaceae* family.

Geographical distribution : The plant is a native of India grown in the orchards in Maharastra, Karnataka, Tamil Nadu and Uttar Pradesh and it is also cultivated in Southern Italy, Spain, Portugal, Australia, etc.

Preparation of Lemon oil : Lemon oil can be prepared by following methods.

(1) **Sponge method** : The fruit is cut and pulp is removed with a sharp knife. The peels are soaked in water for few hours and peel curvature is reversed and oil glands ruptured. Ejected oils are absorbed on the sponge which is squeezed, the oils are separated and filtered.

(2) **Ecuelle a piquer process** : Eucelle a piquer means a " boul for pricking". In this process oil glands present over peels are ruptured with the help of pins about 0.5 cm long. Lemons are rotated by hand and oil is sucked.

Characters : The oil is a pale yellow liquid. It has pleasant, agreeable, and characteristic odour; taste is acidulous and bitter.

Constituents : The lemon peels contain 2-4% volatile oil. The main constituents volatile oil are terpenes 94% [limonene (90%); citronellal, pinene, limonene, camphene, citral (4%) geranyl acetate,, etc.]. The chief odourous constituent of oil is citral, geranyl acetate, etc.

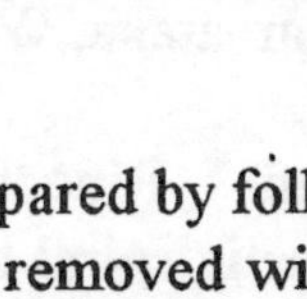

Citral

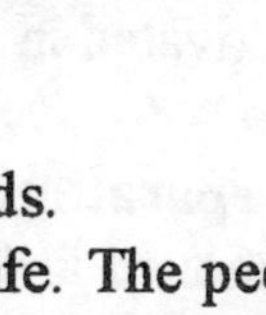

Limonene

Standards

Optical rotation	:	+ 57 to + 65
Refractive index	:	1.4711 to 1.4761
Specific gravity	:	0.849 - 0.855

Uses : Lemon oil is mainly used as flavouring and perfuming agent. It is also used as stimulant, carminative and stomachic and in rheumatism.

ORANGE OIL

Synonym : Oleum Aurantii.

Biological source : Orange oil is obtained from peels of orange fruits of the plant *Citrus aurantium* Linn. It is a member of *Rutaceae* family.

Geographical source : The bitter orange is a native of north eastern India. It is cultivated commercially in Spain, U.S.A., Morocco, Sicily, etc. In India, it is widely cultivated in Maharastra, karnataka, West Bengal, Andhra Pardesh and Punjab.

Preparation of Orange oil : Ripe fruits are collected from the plant and peels are removed in four quarters or in spiral band for the extraction of volatile oil. The volatile oils are extracted from orange peels by sponge method and Ecuelle a piquer method as given in lemon oil.

Characters : Orange oil is an orange-yellow liquid. It has characteristic aromatic odour and taste. It is soluble in carbon disulphide, dehydrated alcohol and glacial acetic acid.

Chemical constituents : Orange peels contain volatile oil (1.0-2.5%). The chief constituents of volatile oil are d-limonene, citral, citronellal, decyl alcohol and methyl anthranilate.

Use : It is used as a flavouring agent.

LEMON GRASS OIL

Synonyms : East India lemon grass, Malabar or Cochin lemon grass.

Biological source : Lemon grass oil is obtained by steam distillation from aerial parts and leaves of *Cymbopogon flexuosus*, *C. citratus*, etc. This is a member of *Graminae* family

Geographical source : Lemon grass (*C. flexuosus*) is indigenous to India and it is available as wild and cultivated plant throughout the country mainly at Tinnevelly, Travancore and Cochin. *C. citratus* is cultivated in Burma, Ceylon, Mauritius, West Indies and South America. In India, it is mainly cultivated in Maharashtra, Gujarat and Punjab.

Description : Lemon grass is mainly cultivated in the well drained sandy loam. Sunshine favours the volatile oil content in the plant while excessive rain fall decreases the content of oil. The two varieties of lemon grass are mainly available (1) red steamed variety- *C. flexuosus* and (II) white variety - *C. flexuosus* lower albescens. The white variety contains lower aldehydic content.

Characters : Lemone grass oil is yellowish brown coloured liquid; odour & taste resembles like lemon. It is soluble in 70% alcohol, fixed oil, mineral oil and propylene glycol but insoluble in water.

Chemical constituents : Lemon grass oil mainly contains citral and citronellal (75-85%). The other terpens are geraneol, nerol, linallol, methyl heptenol, limonene,, etc. ß ionone are derived from citral.

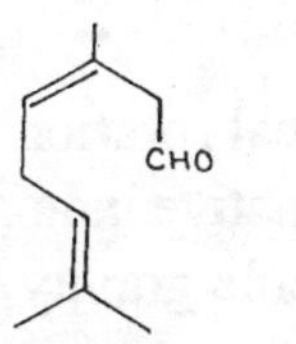

Citral

Standards

Optical rotation	:	-3° to 1°C
Refractive index	:	1.4808 to 1.4868
Weight per ml.	:	0.892 to 0.909

Uses : It is used as flavouring and perfuming agent. It is also used as a mosquito repellent. It is used as a source of citral for the preparation of ß - ionone . The ß ionone is used as precursor of vitamine A.

SANDAL WOOD OIL

Synonyms : Chandan oil, Sandal oil, Yellow sandal wood oil.

Biological source : Sandal wood oil is obtained by distillation of dried heart wood from the plant *Santalum album* Linn. This is a member of *Santalaceae* family.

Geographical source : The sandal tree is available in India & Malaya, In India, the trees are available in Tamil nadu, Mysore, Maharastra, Uttar .Pradesh, Madhya Pradesh, Assam, Bihar, Rajasthan, Gujarat, etc.

Description : It is a medium sized, evergreen, parasitic plant. The 30 year old plant is selected for collection of volatile oil. The plant is uprooted and bark is removed from stem and root. The wood is yellowish to pale red in colour. The wood is cut into small pieces for stem distillation. It contains 2.5% of volatile oil.

Character : Sandal wood oil is yellowish or pale reddish viscous liquid. It has strong fragrance, taste is slightly bitter.

Chemical constituents : Sandal wood oil contains mixture of two isomers α & ß santalol (90%), α & ß santalene, santalone, santanone, santene, isovaleraldehyde, α and ß santalic acids, etc.

Standards

Optical rotation	:	- 15° to - 20°
Refractive index	:	1.499 - 1.506
Specific gravity	:	0.962 - 0.976

Uses : Oil is used as perfuming agent in various cosmetic preparations and in incense sticks. It is used for wounds and blisters caused by small pox vaccination, gonorrhoea, cough & dysuria. Sandal wood oil along with neem oil is used as a contraceptive. Sandal wood oil along with double quantity of mustard oil is used for the treatment for pimples on the nose. Sandal wood oil and sandal wood are considered as cooling, diuretic, diaphoretic and expectorant drugs.

7 - T PHARMACEUTICAL AIDS

The compounds which are therapeutically inert or have little therapeutic value but are used in manufacturing or compounding of various pharmaceutical dosages forms such as tablet, capsule, syrup,, etc. These compounds are obtained from various sources such as plants, animals, minerals and purely synthetic origin.

Pharmaceutical aids are classified as follow.

1. **Diluent** : Cinnamon water, Peppermint water, Glucose, Lactose.

2. Disintegrating agents : Starch, Microcrystalline cellulose, Psyllium husk.
3. Emulsifying agents and suspending agents : Acacia , Agar, Tragacanth, Gelatin, Sodium alginate, Guargum.
4. Flavouring agents : Cardamom, Clove, Fennel, Cinnamon.
5. Lubricants : Cocoa butter, Castor oil, Talc.
6. Sweetening agents : Glycyrrhiza, Honey.
7. Ointment bases : Bees wax, Lanolin.
8. Colour : Cochineal, Caramel, Turmeric, Saffron, Chlorophyll, Indigo.
9. Adsorbents : Kaolin, Pectin,
10. Vehicles : Arachis oil, Olive oil.

HONEY OR MEL

Biological Source : Honey is a saccharine substance deposited by honey bees, *Apis mellifica* Linn and other species of *Apis*. It is a member of *Apidae* family and order Hymenoptera.

Geographical source : Honey is produced mainly in England, California, Chile, West-Indies and some parts of Australia, Africa and Newzealand.

Collection and preparation : The worker bees possess a long hollow tube formed of maxillae and labium, sucks the nector from flower. It passes through the oesophagus into the honey sac. The nectar consists of sucrose (25%) and water (75%) is mixed with salivary secretion. The salivary secretions contain an enzyme invertase which converts nectar into invert sugar. Some part of invert sugar is utilised by the worker bee while the remaining honey is deposited in the content of honey sac in honey comb. The honey comb is smoked to remove bees and comb is cut. Honey is drained or expressed from the comb. The honey collected by expression method is contaminated with the wax. To get the purified honey, it is heated then impurities floats on the surface and filtered.

Characters : Honey is a thick clear syrupy liquid. It is yellow or reddish -brown in colour having sweet taste. The odour depends on the type of flower nectar used in its preparation. On storage honey crystallizes and becomes opaque and granular. Honey collected from *Datura stromonium* is poisonous and honey collected from *Eucalyptus* species or Banksia contains unpleasent odour and taste.

Chemical constituents : Honey consists chiefly a mixture of dextrose and levulose (70-80%) and water (14-20%). It also contains sucrose (1.1-4.4%), dextrin (0.06-1.24%), volatile oil, pollen grains enzymes, vitamins, amino acids, proteins, colouring matters, etc.

Standards

Density	:	1.35 to 1.36 g/ml.
Sp. rotation	:	+ 3° - 10°C
Total ash	:	≤ 1%

Chemical test : To the petroleum ether extract add 1% resorcinol in hydrochloric acid. A transient red colour is formed in natural honey and colour persist in artificial honey.

Uses : Honey used as an important component of linctus and cough mixtures. It is a sweetening agent and used widely due to as its nutritive value. It is also used as demulcent, mild laxative, bactericidal and antiseptic. This is also used as a vehicle in Ayurvedic and Unani preparations.

ARACHIS OIL OR PEANUT OIL OR NUT OIL

Vernacular name : Hindi-Mungphali; Sans. - Buchanaka; Beng. - Chenabadam; Tam. - Varkadalai; Eng. - Groundnut.

Biological source : Arachis oil is obtained by expression of seeds, kernels of *Arachis hypogaea* Linn. This is a member of *papilionoideae* (*leguminosae*) family.

Geographical source : Plant is a native of tropical South America and is cultivated in China, Java, Kenya, Nigeria and India . In India, it is cultivated throughout the country.

Preparation of oil : The underground ripen fruits are collected and seeds are separated. Each fruit contains one to three reddish brown seeds. These seeds are ovoid to ovoid cylindrical in shape, about 10-15 mm long. The taste of seeds is bitter papery and colour is brownish- red. Kernel contain two large cotyledons. They are yellowish white in colour. The kernel contains about 40-50% of fixed oil.

The seeds are separated from fruit. Seedcoat is removed. The kernels are crushed and expressed at room temperature. A low pressure expeller is used initially for the extraction of oil. This oil is used in medicines. The oil cake is again expressed at higher temperature and finally the oil is extracted by solvent extraction process. The oil is filtered with the help of charcoal. The remaining cake is used as cattle food.

Characters : Arachis oil is a pale yellow to greenish yellow non drying oil containing nutty odour and bland taste. At low temperatures, clouds are formed in the oil. On exprosure to air the oil becomes rancid. The oil is generally soluble in organic solvents.

Chemical constituents : Arachis oil consists of glycerides of fatty acid (linoleic, arachidic, palmitic, oleic and stearic acid). Aflatoxins and mycotoxins may be present in raw oil produced by fungal growth which is carcinogenic and damages liver. Aflatoxin B is most active and most toxic member of Aflatoxins. It is a hepatocarcinogen. These toxins can be removed from oil by adsorption on activated kaolin. Oil shows yellow colour due to the presence of carotenoid pigments like ß carotene and lutein. The seeds contain protein (25-30%), starch (15-20%), water (1-1.8%) and high concentration of thiamine. It also contains cholesterol, ß sitosterol, stigmasterol, ß -sitosterol-D-glycoside, ß-amyrin cycloartenol, etc.

Arachidic acid :	$CH_3(CH_2)_{18}COOH$
Palmitic acid :	$CH_3(CH_2)_{14}COOH$
Oleic acid :	$CH_3(CH_2)_7CH{=}CH(CH_2)_7COOH$
Linoleic acid :	$CH_3(CH_2)_4CH{=}CHCH_2CH{=}CH(CH_2)_7COOH$

Standards

Acid value	:	$\leq 2\%$
Iodine value	:	84-100
Saponification value	:	185-195
Density	:	0.911- 0.915
Refractive Index	:	1.4678-1.4698

Uses : It is used as an edible oil. It is an ingredient in various preparations like soaps, paints, liniments, margarine, cooking fat,, etc. The properties of arachis oil are similar to olive oil so it is used as a solvent for vitamin A, vitamin D and in injectables in place of olive oil. Ground nut oil depressed whole blood clotting time in human volunteers.

STARCH

Synonym : Amylum

Biological source : Starch of pharmaceutical use consists of polysaccharide granules. These are obtained from mature grains of

(i) Maize, *Zea mays* Linn.
(ii) Wheat, *Triticum aestivum*

(iii) Rice, *Oryza sativa* Linn.

(iv) Oats, *Avena sativa*, these grains are member of a family *Gramineae*. Starch is also obtained from the tubers of potato i.e. *Solanum tuberosum* Linn. (*Solanaceae*)

Geographical source : Starch is commercially produced in tropical and sub-tropical countries. Argentina, U.S.A., China, India and Japan are the main starch producing countries of the world.

Preparation : A number of methods are used for preparation of starch, it depends upon the nature of raw material used and the degree of purity of starch desired. As starch is present in the endosperm of cereal grains, so they should be freed from oil, cell debris, soluble and insoluble proteins (gluten and glutelins). But in case of potato starch it should be freed from vegetable tissue mineral salts and soluble proteins.

Preparation of wheat starch : A dough is prepared by adding water to wheat flour. It is kept for one or two hours to the gluten to swell. After that, the dough is constantly shaken with water on grooved rollers. The starchy liquid falls down which is separated by centrifugation, then starch is washed and dried.

Preparation of potato starch : Potatoes are washed and freed from dust, soil and other organic and inorganic matters. They are crushed in a rasping machine or in a disintegrator of the hammer mill type. Water is added to remove cell debris by rotary sieves. The white milky liquid falls down which contains starch, soluble proteins, mineral salts and some cell debris. On standing the starch is separated more rapidly and is purified by centrifugation. The starch thus obtained is washed with water and dried.

Preparation of maize starch : First of all the maize grain is softened by soaking it in an aqueous solution of sulphurous acid (0.2%) at 50°C for about 2 to 3 days. In this way the disintegration takes place and the embryo or grains are readily liberated and permitting the separation of starch from fibre. The softened grain is crushed between rollers which partially crush the grains and liberate most of the starch from the embryo or grains, then water is added and milky liquid is filtered through sieves. In this way the cell debris and glutens are separated through starch, as starch is heavier than gluten. The germs are continuously separated from the suspension by liquid cyclones (hydrocyclones) and it is used in the preparation of germ oils. The germ oil is rich in vitamins and possesses unsaturated fatty acids like linolenic and linoleic acids.
The starchy milky liquid contains some proteins which are separated by the use of special starch purification centrifuges. This method is applied again and again till the protein is totally free from starch. Now the starch is washed and dried.

Preparation of rice starch : Broken pieces of rice are softened by shaking in 0.4% sodium hydroxide solution. This causes disintegration and dissolution of insoluble protein gluten. The softened grain is crushed and the ground material is mixed with water. Starch is separated by standing or by centrifugation. The damp starch is cut into blocks and dried at 50-60°C for two days. The outer layer of starch are brown in colour which are scraped from the blocks and dried for 13 to 14 days at lower temperature, then packed.

Macroscopical characters : Starch is found in irregular, angular masses or in form of white powder, it is insoluble in cold water and forms a colloidal solution on boiling. After cooling,the starch solution becomes translucent jelly. When starch is boiled with water, starch granules swell to small several times their original size and become contorted in shape and ultimately burst, thus gelatinization takes place and the process is termed as gelatinization. Starch granules also undergo gelatinization, when treated with concentrated solution of calcium or zinc chloride, chloralhydrate or caustic potash. Potato and wheat starch are slightly acidic while rice starch is slightly alkaline but maize starch is almost neutral.

Table 7.2 : Microscopy of some starches

Variety	Size(μm)	Form	Hilum and striation
1. Wheat	2-45	smaller granules are globular while larger granules are lenticular.	Hilum centrally present, seldom cleft. Concentric but faint striation.
2. Potato	3-110	Simple granules hatchet, wedge or mussel shaped.	Hilum in the form of a point; at the narrower end of the granules and eccentric. Striations concentric and well marked.
3. Rice	2-10	Polyhedral with sharp angles.Compound granules are present with an angular out line.	Hilum minute, centrally pointed. Striations absent.
4. Maize	5 - 25	Polyhedral with blunt angles or rounded.	Hilum - triangular distinct and centrally pointed, 2 to 5 stellate cleft. Striations - absent

Microscopical characters : Microscopically starch granules vary in size from 2 μm to 110 μm. The refractive index of starch is about 1.5. The starch granules contain a central eccentric hilum and striations or concentric rings. The hilum appears as a darker or lighter point, rounded dot or of a simple, curved or multiple cleft. In small starch granules the hilum is not clearly distinguishable. The starch granules are also characterized by the presence or absence of well defined striations.

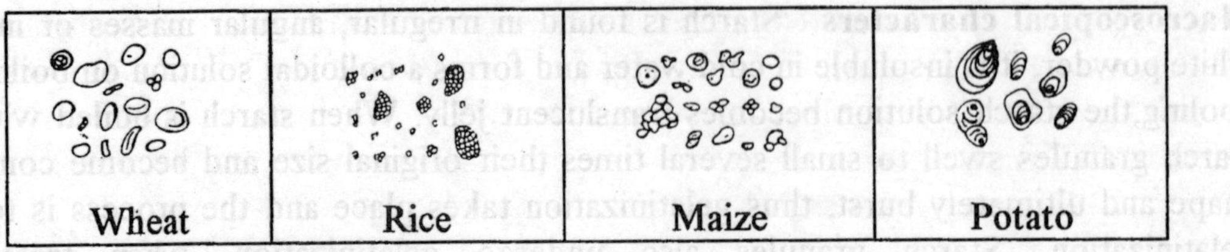

Fig. 7.44 : Starches

Chemical constituents : Starch contains generally a mixture of two polysaccharides, amylopectin (α - amylose) and amylose (β-amylose) .

Amylopectin : It is the main constituent of most of the starches (more than 80%) and is present in outer parts of granules. It contains both stright chained and branched glucose units. It is insoluble in water and is responsible for gelatinizing property. It gives bluish-black colour with iodine solution.

Amylose : Most starches contain 20% amylose . It contains straight chained glucose units and is present in inner part of the granules. It is soluble in water and produces blue colour with iodine solution.

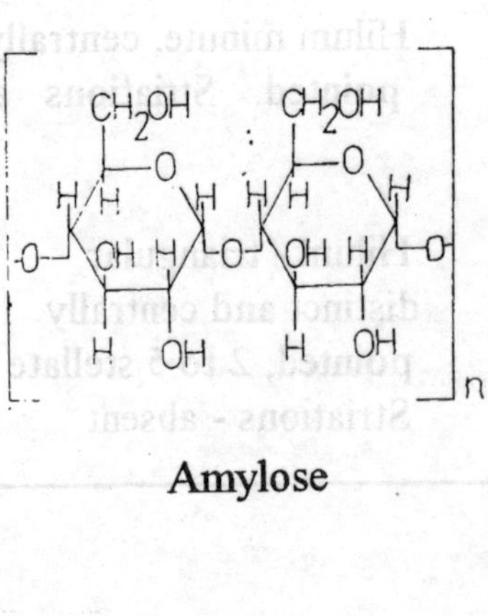

Amylose

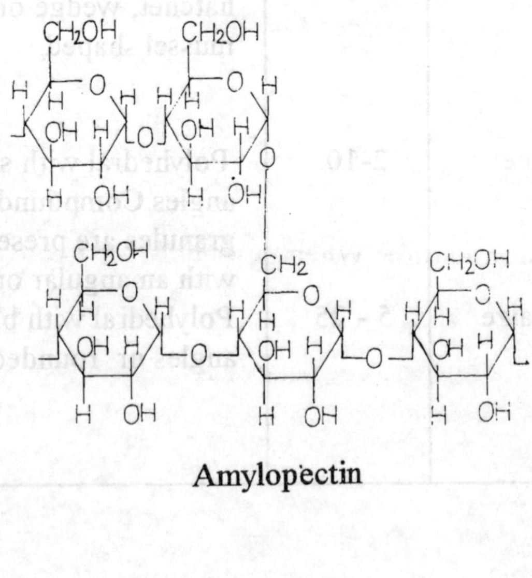

Amylopectin

Uses : Internally, starch is used as mild astringent, nutritive, demulcent, protective and absorbent, externally it is used as skin emollient, absorbent, in dusting powders, ointments and in suppositories. It is used as an antidote in the treatment of iodine poisoning. Starch is also used as a tablet disintegrating agent and diluent.

Identification tests

1. Disslove starch powder in water and boil it in water bath, a viscous translucent Jelly is formed.
2. It gives Molish's test for carbohydrates.
3. Starch solution forms a deep blue colour on addition of iodine solution. The colour disappears on warming and reappears on cooling.

KAOLIN

Synonyms : Kaolinite, China clay.

Source : Kaolin is a pure clay produced by weathering and decomposition from Felspar of granite.

Geographical source : It is mainly found in England. France, USA and India. In India, it is available in Thane (Maharastra), Garo hill (Assam). Rajmahal hill (Bihar). Ranigunj (Bengal),, etc.

Description : Kaolin is fine soft clay, white or white with a yellowish tint in colour. It is insoluble in water. Kaolin is not affected by dilute acids and alkali but strong HCl partially decomposes the kaolin. Heating with H_2SO_4, converts it into insoluble silica and aluminium sulphate. Dry kaolin is odourless but moist kaolin gives clay like odour. Kaolin has slight earthy taste.

Light kaolin : It consists of very fine particles, showing brownian movement. It is colloidal in nature. When suspended in water forms sticky mass. It is used for internal preparation.

Heavy Kaolin : It consists of fine particles when treated with water produced a plastic fluid that is less sticky than light kaolin. When it is suspended in water, settle down and leaving clear supernatant liquid.

Chemical constituents : Kaolin is almost pure aluminium silicate ($Al_2O_3.2SiO_2.2H_2O$). Small traces of Ca, Mg and Fe are also present. The presence of iron gives yellowish tint to kaolin powder.

Standards

Density	:	2.3
Fusion point	:	1700° to 1800°C

Uses : Light kaolin is used in the treatment of certain gastric and intestinal infections because it adsorbs the endotoxins. Heavy kaolin is used as clearing agent, filtering agent, dusting powder, in making poultices and as an excipient in the pills.

Chemical test : It gives blue mass in charcoal cobalt nitrate test due to presence of alumina.

PECTIN

Source : Pectin is a complex carbohydrate found in nature in the middle lamellae of plant cell walls. The middle lamella is pectic in nature containing pectose, pectin, pectic acid and calcium pectate. These are obtained from the inner portion of rind of citrus fruits like lemon, orange,, etc. and vegetative matter like sunflower, papaya, guavas, mangoes, etc..

Geographical source : On commercial scale it is manufactured in USA, India, Switzerland and some other European countries. These countries are producing pectin from citrus peels or apple pomace.

Preparation : Pectin present in the cell wall is insoluble in nature known as protopectin when the fruit pulp is treated with dilute acid at 90°C and pH 3.5-4 for 30 minutes. The solution is filtered and alcohol is added to filtrate, pectin precipitates out. This is separated and dried under reduced pressure.

Characters : Pectin is available as coarse or fine powder. It is yellowish white in colour, taste is mucilaginous and odourless. With water it froms colloidal solution. It is mildly acidic in nature. It is stable at slightly acid pH and depolymerisation takes place in strong acidic or basic conditions.

Chemical constituents : Chemically pectins are polygalacturonic acids in which some of the carboxyl groups are present as methyl esters. Pectic acid is an aldobionic acid which on hydrolysis give galacturanic acid, arabinose, galactose, and methyl pectose. Pectin is a methoxy ester of pectic acid. It is hydrolysed by pectase or dilute caustic soda, produces pectic acid and methyl alcohol. Pectin is soluble in water. Pectin with sugar and acid forms jelly. Pectose is a glycosidal component of pectin and cellulose. It is insoluble in water. Alkaline hydrolysis of pectose forms pectin and cellulose.

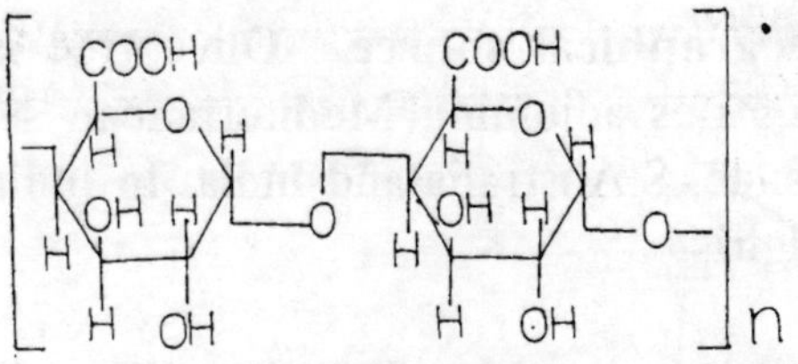

Pectic acid

Standards

Ash value	:	≤ 4%
Acid insoluble ash	:	≤ 0.4%
Loss on drying	:	≤ 10%
Microbial Limit	:	1 gm.is free from *Salmonellae*.

Uses : Pectin is used in the treatment of diarrhoea because it absorbs the toxins from digestive tract. Pectin is stable in acidic medium hence it may be used in combination with gelatin as an encapsulating agent in sustain release formulations. It is also used as thickening, emulsifying and gelling agent. Currently it is widely used in cosmetic preparations.

Chemical tests

1. 10% aqueous solution of pectin forms a stiff gel.
2. To 1% aqueous solution of pectin, add 2% aqueous solution of potassium hydroxide. A transparent gel is formed within 15 minutes, shake well the gel with dilute hydrochloric acid, a gelatinous precipitate is formed which becomes white on boiling.

OLIVE OIL [Salad Oil]

Synonyms : Oleum olivae, Sweet oil, Salad oil.

Biological source : Olive oil is a fixed oil obtained by expression from pericarp of the ripe fruits of *Olea europoea* Linn. This is a member of *oleaceae* family.

Geographical source : Olive tree is native of Palestine. It is also distributed in the countries adjoining Mediterranean sea. The oil is produced in California, Spain, Italy, France, S.Australia and India. In India, plant is found in Himachal Pradesh, Kashmir and Nilgiris.

Collection and preparation : The olive is an evergreen tree, about 12 metre in height. It gives drupaceous fruits about 2-3 cm in length. The unripen fruit is green in colour and turns to purple when ripe. The mesocarp is filled with oil. The fruit is collected in the month of December to April by shaking and beating the tree.

The ripe fruits are crushed in an edge runner mill so that endocarp of fruit break. The pulps are packed in bags and pressure is mounted by screw press. The oil is collected and water is added to remove water soluble impurities. The oily layer is skimmed off and filtered. The first quality oil is called *'Virgin oil'*. The marc is again expressed and finally send for solvent extraction. The second extracted oil is edible oil and last quality of oil is technical quality oil.

Character : Medicinal olive oil (Virgin oil) is pale yellow or greenish yellow liquid. It has slight characteristic odour and bland taste. Olive oil is slightly soluble in alcohol and soluble in carbon disulphide, chloroform and ether.

Chemical constituents : Olive oil contains glycerides of oleic acid (75-85%), palmitic acid, stearic acid, linoleic acid and arachidic acid. It also contains phytosterol, tocopherol and squalene.

Standards

Iodine value	:	79 to 88
Saponification value	:	190-195
Density	:	0.910-0.915 gm/ml.

Uses : Olive oil has demulcent, emollient and laxative properties. It is used as a vehicle for oily parenteral preparations. It is also used in the preparation of lubricants, plasters, textiles, soaps, cosmetics and sulphonated oils.

LANOLIN

Synonyms : Wool fat, Adeps lanae.

Biological source : Lanolin is a purified, anhydrous fat obtained from the secretion of sebaceous glands of *Ovis aries* Linn. This is the member of *Bovidae* family.

Preparation : The crude lanolin is present in the raw wool. The cut wool is wash with alkali or soap and an emulsion is formed in water. Raw lanolin is separated by cracking the emulsion with sulphuric acid. Fatty acids are dissolved in lower layer and wool grease floats. Lanolin is purified by treatment with bleaching agent sodium peroxide and by centrifuging with water.

Characters : Lanolin is a pale yellow tenacious, mass having characteristic odour, and bland taste. It is insoluble in water but soluble in chloroform and ether. It is not saponified by aqueous alkali but saponification takes place with alcoholic alkali solution. Anhydrous wool fat or lanolin consists 70% of wool fat.

Chemical constituents : The main constituents of wool fat are cholesterol and isocholesterol, carnaubic, lanopalmitic, oleic and other fatty acids. The wool alcohol is unsaturated monohydric alcohols of formula $C_{27}H_{45}OH$, both free and combined with carnaubic, lanoceric, lanopalmitic and other fatty acids. It also contains aliphatic alcohols such as cetyl, ceryl and carnaubyl alcohols obtained by saponification of crude lanolin and separations of alcohol fractions.

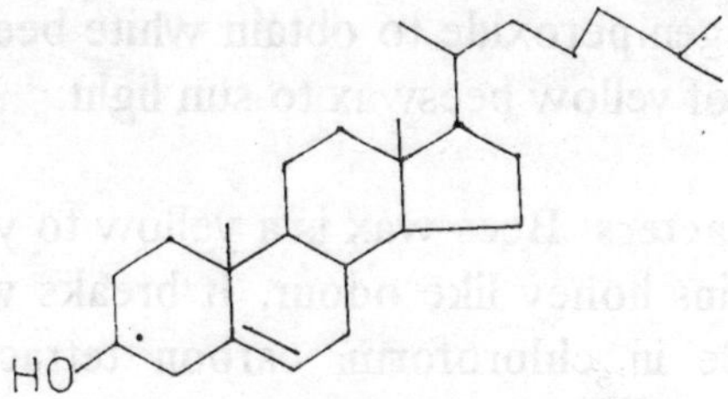

Cholesterol

Standards

Acid value	:	≤ 1
Saponification value	:	94 to 106
Iodine value	:	18-32
Ash value	:	≤ 0.15%
Melting point	:	34-40°C.

Uses : Lanolin is used as absorption ointment base. It is a common ingredient used as an emollient base in various ointments and cream preparations.

BEESWAX

Synonyms : Yellow bees wax; White beeswax; Cera flava; Cera alba.

Biological source : Beeswax is separated from the honeycomb of the hive bee, *Apis* *mellifica* and other species of *Apis* by purification. The hive bee is the member of *Apidae* family.

Geographical source : Beeswax is prepared in California, Chile, Africa, Madagascar, France, Italy, West Africa and India.

Preparation : Combs and capping of honey comb is kept in the boiling water, for melting. The water soluble impurities are dissolved and other impurities sinks in the water. On cooling, the melted wax get solidify and floats on the water surface. Wax is removed and process is repeated several times to get pure yellow beeswax. This is bleached with charcoal, potassium permanganate, chlorine, ozone, chromic acid or hydrogen peroxide to obtain white beeswax. Natural bleaching is done by exposing thin layer of yellow beeswax to sun light.

Characters: Bees-wax is a yellow to yellowish brown or white soft plastic solid mass. It contains honey like odour. It breaks with granular fracture. It is insoluble in water but soluble in chloroform, carbon tetrachloride, benzene, ether, carbon disulphide, hot alcohol and volatile oils.

Chemical constituents: Beeswax mainly contains myricin (myricyl palmitate)-80% ;free cerotic acid (about 15%) and small quantity of melissyl sterate, melissic acid, hydrocarbons, higher alcohols and ceroleine. Pollen and propolis are responsible for yellow colour of bees-wax.

Standards

Acid value	:	5 - 8
Sap. value	:	90-103
Ester value	:	80-95
Density	:	0.958-0.967gm/ml.
Melting point	:	60-65°C

Uses: Bees-wax is used in the preparation of cosmetics, suppository bases, ointments, cerates, wax paper, candles, shoe polishes, molding of artificial fruits.

ACACIA

Synonyms : Gum Arabic; Gum Acacia.

Vernacular name : Sans: Sneta khadira , Punjab and Rajasthan : Kumata, Gujarat : Garadio - babul.

Biological source: Acacia gum is a dried gummy exudate obtained from the stem and branches of *Acacia senegal* wild and some other species of *Acacia.* It is a member of *mimosaceae(leguminosae)* family.

Geographical source: The plant *A. senegal* is available in Africa, Sudan and North-Western India.

Collection: *Acacia senegal* is a thorny tree, 6 metre in height. Generally gum is obtained from about 6 year old plant. Some amount of gum exudes from the cracking of the bark. A transverse incision is made on the bark and loosen bark is pealed off, above and below the incision. The incision is made carefully so that cambium and xylem are not injured. Due to injury, gum is exuded till new phloem is formed, which takes about a month. The tears of gum are formed in the exposed surface & are collected every week till exudation of gum ceases. The gum is garbled to keep it free from sand and vegetable debris and at the same time exposed to sun light for 3-4 month to bleach. In these process gum losses its weight about 30%, minute cracks formed on the tears and surface becomes semiopaque. The tears are graded on the basis of external appearance, packed and send to the market.

Characters: Bleached acacia is available in the rounded or ovoid tears about 1-3 cm in diameter. The outer surface bears numerous cracks and is opaque in appearance. It is white or pale yellow in colour, breaks with a glassy fracture and is odourless. Taste is bland or mucilaginous. It is freely soluble in water and forms acidic viscous solution but insoluble in alcohol and other organic solvents.

Chemical constituents: Acacia contains mainly arabin that is a mixture of calcium, magnesium and potassium salt of arabic acid. In this calcium salt is found in abundance. Arabic acid on hydrolysing with dilute sulphuric acid forms L-rhamnose, L-arabinose, aldobionic acid and d-galactose. It also contains enzyme oxydase, pectinase, peroxidase and diastase. The water content is about 14%.

Uses: Acacia gum is used as an emulsifying agent, suspending agent, emollient, demulcent, binder and adhesive in tablets and lozenges. The gum acacia solution is given as a plasma substitute in hemolysis. This is incompatible with readily oxidizable substances like phenol, cod liver oil,, etc. It is also used in lithographic printing and in the sizing of paper and cloth. It is also applied externally on inflammations, such as burns, sores and nodules in leprosy.

Table 7.3 : Chemical tests for some unorganised drugs

Chemical test	Acacia	Agar	Guar gum	Tragacanth
1. Solubility	Soluble in water	In soluble in cold water, swells but soluble in hot water	Soluble in water	Soluble in water
2. With lead subacetate	White ppts. (heavy)	—	—	Slight ppts.
3. With lead acetate	Negative	—	Flocculent	ppts.
4. With aqueous potassium hydro-oxide	—	Cannary yellow colour	—	Cannary yellow colour
5. With ruthenium red	Negative	Pink colour	Negative	Negative
6. With barium chloride	Negative	White ppts.	Negative	Negative
7. With iodine solution	Negative	Deep crimson to brown colour	Olive-green colour	Green colour
8. With guiacum resin in alcohol	Blue colour	Negative	Negative	Negative
9. Fehling's test.	Red ppts.	Red ppts.	Red ppts.	Red ppts.

Substituents or Adulterants

(1) **Indian Acacia Gum** : It is obtained from *Acacia arabica*. This is a member of *mimosaceae*(*leguminosae*) family. Its Hindi name is babul. The gum is yellow to dark brown in colour and resembles with gum acacia. The solution of Indian acacia is dextro rotatory and Acacia gum is levo rotatory. The Indian acacia is inferior in quality.

(2) **Ghattigum (Indian gum)**: It is obtained from *Anogeissus latifolia* (family-*combretaceae*). The gum contain tears in various colour. Some tears are vermiform showing few cracks in the surface. Its viscosity is in between that of **Acacia** and **stericulia** gum.

TRAGACANTH

Biological source: Tragacanth is a dried gummy exudate obtained by incision on stem of *Astragalus gummifer* Labill and other species of *Astragalus*. This is a member of the *papilionaceae* (*fabaceae*) family.

Geographical source: Tragacanth is a native of Southern and Eastern Europe. The plant is widely distributed in Iran, Afganisthan, Iraq, Syria, Anatolia and India. In India, few species of *Astragalus* are available in Garhwal, Shimla, Kashmir and hilly region of Kumaon.

Collection & preparation: Tragacanth plant is a small, branching, thorny shrub about 1 metre in height. Incisions are made on the stems of two year old plant; gum exudes and dries. The shape of gum may be flat, ribbon like or vermiform depending upon the type of incisions. Gum is produced by the transformation of medullary rays and cell wall of pith and process is called gummosis. The gum is collected every week and new incisions are made. These gums are collected and packed.

Characters: Tragacanth occurs in thin, curved flattened ribbon shaped flakes. It is horny in appearance, translucent, colourless or pale yellow. The gum contains numerous concentric, longitudinal and transverse ridges. It indicates successive exudation and solidification of gum. The gum break with a short fracture. It is odourless and almost tasteless, gum swells when soaked in cold water forming a gelatinous mass. Tragacanth is insoluble in alcohol and organic solvents.

Chemical constituents : The gum tragacanth is a polysaccharide. It contains water soluble component tragacanthic acid, neutral polysaccharides and water insoluble component bassorin. The tragacanthic acid contains galactouronic acid, xylose, galactose and fucose; neutral polysaccharide contains arabinose and galactose. The bassorin is responsible for gelatinising and swelling properties. The other constituents are starch, cellulose, nitrogenous substance and water but enzyme oxidase is absent.

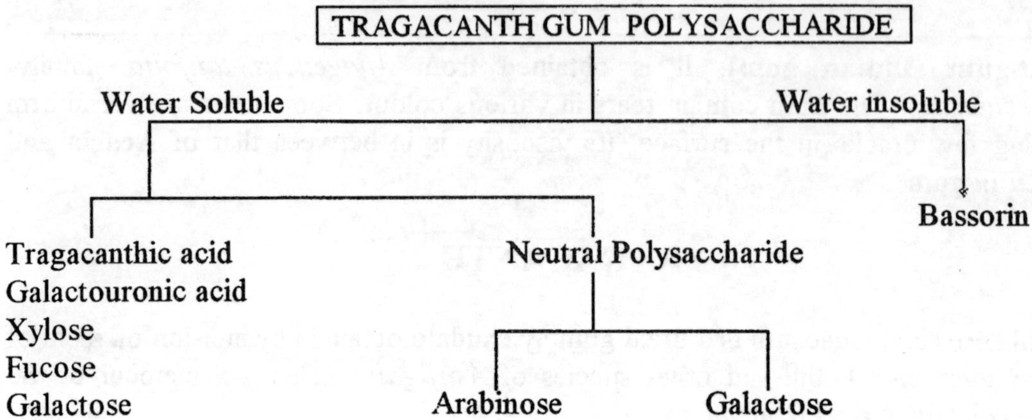

Standards:

Moisture	: ≤	1.5%
Foreign organic matter	: ≤	1%
Sulphated ash	: ≤	4%

Uses: Tragacanth is used as an suspending and emulsifying agent for oils. It is also used as a stabilizer, thickening agent in various pharmaceutical preparations due to its demulcent and emollient properties, it is used in cosmetic preparations. It is used in adhesive and in textile industry. It is resistant to acid hydrolysis & can be used in acidic medium

Chemical test : See table 7.3

SODIUM ALGINATE

Biological source: Sodium alginate is a salt of alginic acid. Alginic acid is prepared from brown algae of the *Phaeophyceae* family. The main species of this seeweeds are *Ascophyllum, Laminaria* and *Fucus*.

Geographical source : These algae are found on the coast of U.S.A., Japan, Canada, Australia, U.K., South Africa, Norway, China and India. In India, it is available on coast of Gujarat.

Preparation: The seeweeds are dried washed with dilute acid to remove most of the salt present with seeweeds. This mass is chopped and bruised in the hammer mill. The prepared seeweed is macerated with sodium carbonate solution at pH 10, liquid is filtered while hot and calcium chloride solution is added. The precipitate of calcium alginate floats on the liquid, filtered, treated with hydrochloric acid and alginic acid is collected. This acid is neutralized with sodium carbonate to form sodium alginate.

Characters : Sodium alginate is a white or cream colour powder, odourless, tasteless, freely soluble in hot and cold water, but insoluble in alcohol, ether & chloroform. A solution of sodium alginate(4 %) gives a thick viscous fluid. The solution dose not gel on cooling and is not coagulated by heat.

Chemical constituents: It is a sodium salt of alginic acid which is composed of straight chain of D-mannuronic acid and L-guluronic acid (Polyuronic acid).

Uses: Sodium alginate is used as an emulsifying, deflocculating, gelling, thickening, stabilizing and film and filament forming agent in textile, rubber, paint, food, cosmetics, dental and pharmaceutical industries. It is used in formulation of creams,pastes, jellies, ointment, and tablets in pharmaceutical and cosmetic industries. It is also useful as homeostatic.

Chemical tests

(1) Solution of sod. alginate is precipitated by the addition of calcium chloride sol.

(2) 1% solution of sodium alginate forms heavy gelatinous precipitate with dilute sulphuric acid.

AGAR

Synonyms: Japanese Isinglass, Agar-Agar.

Biological source: Agar is the dried and bleached colloidal concentrate substance obtained from decoction of various species of red algae like *Gelidium*, *Pterocladi* and *Gracilaria.* The first two algae are the member of *Gelidiaceae* family and another is a member of *Gracilariaceae* family.

Geographical source: Agar is obtained mainly from Japan, Korea, South Africa, U.S.A. China, Indonesia and India.

Collection and preparation of Agar : The Algae are collected from may to october in Japan and manufacturing of Agar is done in winter. The red algae is grown in the sea, on the support of poles on which they develop. These poles are withdrawn, algae is removed, dried, beaten and shaken to remove shell and sand. The algae is bleached by exposure to sun light or washing with water. The washing with water removes the associated salts. Then these are boiled with acidulated water (one part algae with 55-60 parts water) for few hours. Mucilaginous mass is filtered while hot then cooled. The jelly is formed and cut into bars. These bars are forced through wire netting and strips are formed. These are dried in sun light and moisture is removed by freezing and thawing. Finally Agar is dried at 35°C.

Characters: Agar is found as strips and coarse powder or flakes. Strips are yellowish white in colour, translucent; faint or salty mucilaginous taste and insoluble in cold water but swells. On boiling with water, 0.7%-1% Agar forms colloidal fluid and forms jelly on cooling.

Chemical constituent: Agar is a heterogeneous polysaccharide containing two principal constituents agarose and agaropectin. Agarose is a neutral galactosepolymer (free from sulphate) responsible for gel strength . Agaropectin contains glucuronic acid, pyruvic acid and ester sulphate that are responsible for viscosity of Agar. It also contains traces of protein and nitrogen but does not give any evidence for presence of ammonia, when it is heated with soda lime.

Standards

Water soluble ash	: ≤ 1%
Sulphated ash	: ≤ 5%
Foreign organic matter	: ≤ 1%
Starch	: should not present.

Uses : Agar is widely used in the preparation of culture media. It is used as an emulsifying agent, in chronic constipation, jellies, confectionery and cosmetics. Agarose gel is used for protein separation in electrophoretic separation . It is also used as a clarifying agent in the preparation of beverages and sizing medium for paper and silk industries.

Chemical test : See table 7.3.

GUAR GUM

Synonym : *Cyamopsis psoraloides* DC

Vernacular name : Hindi - Gowar; Sans. - Bakuch; Tam. - Kothaveray; Tel. - Gorchi Kudu.

Biological source: Guar gum is derived from ground endosperm of seeds of *Cyamopsis tetragonolobus* (L) Taub. The plant is a member of *leguminosae* family.

Geographical source: Guar is commercially grown in India, Pakistan and United States of America and to a limited extent in South Africa, Brazil and Australia. In India, Rajasthan is the major guar-gum growing state.

Characters: Guar gum is a white or yellowish white free flowing powder .It is odourless and contains a characteristic taste. It is soluble in cold and hot water and forms neutral colloidal solution. Guar gum is insoluble in alcohol, oils hydrocarbons, ketones, etc.Guar gum contains much thickening capacity than that of starch.

Chemical constituents: Guar gum contains glactomannan (high molecular wt. hydrocolloidal polysaccharide) which is made of galactan and mannan unit through glycosidic linkage. On hydrolysis guargum produces a glactose and mannose. It also contains protein in small amount.

Standards

Ash	:	≤ 1%
Acid insoluble ash	:	≤ 0.5%
L.O.D.	:	≤ 8%

Uses: Guar gum is used as binding agent, disintegrating agent; emulsifying agent thickening and suspending agent and dietary building agent and guar gum also reduces blood glucose concentration in diabetic patients and serum concentration in hyper lipidaemia. It is a good flocculent and is used in many mining applications, which results in rapid settling, reduces the friction and modifies the flow. It is a good emulsion stabilizer and a protective colloid.

Chemical test : See table 7.3

GELATIN

Synonyms: Gelatinum

Biological source: Gelatin is a reversible gel forming protein derived from the hot water treatment of specific animal tissues like skin, bones, tendons, ligament of ox (*Bos taurus* Linn), sheep (*Ovis aries* Linn), etc. These animals are member of *Bovidae* family.

Preparation: Preparations of gelatin depend upon starting material. In the preparation, insoluble collagens are converted into soluble gelatin. It is purified and concentrated to a solid mass under reduce pressure and this gelatin is allowed to set in shallow-tray. These are kept in drying room where moisture is removed successively at temperatures of about 30, 40, 50, & 60°C. Drying takes place in few weeks.

Characters: Gelatin is found as granular powder and strips. It is colourless or pale yellow, translucent and breaks with short fracture. It has little odour and taste. Gelatin is insoluble in cold water but swells and absorbs considerable amount of water. It is soluble in hot water and its 2% solution forms jelly on cooling. Long boiling reduces gelatinizing property of gelatin. This property is the measurement of it's quality and is called Jelly strength or Bloom strength. It is stable in dry condition but produces bacteria in moist condition.

Chemical constituents : Gelatin mainly consists of protein glutin, which on hydrolysis gives a mixture of aminoacids like glycine (25.5%), alanine, leucine, aspartic acid, arginine, lysine, leucine, isoleucine, valine, tyrosine, cystine, cysteine, glutamic acid, arginine, etc. Adhesive property of gelatin is due to the presence of glutin. It is an incomplete protein due to absence of tryptophan. Chondrin is a gelatinizing compound of gelatin.

Uses: Gelatin is used to prepare suppositories, pills coating, pastes, enteric coated capsules, gelatin sponge, adhesive, etc. It is used in preparation of bacteriological culture media. High bloom strength gelatin is used for manufacturing of gelatin capsule.
It is also used as suspending, clarifying, binding agent and as a plasma expander or blood plasma substitute .

Identification tests

(1) When gelatin is heated with soda lime in dry test tube, ammonia is evolved due to the presence of nitrogenous compound in gelaten.
(2) Gelatin gives buff white ppt. with tannic acid solution.
(3) Gelatin gives yellow ppt. with trinitrophenol in aqueous solution.
(4) Gelatin gvies white ppt. with Millon's reagent which turns brick red on boiling.

7 - U. MISCELLANEOUS DRUGS

LIQUORICE OR GLYCYRRHIZA

Vernacular name : Hindi - Mulhatti; Sans. - Madhuka; Bengali - Jashtimadhu; Mar. - Jestha Madhu; Tam. - Atimaduram.

Biological source : Liquorice consists of dried roots and rhizomes (stolons) of *Glycyrrhiza glabra* Linn. and other species of glycyrrhiza. The plant is a member of *leguminosae (Fabaceae or Papilionaceae)* family.

Geographical source : The plant is cultivated in England, Spain, Iran, Iraq, Afghanistan, Germany, France, U.S.A, India, etc. In India, this plant is cultivated in Punjab, Sub Himalayan tract and Andaman Islands.

Cultivation & collection : Liquorice is a perennial herb, about 1 metre in height. It is mainly cultivated in moist soil, near the bank of rivers, Sunny climate and suitable manure favour the growth of plant. It is cultivated by planting root cuttings and rhizomes containing aerial buds. Roots & rhizomes are dug out after 4 years, Buds and rootlets are removed and drug is first dried in the sun light and then in ovens.

Morphology : Liquorice occurs as peeled or unpeeled rhizomes and roots. The unpeeled rhizome is dark brown to yellowish brown externally while internal surface (Peeled) is yellowish in colour. It is straight & cylindrical branched and about 20-50 cm in length, 1-2 cm in diameter. It has a faint characteristic odour, sweet in taste and fracture is fibrous. The unpeeled drug contains longitudinal wrinkles.

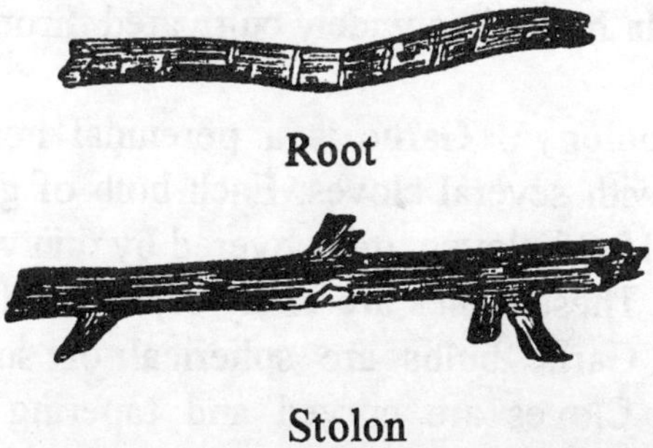

Fig. 7.45 : Glycyrrhiza (Liquorice)

Chemical constituents : It contain triterpenoid saponin glycoside known as glycyrrhizin (6-14%). Glycyrrhizin is 150 times sweeter than sugar. This on hydrolysis produces glycyrrhetinic acid and 2 moles of glucuronic acid. It also contains aspargine, sugar, resin, fat, etc. The yellow

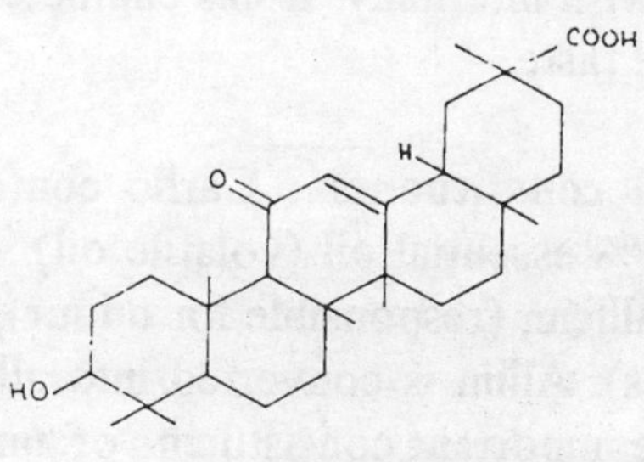

Glycyrrhetinic acid

colour of liquorice is due to the presence of flavonoids like liquiritin, isoliquiritin (charcoal). It also contains other constituents like bitter principle glycycamarin, umbelliferon(coumarin), starch,, etc.

Standards

Extractive value (water soluble)	:	≥ 25%
Total ash	:	≤ 10%
Acid insoluble ash	:	≤ 2%

Uses : Liquorice is used as an expectorant and demulcent,. It is also used for gastric and duodenal ulcers. It is used as a sweetening agent, antispasmodic, antiinflammatory and in Addison's disease. It is not used in alkaline media.

GARLIC

Vernacular name : Hindi & Guj. - Lasan; Sans. - Lashuna; Tel. & Mal. - Velluli.

Biological source : Garlic consists of ripe bulbs of *Allium sativum* Linn. It is a member of *Liliaceae* family.

Geographical source : Garlic is cultivated in central Asia, U.S.A, Southern Europe and India. In India, it is widely cultivated throughout the country.

Morphology : Garlic is a perennial herb containing bulbs with several cloves. Each bulb of garlic contains about 15-25 cloves. It is covered by thin whitish papery scales. These scales are easily separated from bulb and clove. Garlic bulbs are spherical or subspherical in shape. Cloves are curved and tapering at base and apex. It is whitish pink or yellowish white externally and yellowish internally. It has characteristic, alliaceous odour and taste.

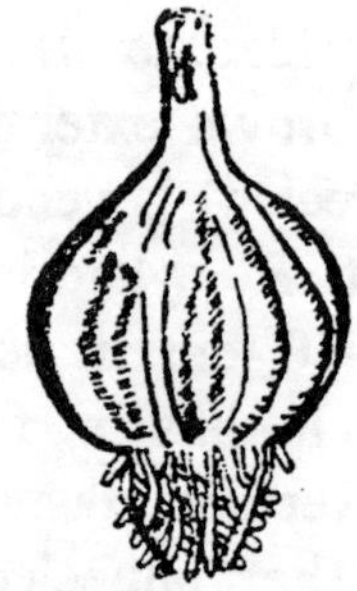

Fig. 7.46 : Garlic (*Allium sativum*) Bulb

Chemical constituents : Garlic contains carbohydrates, proteins, fats, mucilage and 0.06-0.10% essential oil (volatile oil). The volatile oil is the main active constituent. It contains allicin, (responsible for odour), allyl propyl disulphide, diallyl di-sulphide & alliin (odourless). Alliin is converted into allicin by action of enzyme allinase. Ajoene is also one of the important consistuents of garlic formed by self condensation of allicin.

$$CH_2=CH-CH_2-S-\underset{\underset{O}{||}}{S}-CH_2CH=CH_2$$

Allicin

$$CH_2=CH-CH_2\underset{\underset{O}{||}}{S}-CH_2-\underset{\underset{NH_2}{|}}{CH}-COOH$$

Alliin

Standards

Total ash	:	$\leq 5.0\%$
Acid insoluble ash	:	$\leq 2.0\%$

Uses : The allicin and alliin are the potent antibacterial ingredients in garlic. The ajoene is an antithromobotic, aphrodisiac, stimulant, chronic bronchitis and in reduction of hypertension, decreases cholesterol level, etc.

PICRORHIZA [Indian Gentian]

Vernacular name : Hindi & Beng. - Kuru; Sans. - Katuka; Tam, Tel. and Mal.- Katukarogani.

Biological source : Picrorhiza consists of dried rhizomes of *Picrorhiza kurroa* Royle ex Benth., cut into small pieces and freed from attached rootlets. It is a member of *scrophulariaceae* family.

Geographical source : Picrorhiza is well distributed in alpine Himalayas from Kashmir to Sikkim. The drug is also available in China.

Morphology : Picrorhiza is a perennial, low hairy herb with perennial woody, bitter rhizome. The rhizomes are 15-25 cmin length and are cut into pieces of 2-4 cm long and 0.3 to 1.0 cm in diameter. The rhizomes are greyish brown in colour. They are cylindrical, straight or slightly curved in shape. These pieces are longitudinally wrinkled and annulated at the tip. The upper and lower surfaces contain some small root scars and scale leaves on both lower and upper surfaces. Fracture is tough, odour slightly unpleasant and taste is bitter.

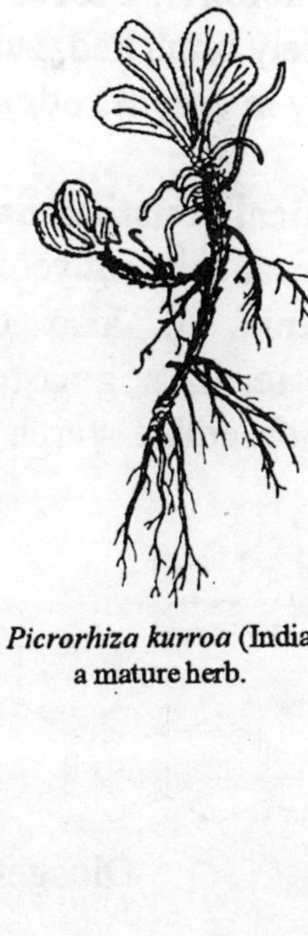

Fig. 7.47 : *Picrorhiza kurroa* (Indian Gentian), a mature herb.

Chemical constituents : Picrorhiza contains a bitter glycoside kutkin, which is a mixture of picroside I, picroside II, and kutkoside. It also contains picrorhizin, kutkiol, kutkisterol, apocynin, d-mannitol, vanillic acid and cathartic acid.

	R	R1	R2
Kutkoside	H	vanilloyl	H
Picroside I	H	H	trans-cinnamoyl
Picroside II	vanilloyl	H	H

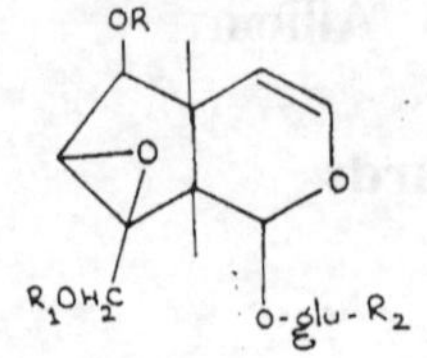

Uses : Picrorhiza is used as a bitter tonic, stomachic, cathartic, antiperiodic, febrifuge, cholagogue and imunogogue. It is also used in the treatment of jaundice, malaria fever, leucoderma and kidney stone.

DIOSCOREA (YAM)

Biological source : It consists of dried tubers of several species of *Dioscorea* like *D. deltoidea, D. composita, D. floribunda, D. spiculiflora, D. prazeri*,, etc. It is a member of *Dioscoreaceae* family.

Geographical source : Dioscorea is available in North America, Mexico, Japan, China, Nepal & India. In India, the plant grows wildly in western Himalayas upto altitude 1000 to 3000 metres.

Morphology : Dioscorea is a climbing plant containing large tuberous roots. These roots are freely branched, surface is rough, bearing fibrous roots. It is slightly brown or whitish creamy in colour, odourless and bitter in taste.

Chemical constituents : The main constituent of dioscorea is steroidal saponin glycoside dioscin and its aglycon is diosgenin. It also contains small quantity of hecogenin, resin botagenin. It also contains alkaloids like dioscorine, levo-epidioscorine, sterols (cholesterol, stigmasterol, ß-sitosterol, etc.) enzyme-sapogenase. Dioscorea contains 75% non edible starch (very bitter in taste).

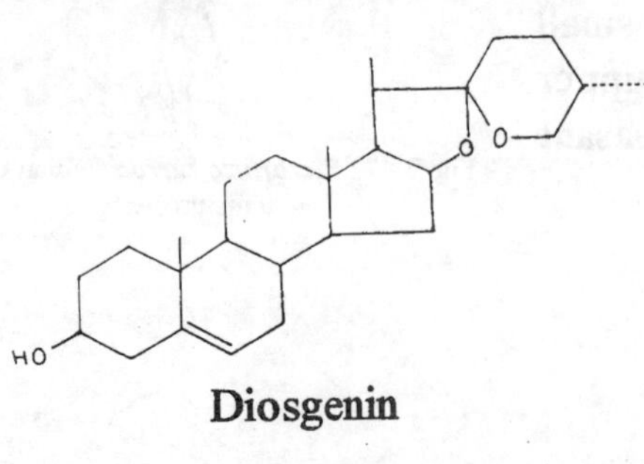

Diosgenin

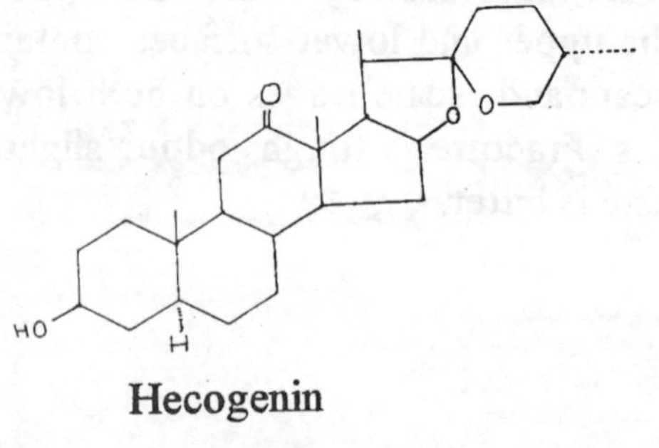

Hecogenin

Standards

Total ash	:	$\leq 7\%$
Acid insoluble ash	:	$\leq 2\%$
Foreign organic matter	:	$\leq 2\%$

Uses : Diosogenin is used as a precursor for the synthesis of many steroidal drugs like corticosteroids, sex hormones and oral contraceptives. The drug is also used in rheumatism.

LINSEED (FLAX SEED)

Vernacular name : Hindi - Alsi, Sans. - Atasi; Beng. - Masina; Tam. - Alivirai.

Biological source : Linseed is a dried ripe seeds of *Linum usitatissimum* Linn. It is a member of *Linaceae* family.

Geographical source : Linseed is cultivated in U.S.A, Canada, England, Russia, Italy, Spain, Greece, Afghanistan and India.

Description : Linseed is an annual herb bearing sky blue and globular capsules about 5-7 mm in diameter containing 10 seeds and five loculi. The plant is cultivated for seeds and fibres. Linseed oil is extracted from the seeds by expression. It contains about 30-35% oil.

Morphology : The seeds are oval flattened and obliquely pointed at one end. They are about 4-6 mm long and 2-2.5 mm broad. The testa is glossy, smooth, brown and finely pitted. Hilum is present at the more acute edge of the seed. The raphae extends as yellowish lines along the acute edge from hilum to the rounded edge of the seed. Endosperm is narrow and surrounded by embryo, which is composed of two large cotyledons and a radical. It is odourless and mucilaginous in taste but becomes oily when chewed. Linseed oil is obtained by cold or hot expression. The oil obtained by cold method is golden yellow while that obtained by hot method is yellowish brown. The oil is neutralized with alkali and bleached with charcoal and fuller's earth. It has a peculiar

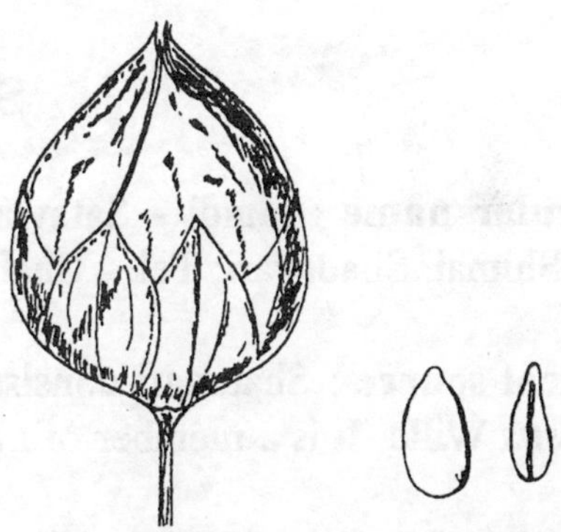

(a) Capsule (b) Seed.

Fig. 7.48 : Linseed (*Linum usitatissimum*)

odour and bland taste. The oil possesses drying property and forms hard varnish. The oil is soluble in organic solvents, turpentine oil and carbon disulphide.

Chemical constituents : Linseed contains about 30-40% fixed oil, 25% proteins, 6% mucilage and a small amount of cyanogenetic glycoside linamarin and enzyme linamerase. The unripe seeds contain starch but after ripening get converted into mucilage, which consists of calcium salt of linseed acids. These on hydrolysis give arabinose, galactose, rhamnose, xylose, galactouronic acid.

Chemical test

(1) Test for mucilage: It gives red colour with ruthenium red.

Standards

Acid value	:	≤ 4%
Sap. value	:	188-195
Iodine value	:	160-200
Unsaponifiable matter	:	≤1.5
Specific gravity	:	0.925-0.935
Refractive Index	:	1.478-1.481

Uses : Crushed linseed is used in poultice and whole seed is used as demulcent. It is used as antibacterial and diuretic. The seed is also used as laxative like Ispaghula and Psyllium. Linseed oil is used as a drying oil in paint and warnish industry.

SHATAVARI

Vernacular name : Hindi - Satawar, Sans. & Beng. - Satamuli; Mar. - Satawarmul; Tam. - Shimai, Shadavari; Tel. - Challagadda; Mal.- Shatavali.

Biological source : Shatavari consists of dried leaves and tuberous roots of *Asparagus racemosus* Willd. It is a member of *Liliaceae* family.

Geographical source : The plant is found throughout tropical Asia, Australia and Africa. In India, it is found throughout the country specially in the tropical and subtropical regions.

Description : The plant is a climber, branched and spinous, undershurb. Roots are tuberous inflorescence is in simple receme; flowers are white; fruit is globose, berry,

4mm in diameter, turns red when ripe. It is cultivated in garden as a potted plant due to its graceful feathery leaves and flowers.

Morphology : Roots are adventitious and fasciculated. The commercial samples of roots are peeled, dried, cylindrical, straight or slightly curved. Roots are swollen in the middle and tapering at apex and base. The fresh drug is smooth but becomes longitudinally wrinkled on drying. Occasionally transverse cracks and scars are present. The drug is white to buff in colour, 5-15 cm in length and 1-2 cm in diametre, fracture is short and irregular. It is odourless and slightly bitter in taste. The dried drug is very hard but swells in water and becomes soft and fleshy. The leaves are linear, green, needle like in shape and bear a tuft of cladodes.

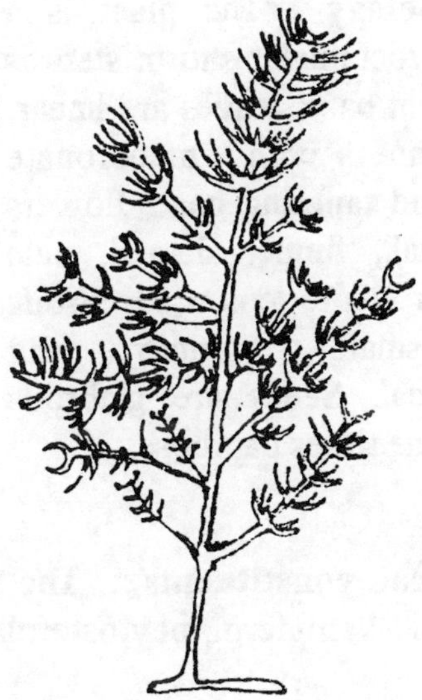

Fig. 7.49 : Shatavari (*Asparagus racemosus*).

Chemical constituents : Shatavari contain steroidal saponin glycosides Shatavarins 1 to 4 (0.1-0.2%). The aglycone moiety of shatavarin is sarsapogenin and glycon moieties are glucose and rhamnose while shatavarin I contain one additional glucose.

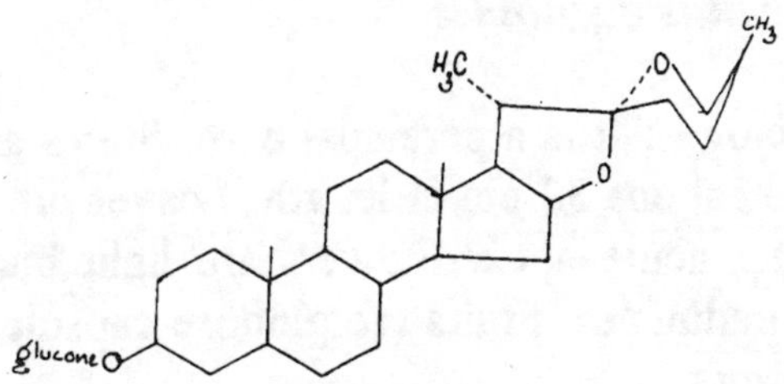

Shatavarin I

SHANKHPUSHPI OR SHANKHAVALI

Biological source : Shankhpushpi consists of whole aerial part of following different plants.

(i) *Convolvulus pluricaulis* (syn. - *C. microphyllus*) (Family - *convolvulaceae*)

(ii) *Evolvulus alsinoides* (syn. - *C. alsinoides*) (Family - *convolvulaceae*)

(iii) *Canscora decussata* (Family -*Gentianaceae*)

Geographical source : The plant is found in all parts of India.

A. *Convolvulus pluricaulis*

Morphology : The plant is a small procumbent shurb, stem is woody at base, leaves are linear, lanceolate, with mucoronate apex and tapering base, flowers are small, funnel shaped, pale pink or white coloured. Fruits are small, smooth and ellipsoidal. Seeds are glabrous and some times papillose.

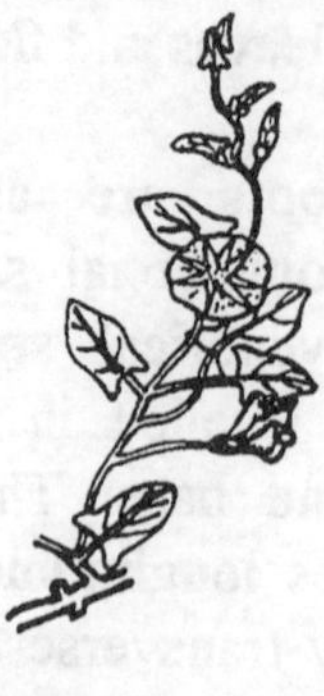

Fig. 7.50 : Shankhpushpi (*Convolvulus pluricaulis*), a mature herb.

Chemical constituents : The drug contains alkaloid shankhpushpine, volatile oil, flavonoid-kampferol, phytosterols, ß sitosterol, carbohydrates-glucose, rhamnose, starch, etc.

B. *Evolvulus alsinoides*

Morphology : It is a perennial herb. Stems are prostrate, cylindrical, wiry, with densely silky hair, about 30 cm in length. Leaves are simple numerous, sessile, hairy, lanceolate containing acute apex. Flowers are light blue in colour, solitary, with, very long and filiform peduncles. Fruits are globose capsules, bearing four walls and four seeds. Seeds are glabrous.

Chemical constituents : The drug contain alkaloid evolvin. It also contains betaine, pentatriacontane, triacontane and ß sitosterol.

C. *Canscora decussata*

Morphology : This is an erect, branching, annual plant about 0.6 metres in height. It bears a four winged stem with decussate branches. Leaves are oblong, lanceolate, acute, about 2.5-3.8 cm in length. The plant bears white flowers with long pedicel, capsules and fruits are larger.

Chemical constituents : The drug contains alkaloids, xanthanons and triterpenoides. The drug also contains a bitter substance and an oleo resin.

Uses : Entire plant and fresh juice of shankhpushpi are used as brain tonic and in various nervine disorders like epilepsy insanity,, etc. The drug is very useful in improving and strengthening memory. Alcoholic extract of drug is used as antiviral activity. Shankhpushpi is also effective in thyrotoxicosis.

PYRETHRUM (Insect flower)

Synonym : *Pyrethrum cinerariaefolium*

Biological source : Pyrethrum flower consists of dried, fully expanded flower heads of *Chrysanthemum cinerariaefolium* Visiana and other species of *chrysanthemum.* It is a member of *compositae* family.

Geographical source : The plant is indigenous to Dalmatia and is widely cultivated in Africa, Brazil, Equador, Japan, Yugoslavia and India. In India, it is cultivated in Jammu and Kashmir, Kulu, Kodaikanal and Kumaon.

Description : Pyrethrum is generally cultivated by seeds and vegetative means. The vegetative propagation is more satisfactory than seed sowing. The plant becomes mature within four months. The fully expanded flower heads are collected, because at this stage maximum active constituents are present. They are dried under sun light for 3-5 days.

Morphology : The commercial sample of pyrethrum is a compressed mass of flower heads. The colour of flower heads is dull brownish yellow. The individual flower head is 0.9 to 1.1 cm in diameter, containing a short peduncle (straited longitudinally) Receptacle is 0.4 to 0.8 cm in diameter and flat and surrounded by involucre of 2-3 rows of brackets. The brackets are lanceolate, hairy and yellowish in colour. Ray florets are 15 to 23 in number. They are white and are arranged on rim of the disc. Disc florets are about 200-300 in number, yellow coloured, tubular and arranged on disc. The flower possesses a characteristic odour and a bitter taste followed by numbness.

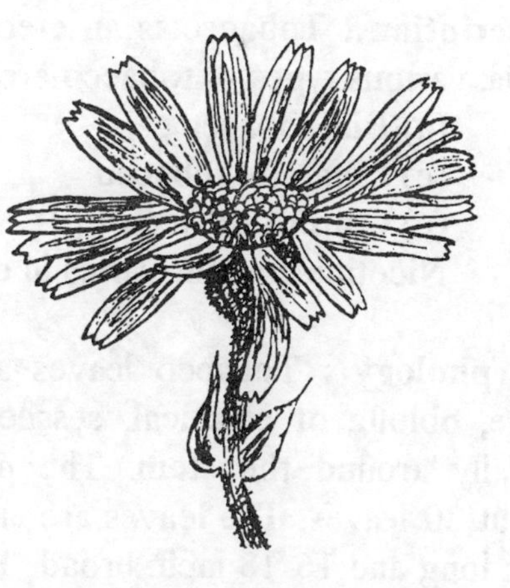

Fig. 7.51 : Pyrethrum flower.

Chemical constituents : The active constituent of pyrethrum flower is pyrethrins. It is a collective term for different organic esters like pyrethrin I, pyrethrin II; cinerin I, cinerin II; Jasmolin I & Jasmolin II. Pyrathrin I, Cincrin I & Jasmolin I are the ester of chrysanthemic acid while Pyrethrin II, Cinerin II and Jasmolin II are the esters of pyrethric acid. They also contain pyrethrol. The synthetic derivative of pyrethrins is known as pyrethroids(rethroids). Allethrin, cyclethrin and furethrin are important pyrethroids.

Uses: It is a contact poison for insects. Insect flower is generally used in the form of powder or extract in organic solvent or kerosine to spray over large variety of pests and insects. It is harmless for warm blooded animals. When mixed with piperonyl butoxide, potency of pyrethrins increases fifteen times due to synergestic action.

TOBACCO

Vernacular names : Hindi, Beng. Mar. & Guj.-Tamaku, Tambaku; Sans.-Dhaumrapatra; Beng. - Tamak; Tam. -pugaiyilai; Eng.-Tobacco.

Biological source : Tobacco consist of dried leaves of *Nicotiana tabacum* Linn. and other species of *Nicotiana.* The plant is a member of *solanaceae* family.

Geographical source : Tobacco is cultivated commercially in China, USA, Brazil, Turkey, USSR and India. In India, the plant is cultivated throughout the country.

Description : Tobacco is an erect viscidly, annual herb. The plant is 4-6 feet high. In India, various types of tobacco are cultivated.

(a) Bidi tobacco (b) Cigar tobacco
(c) Cigarette tobacco (d) Hookah tobacco
(e) Chiroot tobacco (f) Snuff tobacco

Nicotine content varies in different varieties.

Morphology : Tobacco leaves are simple, large, oblong or elliptical, sessile, arranged spirally around the stem. The plant bears about 20 leaves. The leaves are about 24-30 inch long and 16-18 inch. broad. The surface of leaf is pubescent bearing thick midrib. The apex of leaf is acute and base is cuneate. The fresh leaf appears light green to dark green

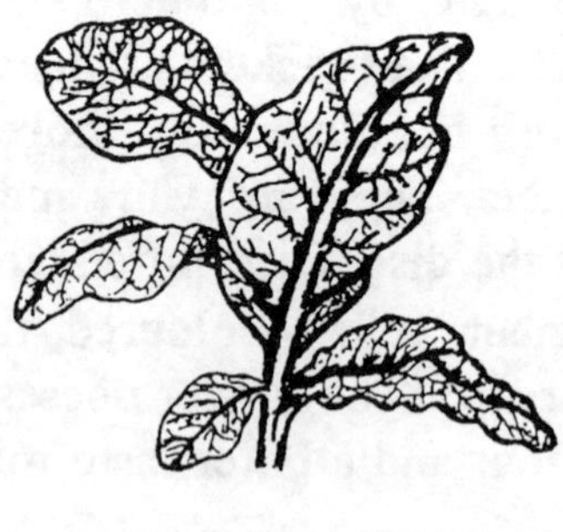

Fig. 7.52 : Tobacco leaf.

in colour but dry leaves are yellowish brown. Tobacco leaf contains sternutatory odour and an unpleasant and sharp bitter taste.

Chemical constituents : The drug contains pyridine-piperidine type of alkaloids. The most prominent alkaloid is nicotine and other are nornicotine and anabasine. These are oily liquids. The minor alkaloids are nicotelline, nicotyrine, nicotimine, piperidine, pyrrolidine,, etc. The other constituents are proteins, organic acids, carbohydrates, amino acids, pigments and inorganic constituents.

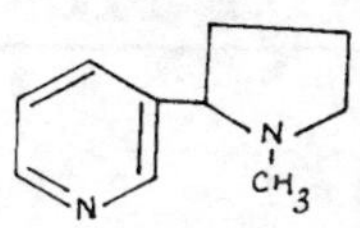

Nicotine

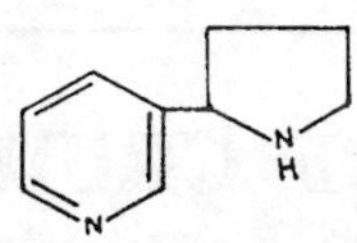

Nornicotine

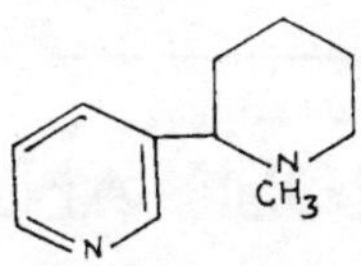

Anabasine

Uses : Nicotine shows stimulant effect on heart and nervous system. It is also used as insecticidal agent to control a wide range of insects. Tobacco leaves are used as antiseptic, antispasmodic, anthelmintic, narcotic and sedative. Decoction of tobacco leaves is applied for muscle relaxation. Tobacco oil is used in gout, lumbago and rheumatism.

CHAPTER - 8

GROSS ANATOMY OF CRUDE DRUGS

MICROSCOPICAL CHARACTERS OF SENNA LEAF

(*Cassia angustifolia*)

The transverse section of senna leaf contains the following tissues in the lamina and the midrib region.

Lamina : The lamina is isobilateral. It has a single layer of palisade beneath the epidermis.

Upper epidermis : It is single layered having polygonal cells and cuticle contains unicellular, conical, scattered, non lignified thick walled, warty hair or trichomes. Some of them contain mucilage. Paracytic type of stomata are found on both surfaces in about equal numbers. The stomata have two guard cells with their long axis parallel to the pore.

Mesophyll : It is also bilateral in structure. It contains upper and lower palisade and spongy parenchyma. It also contains clusters of crystals of calcium oxalate. The upper palisade cells are single layered, compact, columnar and continues over the midrib region. The spongy parenchymatous cells are thin, narrow, loosely arranged cells between lower and upper palisade. It may contain sphaeraphides and vascular strands. The lower palisade cells are single layered and loosely arranged, with wavy walls but are smaller than the upper palisade cells. It is found in lamina region only.

Midrib : The midrib is biconvex in structure. A zone of parenchyma is found below the midrib. Collateral vascular bundles are found in the centre of the midrib which show xylem towards the ventral surface and phloem towards the dorsal surface. The vascular bundle is surrounded by two to three layers of sclerenchymatous fibres and a single layer of parenchymatous cells. The parenchymatous cells contain prisms of calcium oxalate. Collenchyma is also present in midrib.

Lower epidermis : It is similar in structure to the upper epidermis.

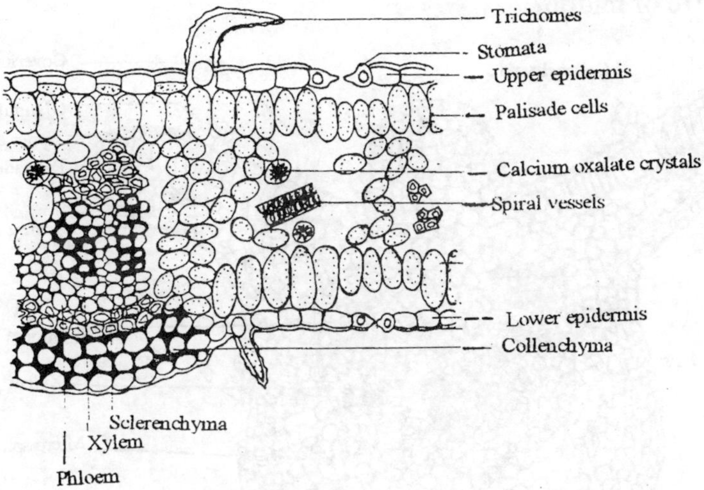

Fig. 8.1 : Transverse section of senna leaf let (cellular)

MICROSCOPICAL CHARACTERS OF DATURA LEAF

(Datura stramonium)

The transverse section of Datura leaf shows the following structures.

Lamina : It is bifacial or dorsiventral in structure.

Epidermis : It is single layered with small cuticle containing both stomata and hairs. The trichomes are uniseriate, multicellular and warty. The hairs are blunt at the apex. Small glandular hairs having one or two celled pedicel and an oval head of 2-7 cells are also present. Anisocytic type of stomata is also present. The lower epidermis possesses wavy walls.

Mesophyll : The mesophyll is composed of palisade cells and spongy parenchyma. The palisade cells are single layered and radially elongated. The spongy parenchyma consists of 6 to 8 layers in numbers that are loosely arranged having intercellular spaces. The spongy parenchyma contains vascular strands, sphaeraphides and microsphenoidal crystals.

Midrib : The midrib has a bicollateral structure. It contains 2 to 3 layers of collenchyma on both surfaces. Sclerenchyma is not present. Cortical parenchyma contains microsphenoidal crystals with prisms of calcium oxalate. The vascular bundles are present in the centre of midrib.

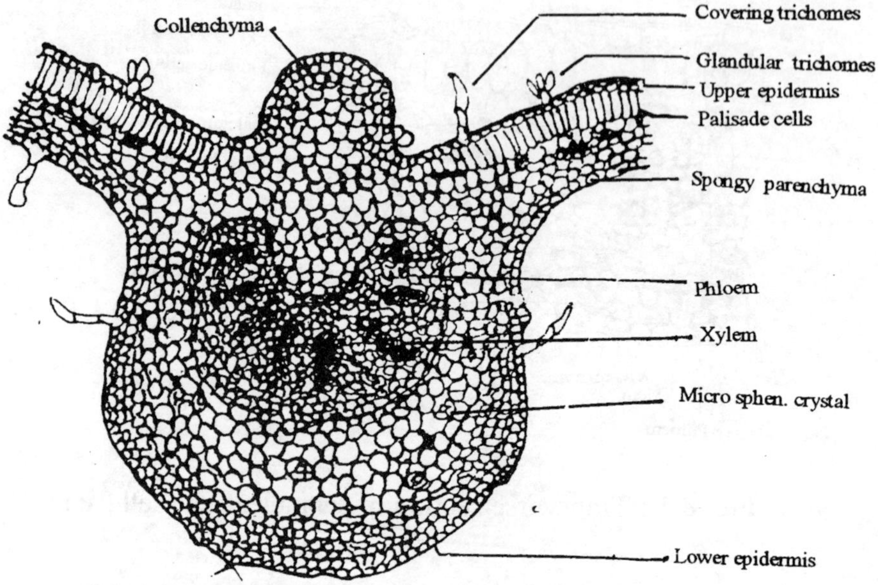

Fig. 8.2 : Transverse section of Datura leaf (cellular)

MICROSCOPICAL CHARACTERS OF CINNAMON BARK

(Cinnamomum zeylanicum)

The transverse section of cinnamon shows the complete absence of epidermis and cork. It consists of an inner bark. The outermost layer of the bark is pericycle that is composed of a continuous ring of 3-4 layers of sclereids. Small groups of pericyclic fibres are present on the outer side of sclereids. The sclereids are thickened, lignified, pitted and show clear lumen. The outer wall is less thickened than the radial and inner tangential walls. The lumen sometimes contains starch. The pericyclic fibres are strongly thickened, lignified walls showing stratification and pit canals. Primary phloem is not seen clearly.

The secondary phloem consists of phloem parenchyma, phloem fibres, medullary rays and obliterated sieve-tubes. The cells of sieve tube are embedded in the phloem parenchyma and arranged in tangential bands which are completely collapsed in the outer layer. The sieve plates are present on the transverse wall. The phloem parenchyma consists of thin walled cells with yellowish brown walls. It contains starch grain, numerous acicular crystals of calcium oxalate, tannin, secretion cells containing volatile oil or mucilage. The phloem fibres are axially elongated. The phloem fibres are thick walled with lignified stratification which occurs either in isolated or in tangential rows and are found in abundance towards the inner part of the bark.

The secondary phloem is divided by the radial medullary rays. The medullary rays are uniseriate or biseriate near the cambium and broader towards the outerside by tangential growth of the cells. The rays are 7-14 cells in height. The medullary rays cells are radially elongated and thin walled. The medullary ray contains yellowish brown content and numerous acicular crystals of calcium oxalate.

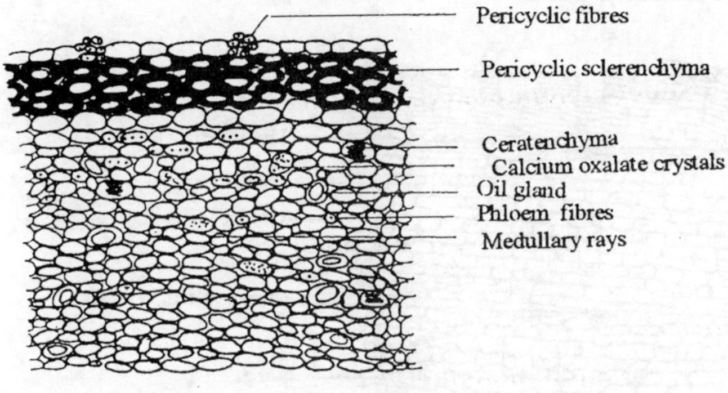

Fig. 8.3 : Transverse section of Cinnamon bark (cellular)

MICROSCOPICAL CHARACTERS OF CINCHONA BARK

(Cinchona succirubra)

General microscopical characters are found in cinchona bark. The transverse section of bark represents the following characters.

Periderm: Periderm is composed of cork phellogen and phelloderm. Multilayered thin walled cork cells which are arranged in regular radial rows, present in the cork. The contents of these cells are dark brown in colour. Phellogen consists of two to three layers of thin walled, rectangular cells. The phelloderm is found within the cork cambium having several layers of regular cells with dark walls.

Cortex : The cortex is composed of thin walled, multilayered, tangentially elongated cells. Many of them contain amorphous reddish brown matter or small starch grains, prisms of calcium oxalate are also present. Secretion cells are also scattered in the cortex.

Phloem : The phloem consists of narrow sieve-tubes, phloem parenchyma, spindle-shaped phloem fibres and medullary rays. The phloem fibres are numerous, large, isolated or in groups, round to oval spindle shaped, thick walled, striated and pitted. Phloem fibres may occur in irregular radial rays.

Medullary rays : Medullary rays are bi or tri-seriate, the cells are thin walled and radially elongated.

Sclereids are absent in cinchona bark.

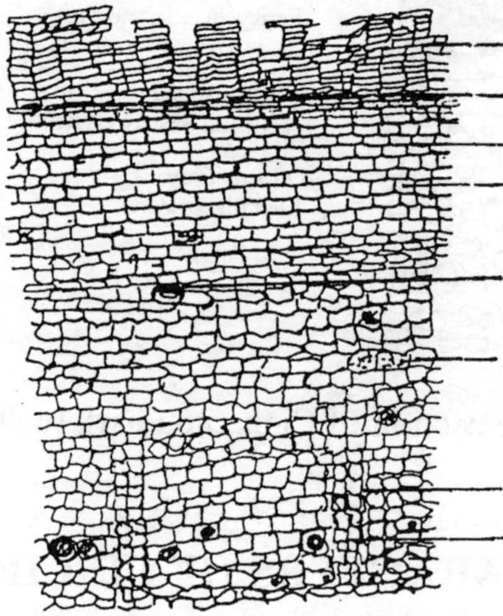

Fig. 8.4 : Transverse section of Cinchona bark (cellular).

MICROSCOPICAL CHARACTERS OF FENNEL FRUIT
(Foeniculum vulgare)

The transverse section of Fennel fruit shows two surfaces, dorsal and ventral. The dorsal surface is grooved, having five ridges. The ventral surface is flat and a carpophore is present in the middle. The mericarp is divided into three parts, i.e., pericarp, testa and endosperm.

Epicarp : The epicarp is composed of polygonal tangentially elongated thin walled cells with smooth cuticle. Anomocytic types of stomata are found which are covered by two to four radiating cells.

Mesocarp : The mesocarp contains thick walled, lignified, bicollateral, parenchymatous cells, six vittae are present, four on the dorsal surface and two on the ventral surface. The colour of the vittae is brown and the shape is oval. The vascular bundles are seen below the primary ridges.

Endocarp : Endocarp contains parquetry arrangement of cells. It is found in a single layer between mesocarp and testa.

Testa : Testa is composed of narrow tangentially elongated cells and is brown in colour.

Endosperm : The endosperm is composed of polyhedral thick walled, polygonal colourless parenchymatous cells. They contain aleurone grains, fixed oil and microrosette crystals of calcium oxalate. In front of carpophore, raphae is present in the middle of commisural surface.

Embryo : Embryo is present in the upper one third part of the fruit.

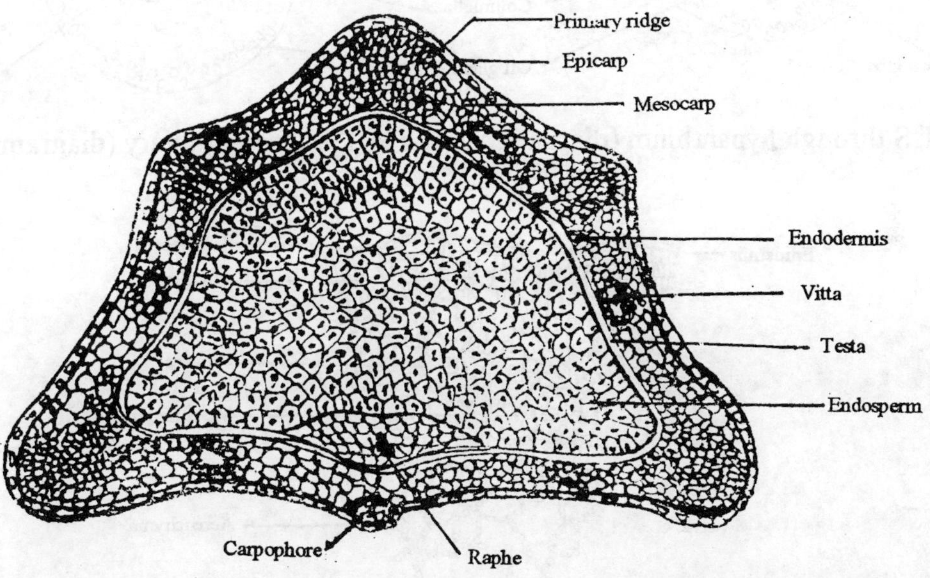

Fig. 8.5 : Transverse section of mercarp of Fennel fruit (cellular).

MICROSCOPICAL CHARACTERS OF CLOVE BUD

Syzgium aromaticum(Eugenia caryophyllus)

The transverse section of the clove hypanthium in the region below the ovary shows the following characters.

Epidermis : The epidermis is thick walled, single layered, consisting of heavily cuticularized cells with straight walls. The stomata are anomocytic type having well defined substomatal spaces.

Cortex : The cortex contains three layers, the outermost, the central and the innermost layers. The outermost layer is composed of 2-3 layers of large ellipsoidal schizo-lysigenous oil glands embedded in the radially elongated parenchymatous cells.

The oil glands are ellipsoidal in shape with the long axis radial and show an epithelium made of two to three layers of flattened cells. A zone of cells with thickened wall

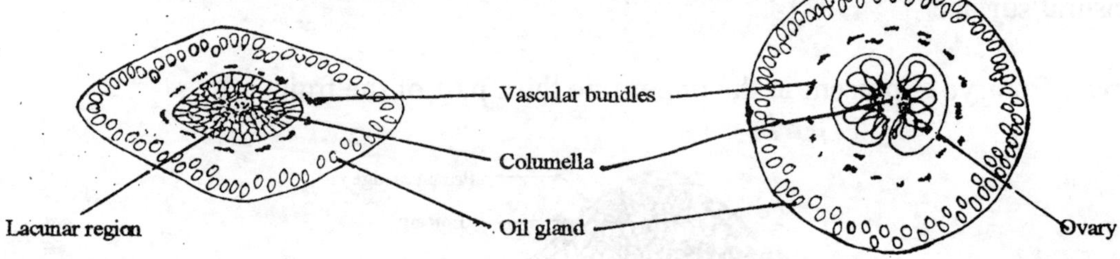

(a) T.S through hypanthium (diagrammatic) (b) T.S through ovary (diagrammatic)

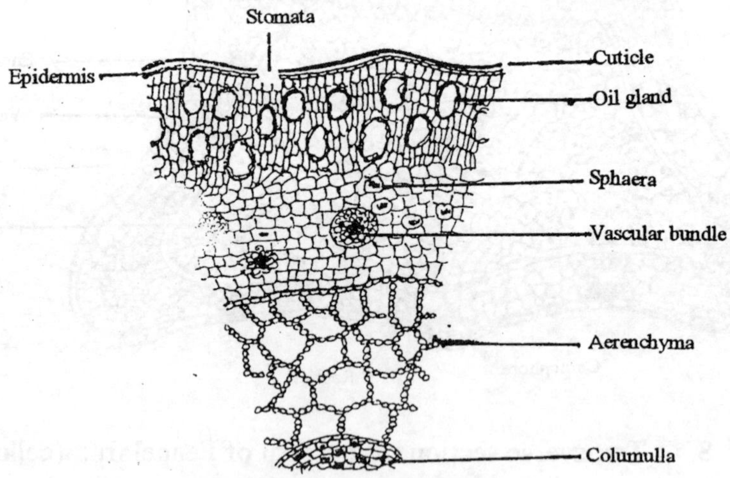

(c) hypanthium (cellular)

Fig. 8.6 : Transverse section of Clove buds

embedding a ring of bicollateral vascular bundles are found within the oil gland layer. Cluster crystals of calcium oxalate are present throughout the tissues.

Central region : The central region consists of one or two rings of bicollateral vascular bundles which are enclosed by lignified pericyclic fibre. The xylem contains 3 to 5 lignified spiral vessels. A zone of parenchyma is found below the vascular bundle. The inner most layer contains loosely arranged aerenchymatous cells. The aerenchyma is composed of air spaces separated by lamellae. The columella contains thick walled parenchymatous cells with a ring of bicollateral vascular bundles. It is rich in cluster crystals of calcium oxalate.

The transverse section of hypanthium in the region of ovary shows epidermis, oil gland layer and a ring of bicollateral bundles. The ovary is parenchymatous, ovules contain axile placentation. The placenta is rich in cluster crystals of calcium oxalate and vascular bundles. Stone cells are absent.

MICROSCOPICAL CHARACTERS OF GINGER RHIZOME
(Zingiber officinale)

The transverse section of Ginger rhizome shows the following tissues.

Cork tissue : The cork tissue is differentiated into outer cork and inner cork. The cells of outer cork are irregularly arranged and dark brown in colour. The inner cork cells are arranged radially and produced by tangential division of the cortical cells. Cork cambium is not differentiated.

Cortex : The cortex is composed of thin walled parenchymatous cells with intercellular spaces. It is rich in starch, grains, oleo resins and numerous oil. The vascular bundles are conjoint, collateral, closed and enclosed in a sheath of non lignified fibres. The nonlignified fibres are known as fibro - vascular bundle and it is the main characteristic of ginger.

Each vascular bundle contains phloem, xylem and sieve-tube. The xylem is composed of 1 to 14 vessels with annular, spiral or reticulate thickenings.

Endodermis : The endodermis is thick walled, single layered having radial cells, containing no starch grains.

Ground tissue : The ground tissue is composed of thin walled rounded polygonal cells rich in starch, oleo resins, large cellulosic parenchyma cells and vascular bundles. The vascular bundles are arc shaped, conjoint, having non lignified fibres. The xylem vessels are annular, spiral or reticulate and the thickenings are non lignified.

Each vascular bundle is composed of phloem having distinct sieve tubes. The ground tissue is composed of parenchyma similar to the cortical parenchyma and is rich in starch and numerous oils. The stone cells (sclereids) and calcium oxalate crystals are absent.

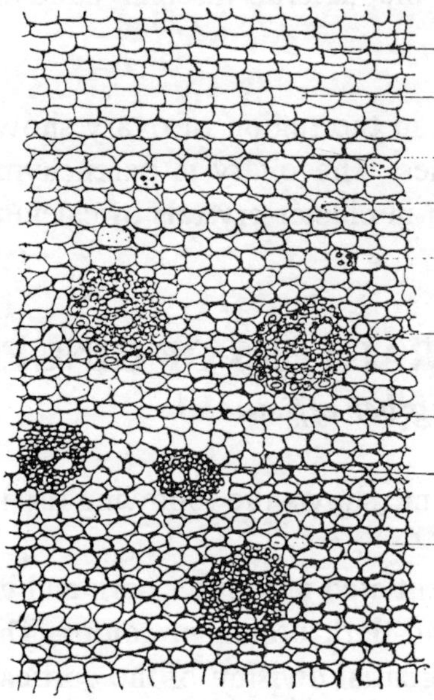

Fig. 8.7 : Transverse section of Ginger rhizome (cellular).

MICROSCOPICAL CHARACTERS OF NUX-VOMICA SEED

(Strychnos nux-vomica).

The transverse section of Nux-vomica seed reveals the following tissues.

Epidermis : The epidermis is single layered with a long thick walled lignified trichomes or hairs. The trichome is composed of pitted bulbous base and a projection. Ten longitudinal ridges like thickenings are found on the upper part of the wall of a hair. On the ridge, the hairs are irregularly arranged. The upper portion of the hairs is arranged in a right angle to the bases and all radiate out side towards the margin of the seed, giving the testa a silky appearance. The inner region of the thin testa is composed of collapsed parenchymatous cells which contain yellowish brown content.

Endosperm : The endosperm is composed of large thick walled cellulosic parenchyma. The walls are composed of hemicellulose, non lignified and are carbohydrate in nature. The outer cells are longer while the inner cells are polyhedral, thick walled and nonlignified parenchyma cells. Well marked protoplasmaic threads (plasmodesma) are present which are clearly seen by staining the section with dilute iodine. Aleurone grains, oily plasma, fixed oil and alkaloids like strychnine and brucine are also present in endosperm. The inner part of endosperm is rich in strychnine while the outer layer is rich in brucine.

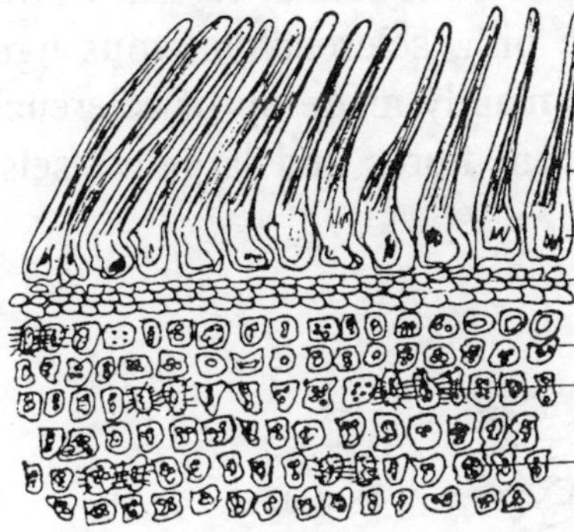

Fig. 8.8 : Transverse section of Nux-vomica seed (cellular).

MICROSCOPICAL CHARACTERS OF IPECAC ROOT

(Cephaelis ipecacuanha.)

The transverse section of root of Ipecac shows the following tissues.

Cork : It is 3-5 layered and consists of thin walled tangential cells which contain brown granular material.

Phellogen : It is one to two layered found below the cork. The cells are tangentially arranged.

Cortex : It is multilayered, thin walled, wide, parenchymatous cells that contain starch grains and raphides of calcium oxalate. The individual starch grains are muller-shaped. The raphides of calcium oxalate are found either scattered or in bundles.

Phloem : Phloem is made of parenchymatous cells in which sieve tubes are embedded. It has no sclerenchymatous cells or fibres.

Xylem and medullary rays : The xylem is composed of small tracheidal vessels, tracheids, xylem fibres, xylem parenchyma and substitute fibres. Xylem is found in the centre but some times triarch primary xylem is surrounded by secondary xylem. The arrangement of the xylem is alternate with medullary rays. The cells of xylem and medullary rays are lignified hence it can not be easily differentiated. Starch is present in the xylem parenchyma and the substitute fibres also contain starch. The tracheids and vessels are bordered pitted and xylem parenchyma is simple pitted. Sclereids are not present in the root.

The transverse section of ipecacuanha rhizome is similar to that of the root. But it shows the presence of a ring of xylem, a large pith, sclerenchymatous lignified continuous or discontinuous pericycle. The pericycle is mainly made up of sclerenchymatous cells. The protoxylem contains spiral vessels. Phloem fibres and large vessels are absent in both root and rhizomes of ipecacuanha.

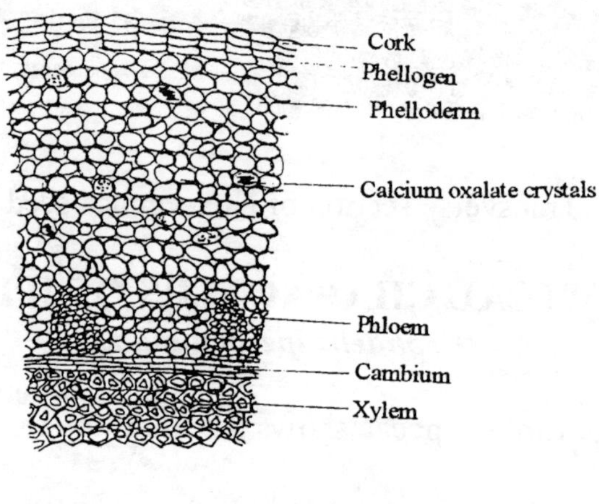

Fig. 8.9 : Transverse section of Ipecac root (cellular).

CHAPTER 9

FIBRES, SURGICAL DRESSINGS AND SUTURES

FIBRES

Fibres are used in Pharmacy as filtering media and are also used for making, dressings and sutures. It may be natural or artifical. Fibres are classified into four categories.

Natural fibres : Natural fibres are obtained from vegetable origin like cotton, hemp, flex, jute;animal fibres can be obtained from wool and silk.

(1) **Artificial fibres** : Artificial fibres are obtained from regenerated carbohydrate and regenerated protein fibres material or chemically modified fibres. e.g. Viscose,

(2) acetate rayons, cellulose wadding, alginate yarn, fibrolane, etc.

(3) **Synthetic fibres** : Some synthetic fibres are also available like nylon, terelene.

(4) **Mineral fibres** : The example of these fibres are Asbestos and glass.

ABSORBENT COTTON

Synonym : Purified cotton.

Vernacular name : Sans. - Karpas; Hindi & Beng.-Kapas; Mar.-Khapur; English-cotton.

Biological source : Cotton consists of the epidermal trichomes (hairs) e.g. the seeds of cultivated *Gossypium herbaceum* Linn. and other species of *Gossypium*. This is a member of *Malvaceae* family. Absorbent or purified cotton is free from impurities deprived of fatty material, bleached and sterilized product.

Geographical source: Cotton is cultivated in U.S.A., Egypt, Africa, China and India. In India, it is cultivated in Rajasthan, Maharastra, U.P., Bihar,, etc.

Cultivation, collection and preparation : The cotton plant is shrub or small tree (containing woody stem), perennial but grown annually due to their susceptibility to attack of insects and diseases. The plant is cultivated near the rivers, which contain rich alluvial deposits. The plant is cultivated from seed. Initially nitrogenous mannures are used for the growth of plant. The phosphatic mannures are used for the uniform ripening of the bolls or capsules. The plant bears 3-5 celled capsule. Each capsule contain about 36 seeds. The ripe bollsare collected, dried and taken to ginning process to separate the hairs (trichomes) from seeds. Long and small hairs are separated by various devices. Short length hairs are known as linters. It is used in the manufacture of adsorbent cotton, wool and rayon. Long hairs are used in fabrics (cloth).

Surgical cotton : Surgical absorbent cotton wool is prepared from linters and cotton waste.

Step I: The impurities are removed from cotton hairs and boiled with 5% caustic soda for 15 hours at 1 to 3 atmospheric pressure.

Step II : Cotton is washed with water and bleached by soaking in 5% chlorinated lime solution for 10-18 hours.

Step III : Bleached cotton is washed with water and soaked in dilute hydrochloric acid for hours.

Step IV : Acidified cotton is washed, dried, loosened and carded into flat sheet. The carding machine gives continuous thin layers of cotton.

Step V : These thin layers is placed one above the other, packed and sterilized by gaseous method or radiation.

The above treatment removes the cuticle containing fatty matter (Wax, Palmitic and Stearic acid.)

Characters : Absorbent cotton consists of thin soft filamentous hairs and is white in colour. The hairs are unicellular, 2-4 cm. in length and 25-40 micron in diameter. The Indian variety contains 75 twists per cm and sea variety island contains 150 twist per cm . The apex of hair is solid and rounded. Cotton hairs are cylindrical when young but become twisted and flattened on maturity. It is odourless and tasteless. Absorbent cotton sinks in water whereas nonabsorbent floats on water (due to presence of fatty material).

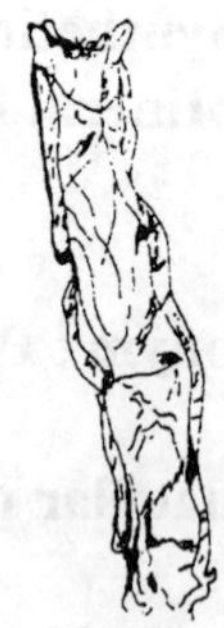

Fig. 9.1 : Cotton fibres

Chemical constituents : Absorbents cotton contains pure form of cellulose. Cellulose molecule is made of glucose residue united by 1,4 ß glucosidic link (contrast to starch).

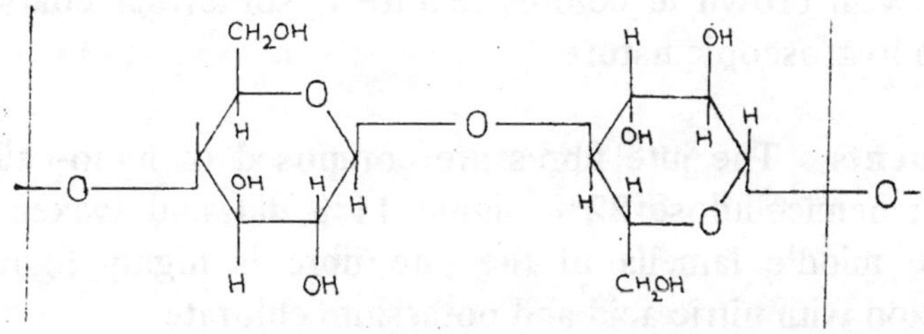

Cellobiose unit

Uses : It is used as surgical dressing. It gives mechanical support to absorb blood, mucous, pus and protects the wound from bacterial infection. It is used in the preparation of cellulose derivatives like methyl cellulose, carboxy methyl cellulose, etc. It is also used as filtering media, absorbent gauze and collodion.

JUTE (GUNNY)

Biological source : Jute consists of strands of phloem fibre from the stem bark of *Corchorus olitorius* Linn. *C. capsularis* Linn.and other species of *Corchorus*. This is a member of *Tiliaceae* family.

Geographical source : Jute plant is cultivated in India, Chiefly in Bengal and Assam, in the basins of Brahmaputra and Ganges.

Preparation : Jute is an annual plant about 3-4 metre in height. Plants are normally collected in the month of July at the flowering stage. The straight branched stems are cut and leaves are removed, bundle of stems are formed and submerged into stagnant water for 10 to 12 days. These are covered with straw to protect from the direct sun light. This process is known as retting. During this process phloem and parenchymatous tissues of bark get separated from the wood. After retting the ends of stem are beaten with a mallet to separate the wood from fibres. The fibres are cleaned by jerking them backwards and forwards on the surface of water. These are hung up in sun light for drying and bleaching. These are graded according to their colour, glossyness and length.

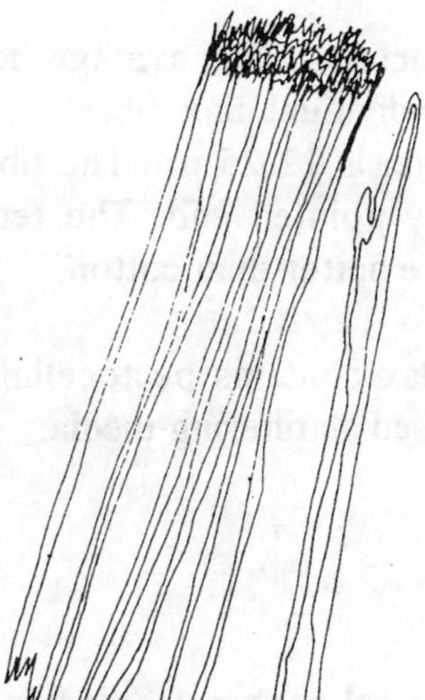

Fig. 9.2 : Jute fibres

Characters : Jute strands are about 1-3 metre in length and 30-140 micrometer in diameter. The individual jute fibre is 0.8 to 5 mm in length and 10-25 micrometer in diameter. It is yellowish brown in colour; texture is somewhat coarse and has a great tensile strength with hygroscopic nature.

Chemical Constituents : The jute fibres are composed of ligno-cellulose. It contains true cellulose 53%; hemicellulose 22%; lignin 11%; fat and waxes 1%; ash 1% and moisture 12%. The middle lamella of the jute fibre is highly lignified and is easily destroyed by oxidation with nitric acid and potassium chlorate.

Uses : Jute is used in pharmacy for the manufacture of medicated tow, padding splints and as straining or filtering media. It is used in making sacking and coarse lages. It is used in manufacturing of yarns and ropes.

Storage : Jute is stored in cool place. Drying makes it brittle and dusty. The tensile strength reduces by bleaching and colour darkens on exposure to sun light.

FLAX

Biolological source : Flax is obtained from pericyclic fibres of the stem of *Linum usitatissimum* Linn. This is a member of *linaceae* family.

Preparation : Flax is prepared by retting process as described under jute.

Characters : The average height of flax strand is 50 cm The individual flax fibre is 25-30 cm long and average diameter is 12-25 μm The fibre is non-lignified containing sharply pointed end. The tensile strength and lusture of flax are better than cotton.

The flax contains pectocellulose as the main constituent. It is used as filtering media.

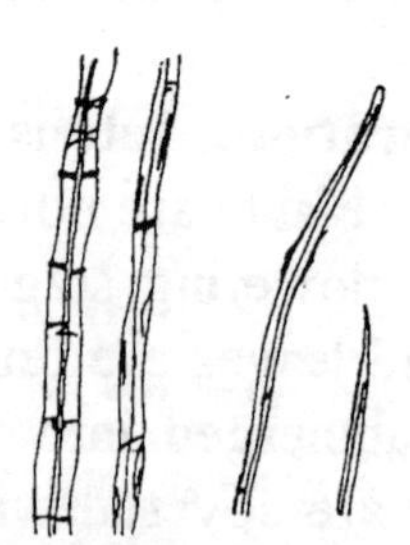

Fig. 9.3 : Flax fibres

SILK

Biological source : Silk fibre is prepared from the cocoons of *Bombyx mori* Linn. and other species of *Bombyx* and *Antheraea*. This is a member of *Lepidoptera* order.

Geographical source : It is produced in India, Japan, China, France, Italy, etc.

Cultivation and preparation : Sericulture is a technique that deals with the cultivation of domesticated silk worm from egg to cocoon stage and production of mulberry trees for worm food. The egg of silk worm is wrapped in fine gauze envelopes and kept at 0°C to prevent premature development. The silk worms eat mulberry leaves and in 4-5 weeks they attain their full size. Before the silk worm passes from the larval or caterpillar to pupal (chrysalis) stage, it secretes an oval cocoon around itself. The cocoons are collected at the chrysalis stage and pupa are killed by heating at 60-80°C for few hours or by exposing to steam. The cocoons are graded. They are placed in hot water to soften the sericin and loosen the fibre. It contains about 1200 metre long thread. The thread consists of two silk fibre joints together by a layer of silk glue (sericin). A single thread of silk is prepared by twisting and reeling from fibres of 2-15 cocoons.

Characters : Silk threads are soft, smooth and solid. They are usually yellow in colour and contain considerable tensile stength. It is soluble in concentrated HCl, ammonical copper oxide solution, cuoxam and 66% H_2SO_4.

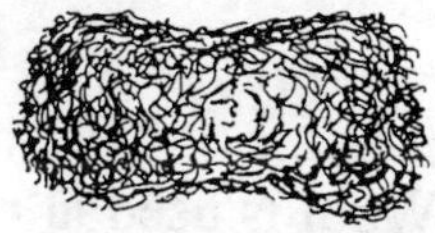

Fig. 9.4 : Cocoon (Silk)

Constituents : Silk fibre is mainly composed of protein known as fibroin, which on hydrolysis produces amino acids like glycine and alanine.

Uses : The silk fibre is used in the preparation of ligatures and seives.

WOOL

Biological source : Wool is prepared from the fleece of sheep *Ovis aries* Linn. This is a member of *Bovidae* family (order-ungulata).

Geographical source : The main wool producing countries are Argentina, America, Australia, Russia and India.

Preparation : The wool is removed from the body of the sheep at shearing time. It is thoroughly cleaned to remove dirt. After this the wool is washed with warm soft soap or alkali to remove wool grease. The fibres are squeezed between rollers, dried and are loosened. This fibre may be bleached with sulphur-dioxide or hydrogen peroxide and washed. It is dried in hot air by spreading over wire natting.

Characters : Wool occurs as elastic, lustrous smooth less curly hairs and loosely felted mass. It is slippery . It is hygroscopic and can absorb 40-50% of moisture. It is insoluble in 66% of sulphuric acid, concentrated hydrochloric acid (HCl) and cuoxan. Wool fibre contains a protein known as keratin which provides elasticity to fibre. The keratin contains cystine amino acid having sulphur group. It gives black precipitate when treated with lead acetate in caustic soda.

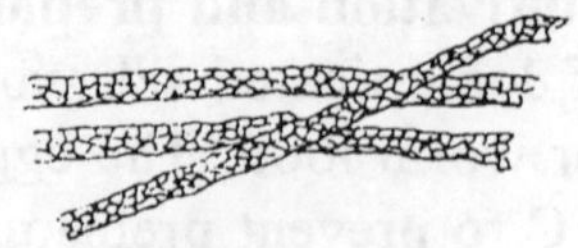

Fig. 9.5 : Wool fibres

$$\begin{array}{l} S\text{-}CH_2\text{-}CH(NH_2).\ COOH \\ | \\ S\text{-}CH_2\text{-}CH(NH_2).COOH \end{array}$$

Cystine

Use : Wool is used in manufacturing of crape bandage, dressing & flannel. It is also used as filtering or straining media.

VISCOSE RAYON

(Regenerated Cellulose or Artificial Silk.)

Regenerated fibres are prepared from naturally produced long chain molecules and modified to give fibre.

Source : Viscose rayon is a regenerated fibre prepared from the wood cellulose or *Picea abies* (Syn. *Picea excelsa*). This is a member of *pinaceae* family. The wood cellulose contains 80-90% cellulose and rest hemicellulose.

Description : Wood cellulose is macerated in 15 to 20% caustic soda solution for 2 hours. This removes hemicellulose from wood. Then wood cellulose squized until its weight is about four times its original weight. The alkaline cellulose is broken into pieces and kept in closed vessels for 24 hours. Then it is treated with carbon disulphide. The cellulose becomes deep orange in colour and start smelling. It becomes gelatinous after 3-4 hours. It is converted to viscous fluid after 24-48 hours. This is called cellulose-xanthate. The rayon is derived from this viscous mass, hence called viscose. The fluid is filtered and clear solution is forced through metal nozzle into a coagulating bath of sulphuric acid and sodium sulphate. This process gives filaments of regenerated cellulose.

Rayon is a white, highly lusturous fibre. Its tensile strength varies from 2/3 to 1 and is about half of that of cotton. On wetting the tensile strength is decreased to about 60%. Rayon is a very pure form of cellulose. It also contains traces of sulphur.

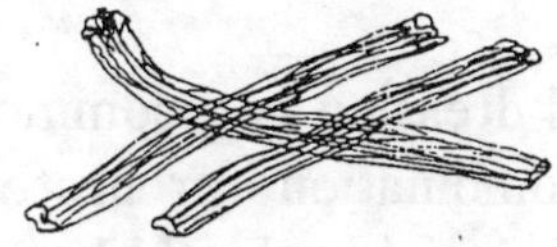

Fig. 9.6 : Viscose rayon

Uses : Vicose rayon is used in the preparation of surgical dressings and fabrics. Its absorbency does not change with time.

Table : 9.1 Identification tests for vegetable and animal fibres

Identification Test	Vegetable and Regenerated Carbohydrate fibres	Animal and Regenerated Protein fibres
1. On boiling with aqueous picric acid solution.	No permanent yellow stain	Permanent yellow stain
2. With Molisch's reagent (α-napthol and sulphric acid)	Violet colour formed	Negative
3. On ignition	No foul odour or fumes, formed white ash.	Burns with foul odour, giving beads. Fumes are alkaline to litmus
4. With iodine solution	Blue colour produced	Yellow colour produced
5. With Cuoxam (Copper oxide ammonia solution)	Dissolves and forms blue colour	Negative
6. On boiling with Millon's reagent	No red stain produced	Red stain produced
7. Boil with 5% sodium hydroxide then adds lead acetate	Negative test	(a) Wool produces black precipitate. (b) Silk produces white precipitate

SURGICAL DRESSINGS

Surgical dressing is a common word which includes wide range of materials used alone or in combination for protections, coverings, absorbents or supports to the wound. Surgical dressing should be easy to handle, sterilizable and free from any loose threads and fibres.

Surgical dressings are classified as

(a) Primary wound dressings
(b) Absorbents
(c) Bandages
(d) Adhesive tapes
(e) Protectives

a) **Primary wound Dressings**: These dressings are placed over the wound surface to absorb wound secretions (Pus, blood, mucus). Since long gauzes of suitable mesh size and thickness are used for primary wound dressings. These dressings adhere to the wound surface and cause pain on removing. Non adherent dressings have been developed to minimize this problem, such as petrolatum-impregnate gauze. Hydrophilic oil in water emulsion, viscose gauze impregnated with blend or an absorbent pad faced with soft plastic film having minute openings, etc.

b) **Absorbents** : Absorbent cotton is basically used to absorb wound secretions, such as blood, pus, mucous, etc.

There are some other absorbent materials like cotton wool, gauze pads, laparotomy sponges, sanitary napkins,eye pads, nursing pads, cotton tipped applicators , disposable cleaners, etc.

c) **Bandages** : The bandages are used to hold dressings and provide pressure or support at proper site. It may be elastic or non-elastic in nature. Common gauze roller bandage and muslin bandage rolls are generally used. Crepe bandage, conforming bandage and woven elastic bandage is examples of elastic bandages.

d) **Adhesive Tapes** : Two types of surgical adhesive tapes are available. Rubber adhesive and acrylate adhesive tapes. Rubber adhesive tapes are cheap, superior in adhesion, provide strength of backing and are commonly used where as an acrylate adhesive tapes are used mainly in the operations or after the operation, to reduce skin trauma.

e) **Protectives** : Protectives are used to cover wet dressings, for poultices and retention of heat. They prevent the loss of moisture from the dressing. Plastic sheets, wax, oil or plastic coated papers, rubber sheets are commonly employed on protectives.

SUTURES

Sutures and ligatures are the same material. Suture is a thread used to stich together the edges of various tissues with the help of needle e.g. skin, muscle, tendon, etc., but when material (thread) is used to seal off blood vessels, vein or artery by tieing then the thread is known as a ligature.

Sutures are classified into two main groups

(a) Absorbable

(b) Non-absorbable

(a) **Absorbable** : Absorbable sutures are absorbed or digested by tissues in which they are implanted. Surgical catgut is one of the important example of absorbable sutures. Surgical catgut is prepared from collagen derived from connective tissues obtained from healthy mammals like sheep and cattle.

Preparation : Catgut is prepared from the submucosa of the small intestine of sheep or lamb. First 8 meter long intestine measured from the duodenum from freshly killed animal is cleaned and split longitudinally into ribbons. The inner most mucosa and two outer most layer of submucosa, muscularia and sersal layers is removed mechanically leaving the submucosa. These ribbons from one to five in numbers are stretched, or spun undertension and dried to get a uniform strand. These strands are polished to get neither whiskery nor so smooth strings, gauzed for their suitable diameter, cut into suitable length and sterilized either by dry heat or by irradiation.

Chromicized surgical catguts are prepared by soaking the ribbons in the solutions of chromium salts. In this solution tanning of the tissues take place. These catguts are resistant to proteolytic enzymes in the body. These are not absorbed rapidly in the body. Fascia lata, prepared from bovine thigh muscles or excised from the patient are used for hernia repair, urethral slings, etc. Kangaroo tendons are also used for hernia repair and bone surgery. Ribbon gut prepared from bovine esophagus is use for large ventral hernia repair and for closure of kidney after nephrotomy.

Synthetic absorbable sutures : Certain synthetic absorbable sutures are prepared by polymerization of lactides, hydroxy acids, etc. These sutures have high tensile strength. They are completely broken down by hydrolysis and absorbed in the tissue.

Non-absorbable Sutures : Non-absorbable sutures are not absorbed by tissue, they are not affected by body fluid and remain unchanged for long period. After healing of the wounds, they are removed after the incision. Silk, cotton, linen, nylon, polyester and stainless steel wire are used as non-absorbable sutures.

Silk sutures : These are prepared by twisting silk fibres into single strand. In large scale, plaited or braided silk is used in modern surgery. Number of strands is braided together into a compact mass. Silk sutures are smooth, strong and sterilized by autoclaving, radiation or ethylene oxide.

Cotton Sutures : These sutures have uniform size and reproducible strength. Cotton sutures are not used in the critical area where the strength of the sutures is required for long period of time.

Nylon sutures : Synthetic polyamide is known as Nylon. It is formed by polymerization of an acid and amine. It is available in the form of monofilament or multifilament fibres braided into strands. Nylon sutures are strong and water resistant used in skin suturing and plastic surgery. These are sterilized by autoclaving, by ethylene oxide or by radiation.

Linen sutures : Linen suture consist of flax fibres. Normally strands are prepared by spinning three cords together. Linen sutures are cheap and very strong.

Polyester sutures : These are prepared in plaited or braided form. It consists of filaments that is prepared by polymerizing the ester formed by ethylene glycol and terephthalic acid.

Metallic sutures : Metallic sutures consist of wires of silver or stainless steel. These are used in the forms of monofilament which are twisted and plaited or braided.

GLOSSARY

BOTANICAL TERMS

Accentric hilum : Hilum not present centrally.
Acene : Dry indehiscent and one-seeded simple fruit having superior ovary.
Acicular : A needle like projection.
Acuminate : When leaf narrows down into an acute angle.
Acute : Forms acute angle, pointed.
Adventitious : Arising from abnormal position.
Albuminous cell : Seeds containing endosperm, cells rich in nitrogenous content.
Aleurone grains : Protein granules of globulins and peptones found in seeds.
Alluviol soil : Made of soil and sand left by rivers or floods.
Annual : Yearly.
Annual ring : The layer of xylem formed by one years.
Annulate : Ring shaped.
Anther : A stamen that bear pollen.
Apical : Apex tip.
Aril (arillus) : Succulent development of stalk.
Ascospore : A spore produced by sac.
Axil : Situated into an axis.
Axillary bud : A lateral bud situated in the axil of a leaf.
Bicarpellary : Having two carpels
Bicollateral : Having two similar sides
Biennial : A plant that completes life cycle in two years
Bifacial : Possessing two faces.
Bracteole : A leaf or leaf like structure born upon the pedicel of a flower.
Bud : Undeveloped shoot having no internode covered wholly or partly by overlapping leaves.
Bulbous base : Swollen base.
Cambium : Meristematic cells between xylem and phloem.
Carpels : A female floral organ that bears simple or compound gynoecium of the flower.
Carpophore : A central stalk.
Caruncle : A massive out growth of the tip of the outer integument.
Chalaza : The place where the seed coat unites with the ovules.
Collateral : Phloem occurs only on the outer side of the xylem.

Collenchyma : A partially mechanical tissue having living cells, thickened at the corner with cellulose.

Columella : A small column.

Commissure : The line separating the mericarp.

Conspicuous : Clearly seen.

Cordat : Heart shaped.

Crenate : When the margin is cut into rounded teeth.

Deciduous : Duration of leaf last for one seasen only.

Dehiscence : A process of releasing seeds or spores.

Dentate : A toothed margin.

Dioecius : Unisexual.

Dorsal : Outer surface of an organ.

Drupe : A simple fruit in which pericarp is differentiated into thin epicarp, a fleshy mesocarp and stony innercarp.

Endocarp : Innermost layer of the pericarp of the fruit.

Epicarp : Outermost layer of the pericarp of the fruit.

Exalbuminous : Having no albumin.

Glabrous : Without hairs.

Guardcell : A pair of chlorophyllous cell that encloses stoma.

Gymnosperm : Naked seeded plants.

Hilum : Scar on a seed coat making the place of an attachment of the seed stalk to the seed.

Hydothode : Water stomata, water excrecating gland occurring at the tips of leaves of many plant.

Hypha : A fungal filament.

Hypodermis : The tissue just below epidermis.

Hypogynous : When the stamen's petals and the sepales are attached upon the thalamus below the gynoecium.

Inconspicuous : Structure not easily seen.

Indehiscent : Not releasing seeds or spores.

Integument : Coating of an ovule.

Isobilateral : A structure that can be devided into two planes at right angle, having similar structure.

Kernel : Seed within the strong endocarp.

Lamina : Blade of the leaf.

Lenticel : A pore through which breathing takes place in the bark of trees.

Lichen : An organism formed by the close association of a fungus and an alga.

Lignin : Hardening of cell wall by the deposition of a complex aromatic compound in sclerenchyma, xylem vessels and tracheids.

Lumen : Cavity of the cell.
Mericarp : One seeded portion of a schizocarpic fruit.
Meristem : Capacity of unlimited cell division.
Mesocarp : Middle portion of the pericarp of the fruit.
Micropyle : An opening in integument of an ovule or seeds.
Monoceious : Having both sexes on the same plant.
Napiform : Turnip like structure.
Oblong : Similar to rectangle.
Obtuse : Rounded apex.
Ovate : When the leaf is braod and rounded at the base and tapers wards the apex.
Perennial : A plant living for many years.
Pericarp : The mature ovary wall that enclose the seed.
Periderm : Cork, cork cambium and phelloderm is collectively termed as periderm.
Perisperm : Nutritive tissue or albumen of the seed.
Pinnate : When the incision extend from the margin towards the midrib.
Pith : A central core of cells in dicotyledonus stem.
Placenta : The part of the ovary through which the ovules are arise.
Plumule : The embryonic shoot present in the seeds.
Polygamous : Possessing unisexual and bisexual flowers on the same plant.
Radicle : The embryonic root below the cotyledon.
Raphe : Portion of the funiculus, fused with the body of the ovule which is usually in the form of a ridge.
Reniform : Kidney shaped.
Rosette : A dense, imbricated collection of leaves growing close together.
Scar : A mark left by natural separation.
Sclerotium : A compact and hard tuber like structure.
Sclerenchyma :Thick walled elongated or shorter cells provides strength.
Sclerotium : A compact and hard tuber like structure.
Serrate : The margin is cut thin fine teeth directed towards leaf apex.
Sessile : Stalkless.
Stamen : Male sex organ of a flower.
Stigma : Female sex organ of a flower
Stolon : A creeping stem.
Striation : A marking due to formation of the bands.
Testa : Seed coat.
Tortuous : Flashy

Tracheids : A non perforate conducting and strengthening cell in xylem tissue.
Turgidity : Plump state.
Umbelliferous : Umbellate flowers.
Viscid : Adhering
Vitta : An oil tube.
Wrinkle : A small furrow or ridge in the skin
Xerophyte : The plants growing in the regions where the supply of water available to the plant is deficient.

MEDICAL TERMS

Abrasion : Any rubbing or scraping action that produces surface wear.
Abortifacient : An agent that causes abortion.
Amenrrhoea : Absence of abnormal cessation of menses.
Analgesic : A drug that relieves pain.
Anesthetic : An agent that reduces or abolishes sensation.
Anorexia : Loss of appetite.
Antacid : A drug which counter act acidity.
Anthelmintic : A substance that destroys or expels intestinal worms.
Antidote : An agent that counteracts poison.
Antiemetic : A drug that arrests vomiting.
Antifungal : An agent which destroy or supress the growth or reproduction of fungi.
Anti-inflammatory : An agent which contract or supress the inflammation.
Anti-rheumatism : An agent that prevents or relieves the pain of rheumatism.
Antiseptic : An agent that inhibits and destroys the growth and development of microorganisms.
Antispasmodic : A substance that prevents or relieves spasm.
Antitussive : An agent that relieves cough.
Aperient : Mild purgative.
Aphrodisiac : An agent that stimulates sexual exitment.
Appetizer : A substance that stimulates appetite.
Arthritis : Inflammation of a joint.
Astringent : A drug that causes cells to shrink by precipitating proteins from their surfaces.
Bronchitis : Inflammation of bronchi.
Bronchodilator : An agent that dilates the bronchi.
Carminative : An agent that relieves flatulence.

Cathartics : Strong purgative.
Chronic : A disease of long duration.
Contraceptive : An agent that prevents pregnancy.
Colitis : Inflammation of the urinary bladder.
Constipation : A condition in which bowel evacuations occur infrequently or where passage of feces causes difficulty or pain.
Contraceptive : An agent that prevents pregnancy.
Counter-irritant : An agent that causes irritation when applied to the skin and is used in order to relieve some other irritation.
Convulsion : A violent contraction of voluntary muscles.
Cystitis : Inflammation of the urinary bladder.
Demenorrhoea : Painful menstruation.
Demulcent : A soothing agent that protects the mucous membrane.
Dentifrice : A powder or paste for cleaning the teeth.
Depressant : An agent that reduces the functional activity of an organ.
Dermatitis : Skin lesion.
Diaphoretic : An agent that promotes sweating.
Diarrhoea : Frequent discharge of fluid fecal matter from bowel.
Digestive : A drug that permotes the digestion of foods.
Diuretic : An agent that promotes the flow of urine.
Dropsy : Abnormal accumulation of serous fluid in cellular tissue or in body cavity.
Dysentery : An infection of the intestinal tract causing severe diarrhoea with blood and mucus.
Dysuria : Difficulty and pain in urination.
Edema : Excessive accumulation of fluid in the body tissues.
Emetic : An agent that causes vomiting.
Emmenagogue : A drug that promotes menstrual flow.
Emollients : A substance that softens the skin and soothes irritation of the skin and mucous membrane.
Epilepsy : A nervous disorder characterized by sudden loss of consciousness.
Euphoria : A state of optimism cheerfulness and well being.
Expectorants : An agent that increases bronchial secretion and facilitates its expulsions.
Febrifuge : A remedy for fever
Febrile : Affected with fever.
Flatulence : Excessive formation of gases in stomach and intestine.

Glactogogue	: An agent that promotes the secretion and flow of urine.
Gonorrhoea	: A venereal disease that affects the genital mucous membranes of either sex.
Gout	: Inflammation of joints due to excessive accumulation of uric acid in the blood stream.
Haemolysis	: Disintegration of R.B.C. in the blood.
Haemorrhage	: Bleeding.
Haemostatic	: Arrest of bleeding.
Hallucinations	: A false perception.
Hayfever	: Inflammation of the mucous membrane of eye, nose and air passage due to allergy.
Hemorrhoid	: Piles with painful swellings at the anus.
Hepatitis	: Inflammation of the liver.
Hodgkin's disease	: Painless enlargement of lymphatic glands in the neck, groin, chest.
Hypertension	: High blood pressure.
Hypnotics	: Causing sleep.
Hypoglycemic	: An agent which lowers the blood sugar level.
Hypertension	: Low blood pressure.
Immunity	: The body's ability to resist infection, disease and poison.
Influenza	: A highly contagious virus infection that affects the respiratory system.
Insanity	: Mental illness.
Insecticides	: A preparation used for killing insects.
Insectifuge	: A preparation use to repell insects.
Insomnia	: Sleeplessness.
Intoxication	: The symptoms of poisoning due to ingestion of any toxic material.
Labour	: Delivery
Lactogogue	: An agent that promotes the secretion and flow of milk.
Laxative	: A drug used to stimulate or increase the frequency of bowel evacuation.
Leprosy	: A chronic disease that affects the skin nerves and mucous membrane.
Leucoderma	: Depigmentation of skin.
Leucorrhoea	: A whitish yellowish discharge of mucus from the vaginal opening.
Malaria	: An infections disease due to the presence of parasitic protozoa of the genus plasmodium.

Mania : A state of mind characterized by excessive excitement.
Menorrhagia : Excessive or prolonged menstruation.
Migraine : Pain on one side of the head.
Mydriatics : A drug that causes the dilation of the pupil.
Narcotic : A drug that induces stupor and insensibility and relieves pain.
Nausea : Feeling of vomiting sensation.
Nephritic : Inflammation of the kidney.
Nuralgia : Nerve pain.
Nyctalopia : Night blindness.
Obese : Overweight.
Oedema : An accumulation of an excessive amount of fluid in intracellular space of the body.
Ophthalmia : Inflammation of the eye.
Oxytocin : A harmone that releases by the pituitary gland which imulates the uterine muscle to contract and stimulates ejection of milk from the brests.
Paralysis : Partial impairment of muscular or sensory functions.
Pathogenic : Capable of causing disease.
Piles : Enlarged veins in the wall of the anus.
Prophylactic : An agent that prevents the development of a condition or disease.
Pruritus : Itching.
Purgative : An agent that produces evacuation of the bowels.
Pylemia : Presence of pus cells in the blood stream.
Pyorrhea : A dental disease in which inflammation of the gums take place and bleeds easily.
Refrigerants : Cooling effect.
Rheumatism : Any disorder in which aches and pains effect the muscles and joints.
Rickettsiae : A group of very small non motile spherical or rod like rasitic organisms.
Rubefacient : An agent that reddens the skin producing a local congestion.
Scurvy : A disease cause due to deficiency of vitamin C.
Sedative : A drug that has a calming effect relieving anxiety and tension.
Spasmodic : Resembling a spasm.
Spasmolytic : An agent that relieves spasm.
Sprain : Injury to a ligament, caused by sudden over stretching.

Stomachic : A agent that improves appetite and digestion.
Trachycardia : An increase in heart rate above normal.
Tranquillizer : A drug having calming effect.
Tuberculosis : An infectious disease caused by bacillus *Mycobacterium tuberculosis*.
Ulcer : A wound with superficial loss of tissue that fails to heal and is often accompanied by inflammation. .
Urethritis : Inflammation of urethra.
Vaginitis : Inflammation of the vagina.
Venereal disease : A sexually transmitted disease.
Vertigo : Dizziness (feeling confused).

INDEX

Absorbent cotton, 209
Acacia arabica, 181
A. catechu, 101
Acacia gum, 178, 181
A. senegal, 179
Aconite, 109
Aconitic acid, 110
Aconitine, 110
Aconitum napellus, 109, 110
Adhatoda vasica, 123
Adulteration, 30
Agar, 180, 183
Agaropectin, 184
Agarose, 184
Ailanthus glandulosa, 108
Ajmalicine, 122
Ajmaline, 122
Ajowan, 83
Alginic acid, 183
Alkaloids, 40
  classification, 41
Allicin, 189
Alliin, 189
Allium sativum, 188
Aloe, 64
A. barbandensis, 64
A. ferox, 64
A. perry, 64
Aloe emodin and related glycosides, 65, 73
Amla, 156
Amomum aromaticum, 89
Amygdalin, 49
Amylopectin, 172
Amylose, 172
Anabasine, 197
Anaferine, 112
Anahygrine, 112
Anethole, 83
Anethum graveoleus, 85
A. sowa, 85
Anethole, 88
Anisaldehyde, 88
Anise, 87
Aniseed, 87
Anthraquinone glycosides, 86, 89, 97
Apidae, 167, 178
A. mellifica, 167, 178
Arabic acid, 179
Arabin, 179
Arachidic acid, 169
Arachis hypogaea, 168
Arachis oil, 168
Arjuna bark, 78, 79
Arjunine, 79
Arjunolic acid, 79
Asafoetida, 93
Ashwagandha, 111
Asparagus racemosus, 112, 192
Astragalus gummifer, 181
Atropa acuminata, 106
A. belladonna, 106, 107
Atropine, 106
Avena sativa, 170
Ayurveda, 4
Azadirachta indica, 146

Balsam of Tolu, 124
Barbaloin, 65
Beeswax, 177
Belladonna, 106
Benzoin, 143
Bhang, 16
Bitter orange peel, 164
Black catechu, 106
Black pepper, 91
Boerhaavia diffusa, 139
Bombyx mori, 212
Bovidae, 186, 213
Brucine, 119

Cannabidiol, 117
Cannabidiol carboxylic acid, 117
Cannabinaceae, 116
Cannabinol, 117
Cannabis sativa, 116
Canscora decussata, 193-194
Caraway, 84
Carbohydrates, 61
Cardamom, 88
Cardiac drugs, 75
Cardiac glycosides, 52, 75
Carica papaya, 158
Caricaceae, 158
Carum carvi, 84
Carvone, 85, 86
Cassia acutifolia, 72
C. angustifolia, 72, 198
Castor oil, 68
Catechin, 102
Catharanthus roseus, 131
Cellulose, 211
Cephaeline, 141-142
Cephaelis acuminata, 140
C. ipecacuanhana, 140
Charas, 116-117
Chaulmoogra oil, 133
Chaulmoogric acid, 134
Cholesterol, 50, 177
Chondrin, 186
Chrysanthemum cinerariaefolium, 19
Cinchona bark, 149
Cinchona calisaya, 149
C. ledgeriana, 149
C. officinalis, 149
C. succirubra, 149
Cinchonidine, 152
Cinchonine, 152
Cinchotannic, 152
Cineole, 126
Cinnamic acid, 125
Cinnamic aldehyde, 97
Cinnamomum zeylanicum, 200
Cinnamon, 96
C. aurantium, 164
Citrus limon, 163
Classification, 7
  alphabetical, 7
  chemical, 10

morphological, 8
pharmacological, 9
taxonomical, 7
Claviceps purpurea, 151
Clavicipitaceae, 151
Clove, 98
Codeine, 115
Colchicine, 130
Colchicum autumnale, 129
Colchicum corm, 129
Commiphora molmol, 145
C. mukul, 127
C. weghtii, 127
Commiphoric acid, 145
Compositae, 195
Convolvulaceae, 193
Corchorus spp., 211
Coriander, 80
Coriandrol, 81
Coriandrum sativum, 80
Cotton absorbent, 209
Cumin, 86
Curcuma domestica, 147
Curcuma longa, 147
Curcuminoids, 147
Cyamompis tetragonalobus, 185
Cyanogenic glycosides, 49
Cymbopogon flexuosus, 164-165
Cystin, 214

Datura metal, 108
Datura species, 108
Datura stramonium, 108, 167
Degitoxin, 76
Dextrin, 167
Diastase, 159
Digitalis, 75
Digitalis lanata, 77
Digitalis purpurea, 75
Digitoxigenin, 76
Digoxin, 78
Dill, 85
Dioscin, 190
Dioscorea, 190
Dioscoreaceae, 190
Diosgenin, 190
Dragendorffs reagent, 42
Drug adulteration, 30

Elemicin, 96
Elettaria cardamomum, 89
Ellagic acid, 61, 157
Embelica officinalis, 157
Emetine, 142
Enzymes, 159
Ephedra, 112
Ephedra sinica, 112, 113
Ephedraceae, 112
Ephedrine, 113
Epicatechin, 102
Ergot, 151-152
Ergot alkaloids, 153
Eugenia caryophyllus, 98
Eugenol, 99, 126
Euphorbiaceae, 157
Evaluation of drugs, 32
Evolulus alsinoides, 193-194

Fats, 58
Fehling's test, 72, 180
Fenchone, 83
Fennel, 82
Ferula foetida, 94
Ferulic acid, 94
Fibres, 209
Fibroin, 213
Fixed oils, fats and waxes, 58
Flax, 212
Foeniculum vulgare, 82, 202

Galactomannon, 185
Gallic acid, 61
Gambier, 100
Gambier fluorscin test, 101
Ganja, 116-117
Garlic, 188
Gelatin, 186
Gelidiaceae, 183
Gentianaceae, 193
Ghatti, 181
Ghatti gum, 181
Ginger, 90
Gingerol, 90
Gitaloxin, 76
Gitogenin, 76
Gitoxigenin, 76
Gitoxin, 76
Glucuronic acid, 187
Glutin, 186
Glycyrrhetnic acid, 187
Glycyrrhiza, 187
Glycyrrhiza glabra, 187
Glycyrrhizin, 187
Gokhru, 137
Goldbeater's skin test, 61
Gossipium herbaccum, 209
Gracilaria, 183
Gramineae, 159
Groundnut, 164, 168, 170
Guar gum, 180, 185
Guggal, 127
Gum acacia, 178
Gum resins, 58
Gymnema sylvestre, 134, 135
Gymnemic acid, 136

Hashish, 116
Hecogenin, 190
Hemp, 116
Herpestis monniera, 31
Honey, 167
Hydnocarpic acid, 134
Hydnocarpus wightiana and related species, 133
Hygrine, 111
Hyoscine, 105, 106
Hyoscyamine, 105
Hyoscyamus, 104
Hyoscymus niger, 104
Hypoprion brevirostris, 155

Indian gentian, 189
Indian gum, 181
Indole alkaloids, 44
Ipecac, 140-141
Isoquinoline alkaloids, 44
Ispaghula, 70

Jasmone, 162
Jute, 211

Kaempferol, 73
Kaolins, 173
Kutkoside, 190

Labiatae, 162
Lanolin, 176

Lauraceae, 96
Leguminosae, 168, 179, 181, 185
Lemon peel, 163
Lemongrass oil, 164
Liliaceae, 188, 192
Limonene, 85, 163
Linaceae, 195, 212
Linalool, 46
Linseed oil, 191
Linum usitatissium, 191, 212
Lipids, 58
Liquorice, 187
Loganiaceae, 118
Lysergic acid, 153

Malvaceae, 209
Mayer's reagènt, 32
Meliaceae, 146
Mentha piperita and related species, 162
Menthol, 162
Methyl eugenol, 99, 126
Molisch's test, 62
Morphine, 115
Murexide test, 6
Myricin, 178
Myristica fragrans, 94
Myristicaceae, 94, 98
Myroxylon balsamum, 124
Myrrh, 145
Myrtaceae, 98

Napelline, 109
Narceine, 115
Narcotine, 115
Neem, 146
Nicotiana tabacum, 196
Nicotine, 115
Nutmeg, 94
Nux vomica, 118
Nyctaginaceae, 139

Ocimum sanctum, 112, 125
Olea europoea, 175
Oleaceae, 175
Oleo resins, 58
Olive oil, 175
Opium, 113
Orange oil, 164
Organized drugs, 25
Oryza sativa, 170
Ovis aries, 213

Pale catechu, 100
Papain, 159
Papaver sommniferum, 113-114
Papaveraceae, 113
Papaverine, 115
Papaya, 158
Pectic acid, 175
Pectin, 174
Pedaliaceae, 138
Pedalium murex, 138
Peppermint oil, 162
Pharmaceutical aids, 166
Pharmacological classification, 9
Phyllanthus emblica, 156
Phytolacca decandra, 108
Picrorhiza, 189
Picrorhiza kurroa, 189
Picrosides, 190
Pimpinella anisum, 87
Piper nigrum, 91
Piperaceae, 91
Plantaginaceae, 70
Plantogo ovata, 70
Primula vulgaris, 77
Psyllium seed, 70
Pterocarpus, 134-135
Pterocarpus marsupium, 135
Punarnava, 139
Pyrethrins, 196
Pyrethrum, 195

Quinidine, 150
Quinine, 150
Quinoline alkaloids, 150

Ranunculaceae, 109
Rauwolfia, 120
Regenerated fibres, 200
Resenes, 121
Reserpine, 121
Reserpinine, 122
Resins, 57
Rhapontic rhubarb, 68
Rheum emodi, 66
Rheum officinale, 66
Rheum palmatum, 66
Rheum rhaponticum, 66
Rheum webbiannum, 66
Rhubarb, 66
Ricinoleic acid, 69
Ricinus communis, 68
Rutaceae, 164-165

Safrol, 96
Sandalwood oil, 165
Santalaceae, 165
Santalol, 166
Santalum album, 165
Saponin glycosides, 52
Satawar, 192
Scrophulariaceae, 189
Senna, 71
Sennosides, 72
Shankhpushpi, 193
Shark-liver oil, 155
Shatavari, 192
Siam Benzoin, 144
Silk, 212
Sinigrin, 50
Sodium alginate, 182
Solanaceae, 104, 111, 196
Solonum nigrum, 108
Starches, 169-172
Steroidal alkaloids, 43
Stomata, 12
Stomatal index, 16
Stomatal number, 16
Strophanthus, 71
Strychnos nux-vomica, 119
Styraceae, 143
Styrax benzoin, 143

Sumatra benzoin, 144
Surgical catgut, 217
Surgical dressings, 216
Sutures, 217
Syzygium aromaticum, 98
Tannins, 60
Terpinoids, 55
Thymol, 84
Tiliaceae, 211
Tobacco, 196
Tolu balsam, 124
Trachyspermum ammi, 83
Tragacanth, 180-181
Tragacanthin, 181
Transverse section of
  cinchona bark, 201
  cinnamon bark, 200
  clove bud, 204
  datura leaf, 199
  fennel, 202
  ginger, 205
  ipecace, 207
  nux-vomica, 206
  senna leaf, 205
Trianthema portulacastrum, 30
Tribulus terrestris, 137
T. lanuginosus, 138
Triticum aestivum, 169
Tropane alkaloids, 44
Tulsi, 125-126
Turmeric, 147
Umbellifereae, 84, 85, 87
Umbelliferous fruits, 80, 84, 85, 87
Unani medicine, 6
Uncaria gambier, 100
Unorganized drugs, 24

Vanillin, 99, 144
Vasaka, 123
Vasicine, 124
Vasicinon, 124
Vein islet no., 16
Ven termination number, 16
Vinblastine, 132
Vinca rosea, 131
Vincristine, 132
Viscose rayon, 214
Vitamin
  A, 156
  B, 160
  C, 157
Volatile oil, 52

Wagner's reagent, 42
Waxes, 59
Withania somniferum, 111
Withanolidies, 111
Wool, 213

Yeast, 160

Zea mays, 169
Zingiber officinale, 90
Zingiberaceae, 88, 90, 147
Zingirone, 90
Zygophyllaceae, 140